D1476050

INTEGRATIVE HOLISTIC HEALTH, HEALING, AND TRANSFORMATION

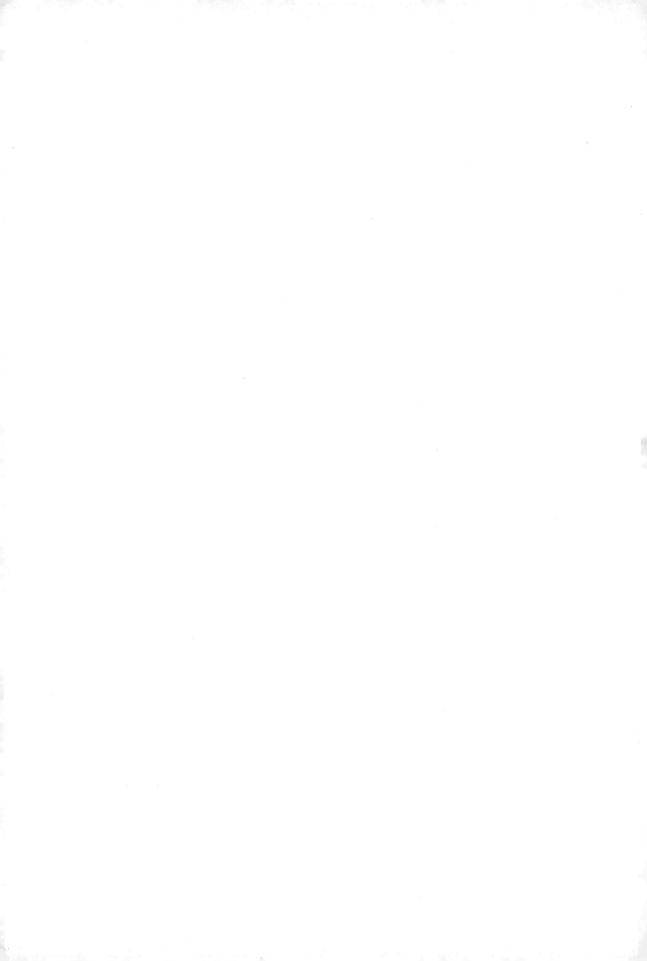

INTEGRATIVE HOLISTIC HEALTH, HEALING, AND TRANSFORMATION

A Guide for Practitioners, Consultants, and Administrators

By

PENNY LEWIS, Ph.D., ADTR, RDT-BCT, OTR, LMHC, NCC, CAMP

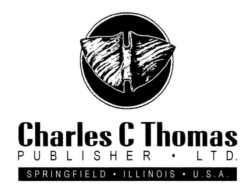

Charles C Thomas
PUBLISHER · LTD.
SPRINGFIELD · ILLINOIS · U.S.A.

Published and Distributed Throughout the World by

CHARLES C THOMAS • PUBLISHER, LTD.
2600 South First Street
Springfield, Illinois 62704

This book is protected by copyright. No part of
it may be reproduced in any manner without
written permission from the publisher.

© 2002 by CHARLES C THOMAS • PUBLISHER, LTD.

ISBN 0-398-07272-8 (hard)
ISBN 0-398-07273-6 (paper)

Library of Congress Catalog Card Number:

With THOMAS BOOKS *careful attention is given to all details of manufacturing
and design. It is the Publisher's desire to present books that are satisfactory as to their
physical qualities and artistic possibilities and appropriate for their particular use.*
THOMAS BOOKS *will be true to those laws of quality that assure a good name
and good will.*

Printed in the United States of America
MM-R-3

Cover photograph from C. Nuridsany and M. Perennou (2002), <u>The Birth of a Flower</u>.
Brussels, Belgium: Graphic de France. Reproduced with permission.

CONTRIBUTORS

Ed Bauman, Ph.D., is a Board Certified Clinical Nutritionist, Founder and Director of Partners in Health, a natural health care clinic and The Institute for Education and Therapy's Nutrition Consultant Training Program. He is co-author of *Holistic Health Handbook, Holistic Health Lifebook, Eating for Health Cookbook, Confronting Cancer in Our Community*, author of *Nutrition and Your Health*, and editor of the quarterly newsletter, *Nutrition Watch*. He is a researcher, consultant and an Associate Dean and faculty member of the University of Natural Medicine in Santa Fe, New Mexico, which offers bachelors, masters and doctoral programs in clinical nutrition and natural medicine.

Christine Caldwell, Ph.D., LPC, ADTR, CMT is Founder and Director of the Somatic Psychology Department at Naropa University in Boulder, Colorado. She lectures and trains internationally, and has authored two books: *Getting Our Bodies Back* and *Getting In Touch*. She offers trainings in somatic evolution (the Moving Cycle), with specializations in addictions, play, movement sequencing, therapist training, and birth and death.

Olivia Cheever, Ph.D., a licensed psychotherapist, is a certified Feldenkrais practitioner. She is on the faculty of the Mind-Body Program for Performers at Longy School of Music and a holistic health practitioner at Wellspace Holistic Health Center.

Charlotte Green, BFA, is a Usui-Tibetan Reiki Master and Teacher; Certified Medium; Commissioned Healer; documented medical intuitive and energy healer; and 15-year Past Board Member of the Massachusetts Federation of Spiritual Healers. She is a teacher of mediumship, spiritual attunement and healing for over 20 years. She is the Visiting Healer at Silverbirch Healing Sanctuary; author, artist, and has a private readings and healing practice in Kingston, New Hampshire.

Nick Hall, Ph.D., M.D., (hc), is the Director of the Wellness Center at Saddlebrook Resort, Wesley Chapel, Florida. He is author of more than 150 articles and book chapters, has appeared on 60 Minutes, NOVA, and Bill Moyers' award-winning program, "Healing and The Mind." He is an award-winning researcher in the mindbody biochemical connection and speaker and consultant in mindbody health and wellness with corporations, the FBI, NASA, and a large number of medical organizations.

Penny Lewis, Ph.D., ADTR, RDT-BCT, LMHC, NCC, CAMP (Board Certified Alternative Medicine Practitioner), is the Coordinator of Integrative Holistic Health Interdisciplinary Graduate Programs, Lesley University, Cambridge, Massachusetts. Founder and Senior Faculty: Antioch-New England Graduate School's Dance-Movement Therapy MA Program; Director: Institute for Healing and Wellness, Inc.; Co-Director: Certificate in Transpersonal Drama Therapy. Author: *Creative Transformation: The Healing Power of the Arts, Theoretical Approaches in Dance-Movement Therapy* Vols. I & II, Co-author: *The Meaning of Movement* and Co-editor: *Current Approaches in Drama Therapy.* International lecturer, consultant and depth therapist in mindbody and spirit education, health, healing and transformation. She is the author and editor of this text.

Wendyne Limber MA, LMFT is Founder and Director of Solutions Center for Personal Growth, Creator of the Imagination Process, and Director of the BA and MA Degree Training at Solutions. She is the author of three workbooks: *Imagination, Transformation and Co-creation, Inspiration: Journey into Power,* and *Intuition: The Journey Deepens*; she is field faculty at Lesley University and Burlington College.

Elaine McNulty, MEd, RPP (Registered Polarity Practitioner), **RCST** (Certified Cranialsacral Therapist), is a Reiki Master; Certified NLP Practitioner, Certified EMF Balancing Practitioner and Trainer; Certified in Guided Self-Healing; Special Education Administrator; former faculty; Polarity Realization Institute and Revier College. She is a National Professional Trainer in Integrative Therapy and private practitioner.

PREFACE

The goal of this book is to begin to present the fundamental body of knowledge which informs current approaches in complimentary and alternative medicine and to explore the role of the new professions of integrative holistic health practitioner, consultant and administrator. This book is designed to compliment, enhance, deepen and broaden the reader's existing expertise through an integrative approach which will improve his/her ability to consult, design programs and work in a variety of settings with various populations including those with medical and psychological conditions as well as those who wish to support their health and well-being.

This book provides the necessary conceptual foundational frameworks for exploring how practitioners in a field of alternative medicine/ holistic health know what they know in support of their work. These core ways of knowing gives them a foundation for evaluating their work, new advances in the field and affords them interrelated frames of knowledge for their continued research, expansion and integrative work in the field. Trained holistic health practitioners who may have applied one or more of these paradigms may now be able to expand their foundational and conceptual base thereby broadening their theory and techniques that are appropriate to their professional arenas.

Section I is designed to explore general ways of knowing and meaning making in holistic health: through for example, mindbody medicine, psychoneuroimmunology, molecular and central nervous system's relationship to emotion and trauma, body posture and movement, nutrition, bioenergy and human energy fields, Eastern, Western and indigenous spiritual traditions and high sense intuition, soul wisdom, and distance intention.

Section I is inclusive of the shifts from the Newtonian Era I medicine to the mindbody Era II, the Einsteinian mind-body-energy paradigm, to Era III medicine with nonlocal consciousness. Various Eastern, Western and indigenous paradigms for experiencing the interconnection among the mind, body, and soul and holistic health are discussed and integrated with the fundamental principles of Western theories of stress, bimolecular research, neurophysiology and the influence of thought and the emotional links to the mindbody experience. Various ways of knowing energy systems such as the chakras and human energy fields and their relationship to stress, the immune system, spiritual path and holistic health are explored. An understanding of the power of the imagination, the arts, embodied somatic experience, and consciousness in healing, health and well-being is addressed. Practitioners explore the various intuitive ways of assessing and healing, and finally the reader/ practitioner is provided with an integrative body of knowledge from which to view a client or population and make programmatic or client-based interventions.

Section II is designed to offer the reader/practitioner methodology regarding the creation and implementation of holistic health centers, programs and integrated consultation practices. Examples of existing successful programs are offered. The authors discuss the genesis, philosophy and workings of the programs.

Finally, Section III offers examples of integrative holistic health clinicians who combine and synthesize a variety of holistic health approaches and paradigms into their practices as practitioners, healers, therapists and consultants.

PENNY LEWIS

CONTENTS

SECTION III: INTEGRATIVE HOLISTIC HEALTH PRACTICES

INTEGRATIVE HOLISTIC HEALTH, HEALING, AND TRANSFORMATION

Section I

WAYS OF KNOWING

Chapter 1

WAYS OF KNOWING:
PARADIGMS IN HOLISTIC HEALTH

The multitude of things which we experience as distinct in reality are but manifestations of the absolute undifferentiated reality that there is an underlying unity among the seeming diversity of existence. It is only the individual, subjective mind—the consciousness informed by the senses—that fragments the world.
(Motoyama, 1978, p. 22)

AT A TIME WHEN CLOSE to half of the population of the United States is engaged in some form of complementary or alternative medicine, it behooves all practitioners in the health and human services to begin to integrate and synthesize the various paradigms that underlie and influence the holistic health approaches being utilized today. Allopathic medicine has its own systems of understanding the body, health and disease. Many individuals are alive today because of the advances that vaccines, antibiotics and surgical procedures have made in the last century. However, I have come to believe that we will look upon the medical procedures and interventions of today, replete with their focus upon pharmaceutical drug remedies and surgical procedures as we now regard the ancient techniques of blood letting.

In 1992, the Office of Alternative Medicine (OAM) was first founded through NIH: The National Institute of Heath. OAM was designed to research and promulgate information regarding what much of the public was already involved. 0AM was charged with evaluating the effectiveness of seven areas: (1) diet and nutrition, (2) mind-body interventions, (3) alternative healing systems, (4) bioelectromagnetic applications in medicine, (5) manual healing methods, (6) pharmacological and biological treatments, and (7) herbal medicine.

I recall listening to a spokesperson for the American Medical Association saying that these forms of healing were nothing more than charlatanism with the public being deceived by con artists liken to those selling snake oil and panacea elixirs two centuries ago. Just five years later the University of Maryland survey showed that 70 percent of the doctors that were questioned were interested in learning more about alternative medicine. In 1998, 0AM was expanded and renamed the National Center for Complementary and Alternative Medicine (NCCAM). Now over 600 specific forms of CAM therapies are reported. Several medical schools and their associated hospitals have been targeted as 0AM centers of research. These sites include Stanford, Harvard, and Columbia as well as the Universities of Michigan, Arizona and Minnesota. These sites as well as others have been supported in longitudinal randomized clinical trials that seek to substantiate various approaches in alternative medicine in relationship to specific diagnostic populations.

In the fifties, chiropractors were seen as "quacks." In the sixties, acupuncturists were looked askance because they did not fit into medical model paradigms. Twenty years later, NIH released a statement confirming that acupuncture is an effective treatment for certain procedures and dysfunctions. In the nineties, energy medicine was addressed as an absolute hoax. Now satellite medical schools and hospital consortiums such as Columbia-Presbyterian and Harvard-Beth Israel are undertaking research which substantiate what was once thought to be hypocrisy resulting in huge shifts and expansions of what is considered to be mainstream health practices.

TWO SHIFTS IN THE WAY MEDICINE, HEALTH AND HEALING IS VIEWED IN THE WEST

Newton Versus Einstein

Alternative and complimentary medicine is based on two major shifts in how the body, medicine and healing is viewed. First, there is a slow expansion from the view of the body from a mechanistic Newtonian frame to an $E=MC2$ Einsteinian frame. With the industrial era came the view of the body as a machine. If part of the body machinery didn't work it was removed, replaced or something was added. Einstein expanded scientific consciousness to view existence as several interfacing phenomena. The human is seen as a multidimensional organism with a physical realm and an energetic realm. In contrast to Newtonian medicine, Einsteinian medicine "attempts to heal illness by manipulating the subtle energy fields" via [clearing, aligning, adjusting and] directing energy into the body "instead of manipulating the cells and organs through drugs or surgery" (Gerber, 1988, p. 69).

The Three Eras of Medicine

Dr. Larry Dossey (1998), one of the leading proponents of alternative medicine, has said that we are moving through several eras of medicine.

Era 1 medicine viewed the body mechanistically as described above within the Newtonian frame.

Era II medicine began to see how the mind affected the body. This resulted in the beginning awareness and research documenting that stress reduced the immune system, and that techniques such as meditation, yoga, and visualization could have a direct result upon affecting reduction of pain and stress and increasing the body's capacity to heal and stay healthy.

Today there is an increasing body of evidence that substantiates that much of the illnesses extant are influenced by emotions. The new field of psychoneuroimmunology has demonstrated that there is more than just proximity to bacteria, viruses, or carcinogens that will result in an individual contracting an illness.

Era III medicine began to understand the concept of the nonlocal mind and its effect on the body of another. Here consciousness is view as separate from the brain and is free from embodied time and space. Thus, individual or group consciousness has the capacity to not only act upon the body of the source of the consciousness, but on distance inanimate objects, life forms, and other individuals. The Harvard Medical School/Beth Israel consortium began to research and substantiate the fact that distant intention, prayer or healing can be sent from the mind of one into the unaware body and psyche of another who was placed in an electrostatically shielded room. The study proved that the moment the healer sent positive healing intention through distance to an unknowing other, that subject's body began immediately to systemically alter in service to health and healing. Clearly the mind is not solely a physical process. It is possible for the mind to transcend the physical world of time and space and to directly affect the external world.

The underlying paradigms which support these three eras in health and healing run the gamut from Western medical model practices, to research in the mind's effect on the immune system and molecular physiology, to indigenous practices in shamanic healing and herbal remedies, to Ayruvedic and homeopathic philosophies, energy medi-

cine, to body-oriented psychotherapy and meditation and to clairvoyants and medical intuitive to name just a few. Practitioners in the field of holistic health, alternative and complementary medicine tend to be trained in one or two approaches, or in a preexisting integrated system such as John Kabat-Zinn's mindfulness based stress reduction and relaxation program (Zinn, 1990). It behooves the mindbodyspirit practitioner/ consultant to begin to grasp, integrate and synthesize an expanding number of paradigms which are influencing this field today. In order to appropriately assess, recommend and/or directly facilitate the client's or diagnostic group's holistic health, the consultant-practitioner needs to see the whole undifferentiated picture (see Figure 1-1, The eras of medicine).

Characteristics	ERA I	ERA II	ERA III
Space-Time	Local	Local	Nonocal
Synonym	Physical medicine	Mindbody medicine	Eternity medicine
Description	Mechanical Cartesian dualism Based upon empirical mechanistic industrial philosophy. If it breaks, remove it, replace it or add something to it.	The mind and the body are an interrelated whole. The mind affects the body and visa versa.	Mind is a factor in healing both within and between persons. Mind transcends time and space and is utimately part of all Consciousness.
Examples	Surgery Drug therapy Radiation	Psychoneuro-immunology Molecular emotions Stress reduction programs Hypnosis Traditional counseling Somatic therapies Movement therapies Beginning mindfulness meditation practices	Somatic Countertransference Distant intentional healing eg. Prayer Noninvasive energy healing Transpersonal imagery Transpersonal dance and drama therapy Channeling and mediumship Advanced meditation Mystical numenous satori experiences

Figure 1-1. The eras of medicine. (From Dossey, 1998, p. 9)

This section explores paradigms for experiencing how we make meaning and know what we know about the mindbodysoul interconnection in growth, health, healing, and transformation. Various paradigms will initially be discussed in distinct areas followed by an example of a synthesized integrative model in the final chapter of the section. It is hoped that holistic health practitioners: be they yoga instructors, massage therapists, somatic psychotherapists, stress reduction and meditation facilitators, transpersonal therapists, nutritionists, herbalists, energy medicine healers, expressive arts therapists homeopaths, osteopaths, chiropractors, holistic health physicians, nurses or those involved with spiritual, mystical, and indigenous practices; may be able to utilize the theoretical and practical knowledge in this book toward expanding and integrating their own frame of reference and work in service to the well-being of others.

REFERENCES

Dossey, L. (1998). Reinventing medicine: Beyond mind-body to a new era of healing. San Francisco: HarperCollins.

Gerber, (1988). Vibrational medicine. Santa Fe, NM: Bear & Co.

Chapter 2

MINDBODY MEDICINE:
ADVANCES IN WESTERN MEDICINE AND SCIENCE

All thought and feelings can affect the immune system on a
cellular, molecular and energetic level.

INTRODUCTION
AND HISTORY

MINDBODY MEDICINE IS AN APPROACH that views the mind–its thoughts and feelings–as having a central impact on the body's capacity to stay healthy and recover from trauma or illness. This construct produced the obvious premise that it is best to treat the whole person not just the physical disease. This is not a new idea. In fact, it was common for all those treating the infirm to uphold this tenant. Unfortunately, the Age of Enlightenment was less than erudite with its analytical reductivist scientific model that brought about the Cartesian split between mind and body. The resurgence of mind-body as an interrelated integrated whole reemerged with the introduction of Asian healing systems into Western medicine in the late twentieth century. The foundational paradigms of these approaches came at odds with the hierarchical, noncommunicative Asclupian scientific medical model. This splitting was reinforced by growing medical specialization and insurance mills that pushed doctors into even greater alienation from their patients.

Along with the realization that the thoughts, feelings and experience of individuals are considered as well as the disease process itself, it is also vital to not only address clients' emotional distress while engaged in psychotherapy, but to take into account the somatic ramifications and manifestations of psychological issues. Similarly, therapists had to begin to expand their verbal techniques to include body–oriented forms of assessment and interventions if they were to be truly effective.

For clients, Era II medicine i.e., the inter-influence of the mind and body means that they needed to expand their understanding of what can influence their health and recovery process. For example, by attending to and clearing negative thinking such as a sense of hopelessness or passivity, an individual can affect their physical health by reducing the severity, frequency, or duration of recovery.

This concept paved the way for a whole field of holistic health with a myriad of practitioners who understood that one needs to both address the overall experience of the wellness including thoughts and feelings as well as the physical distress or disease itself. This premise is not to be confused with the view that suggests that individuals are "responsible" for being ill and that their lack of recovery is "their fault" because of how they think or feel. This destructive supposition often results in individuals' feeling alienated, shamed and guilty that they're not getting better. These feelings then exacerbate the very condition that the person is trying to remediate.

PSYCHONEURO-IMMUNOLOGY

Era II medicine began as early as the sixties and seventies with research on Transcendental Meditation demonstrating that when the mind and body relaxed it affects the autonomic nervous system. Individuals engaged in all forms of meditation, hypnosis as well as biofeedback techniques that were all designed to decrease an overreactive fight/flight sympathetic nervous system response.

The understanding of the relationship between the central nervous system and the immune system began in the seventies with an accidental realization stemming from research with rats. The study inadvertently discovered that a classical conditioning link could occur between an immunosuppressant medication and saccharin. The initial awareness that some aspects of the immune system could be conditioned paved the way for further research and the development of the new field of psychoneuroimmunology.

These key experiments performed in the seventies undertaken by Robert Adler and others (Goleman & Gurin, 1993) have brought about the understanding of the inseparable connection between the immune system and the nervous system. Nerve endings are embedded in the bone marrow and thymus where white cells are manufactured and in the spleen and lymph nodes where they are stored.

The following are the major tenants of this interrelationship:

• The brain monitors and can alter immune responses.
• The stimulated immune responses can cause the hypothalamus (emotional center in the brain) to activate.
• Stress hormones such as adrenaline suppress immune responses through chemical responsivity.
• Lymphocytes can produce hormones and chemicals that the immune system uses to intercommunicate–bypassing the brain.

WHITE BLOOD CELLS. The immune system's main vehicles are white blood cells. Lymphocytes are the primary fighters. They maraud throughout the body attacking viruses and any cells, including cancer cells, that they do not recognize as belonging to the body. The following are some of the most relevant:

B-Lymphocytes produce antibodies that each go after and attack particular viruses and bacteria or (antigens).

T-cells. The, now well-known, cancer fighting T-cells do not produce antibodies but directly attack specific rogue cells by attaching to the invading cell and releasing toxic chemicals. These cells may be cancer cells, viral infected cells, or transplanted tissue cells. All can be affected–either suppressed or encouraged–by the level of stress–real or imagined–to which the body is reacting. Other T-cells are the helper T-cells which stimulate the production of antibodies from B-lymphocytes and the suppressor T-cells which curtail production when enough have been manufactured. These cells communicate through the production of interferons and interleukins.

Individuals may have chronically underactive or overactive T-cells:

Underactive: Individuals with AIDS and other immunodeficient diseases have too few helper cells.

Overactive: People with autoimmune diseases such as rheumatoid arthritis, Multiple Sclerosis, and Lupus have too high an amount of helper cells resulting in patients' connective tissue or nervous system being attacked. Those that are prone to allergic reactions also struggle with this lack of balance. In these situations the immune system is not distinguishing the body from nonself or invasion.

THE EFFECTS OF LIFE STRESSORS AND SOCIAL SUPPORT

Additionally, in the sixties, the Navy researched that serious life changes affected the incidence of serious illnesses of the sample population. The *Diagnostic Statistical Manual for Psychiatric Disorders* began addressing the effect of these stressors in individual's physical health. Giving numerical values to various life stressors such as; death of a loved one, loss of a job, financial difficulties and/or the ending a relationship, psychologists began to predict individuals' susceptibility to trauma and disease (DSM-IVR).

In the seventies, Spiegel studied the effects of support groups for women being treated for breast cancer; and, to his surprise, discovered that the groups not only improved the quality of a woman's life but prolonged her life as well (Goleman, 1996). A recent study confirmed that the more roles a person has (identities such as spouse, parent, job or avocational interests) and their associated social groups, the more likely it is for an individual to survive a serious illness and live longer. Today, it is well known that psychological stressors alter the susceptibility to infections, autoimmune disease and cancer.

The Holmes-Rahe Stressor scale lists life changes along with their numerical rating as to the degree of stress experienced in a year's time. If an individual scores between 150-1999, she/he has a 37% chance of getting sick within the following year. A 200-299 score raises the chances to 79%. Clearly change in and of itself is stressful.

The Stressors of Life	
HEALTH	
An injury or illness that:	
Hospitalized you or kept you in bed a week or more	42
Was less serious than the above	25
Major dental work	40
Major change in eating habits	29
Major change in sleeping habits	31
Major change in usual type of recreation or exercise	30
WORK	
Change to a new type of work	38
Change in work hours and/or conditions	33
Change in responsibilities at work:	
More responsibilities	31
Fewer responsibilities	29
Promotion	31
Demotion	57
Transfer	38
Troubles at work:	
With your boss	39
With your co-workers	35
With persons under you	30
Other work troubles	31

Figure 2-1. Holmes-Rahe Stressor Scale.

Major business adjustment	38
Retirement	49
Loss of job:	
Laid off work	57
Fired from work	64
Taking a correspondence course	29
HOME AND FAMILY	
Major change in living conditions	39
Change in residence:	
Move within the same town or city	28
Move to a different town or state	38
Change in family get-togethers	26
Major change in health or behavior of a family member	52
Marriage	50
Pregnancy	60
Miscarriage or abortion	53
Gain of a new family member:	
Birth of a child	49
Adoption of a child	45
A relative moving in with you	57
Spouse beginning or ending work outside the home	37
Child leaving home:	
To attend college	28
To marry	30
For other reasons	29
Change in arguments with spouse	34
In-law problems	29
Change in marital status of parents:	
Divorce	38
Remarriage	33
Separation from spouse:	
Due to work	49
Due to marital problems	56
Marital reconciliation	42
Divorce	62
Birth of a grandchild	31
Death of a spouse	105
Death of a family member:	
Child	105
Sibling	64
Parent	66
PERSONAL AND SOCIAL	
Change in personal habits	31
Beginning or ending school or college	32
Change of school or college	28
Change in political beliefs	25
Change in religious beliefs	29
Change in social activities	28
Vacation	29
New, close personal relationship	32
Engagement to marry	39

"Girlfriend" or "boyfriend" problems	30
Sexual difficulties	49
Falling out of a close relationship	35
An accident	44
Minor violation of the law	32
Being held in jail	57
Death of a close friend	46
Major decision regarding the immediate future	45
Major personal achievement	33
FINANCIAL	
Major changes in finances:	
Increased income	27
Decreased income	60
Investment and/or credit difficulties	43
Loss or damage of personal property	40
Moderate purchase	26
Major purchase	39
Foreclosure on a mortgage or loan	57

It is clear from human and animal studies that acute high level stress and or chronic stress can compromise the immune system especially if age or an ongoing medical condition such as mono, HIV-AIDs or chemotherapy has already weakened the immune system.

INGESTION AND THE MINDBODY CONNECTION

What individuals put into their body has also begun to be studied as to its effects on health and emotional well-being. Beyond the issues of eating disorders and diet-affected illnesses such as diabetes, researchers began to look at how diet has affected children with specific focus on attention deficit hyperactive disorder. Sugar, dairy, bleached flower products have long been connected to emotional lability.

Conversely, research subjects' minds have been also proven to influence pharmacological drug ingestion. According to Goleman and Gurin (1996) approximately one-third of a tested patient population improves when given a placebo drug if they

were led to believe that it would help them—a reason why double blind studies are required for drug testing.

CHRONIC STRESS: THE AUTONOMIC NERVOUS SYSTEM AND THE SYMPATHETIC RESPONSE

Responses to short-term stress have clearly followed humans through evolution and are a needed part of a natural survival mechanism. Stress is defined as "any challenge to homeostasis" or "a nonspecific automatic biological response to demands made upon an individual" (Hafen, et al., 1996, p. 42). Distress promotes a sympathetic response to danger that helps a person react quickly to, for example, swerve out of the way of an oncoming vehicle. Simply, the body picks up information through the various senses; any phenomena questionable is chemically translated and sent to the limbic system and cortex (see Figure 2-2, The limbic system). Signals are sent from the hypothalamus—a part of the limbic system to the pituitary gland that, in turn, sends a flood of chemi-

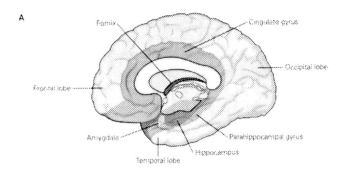

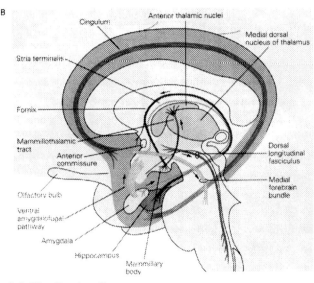

The limbic system consists of the limbic lobe and deep-lying structures.
(Adapted from Nieuwenhuys et al. 1988.)

A. This medial view of the brain shows the prefrontal limbic cortex and the limbic lobe. The limbic lobe consists of primitive cortical tissue that encircles the upper brain stem as well as underlying cortical structures (hippocampus and amygdala).

B. Interconnections of the deep-lying structures included in the limbic system. The predominant direction of neural activity in each tract is indicated by an **arrow**, although these tracts are typically bidirectional.

Figure 2-2. The Limbic System.

cals to the autonomic nervous system. Chronic stress, the protraction of normal responses to danger, can lead to a decreased or deregulated immune system, producing infections, allergies, autoimmune reactions or inflammations; chronic disease such as spastic colon, headaches, hypertension, coronary heart disease; endocrine changes affecting reproductive hormones, insulin and metabolism; or influence the development of a disease.

The result of stimulating the sympathetic nervous system response is one or more of the 4-F's:

Hyperarousal:
fight in which the blood is sent to the upper extremities and jaw for instinctual biting and hitting
flight in which the blood is sent to the lower extremities for escape;

Hypoarousal:
freeze in which the body appears still on the outside but the heart and metabolism is racing on the inside so as not to attract the adversary's attention, or
faint in which the person's "plays dead" with the heart rate and respiration decreasing in deanimation (Caldwell, 2000).

Stress response targets organ-systems and can produce:
• Increased adrenaline and cortisol from the adrenal cortex causing adrenal exhaustion, abdominal fat

• Increased blood cholesterol
• Increased heart rate and blood pressure promoting hypertension
• Increased muscle tension leaving the muscles susceptible to injury or spasm, headaches and aggravated pain
• Closed body posturing leaving a person relationally isolated
• Restricted Upper GI producing stomachaches, nausea, choking feelings
• Volatile Lower GI resulting in diarrhea, constipation or spasm
• Decreased immune system response leaving the individual susceptible to disease or a decreased ability to recover
• Decreased digestive functioning
• Decreased calcium in bones
• Hypocampal impairment producing memory loss and potential brain damage
• Racing thoughts, anxiety, poor concentration and even panic
• Feelings of tension, irritability, depression
• Behavioral symptoms such as sleep disturbances, changes in diet

Conversely, the relaxation response can produce:
• Decreased heart rate and blood pressure
• Natural digestive processes to occur
• Quieted thoughts and emotions
• Relaxed muscle tone
• Opened body posturing allowing a person to be relationally available
• Increased immune system response to disease or recovery (see Figure 2-3, The Stress Stimulus Response and Figure 2-4, The autonomic nervous system and the body's organs).

Techniques in holistic health have tended to focus on increasing the calming or parasympathetic response through increased relaxation and centering. Meditation, visualization, yoga, therapeutic massage, creative expression and self-hypnosis have been proven effective.

EARLY CHILDHOOD TRAUMA AND THE SENSORIMOTOR BRAIN LEVEL

The brain can be seen as developing hierarchically (LeDoux, 1996; Ogden & Minton, 2001). The sensorimotor level of experience is seen as the most basic followed by the emotional level and finally the cortical cognitive level. Individuals who experience physical trauma such as sexual abuse, battering and other energetically and physically invasive abuse early on in life receive this information and store it on a sensorimotor level. This level includes the autonomic nervous system, the limbic system, as well as elements of the peripheral nervous system on both physical and chemical levels. D.W. Winnicott has said that often "early memories are preverbal, nonverbal, and unverbalizable" (Winnicott, in Lewis, 1994). Those who suffer early childhood abuse are riddled with the repetition of isolated, fragmented, and incomplete sensorimotor somatic responses that can be triggered by outside stimuli such as sounds, smells, bodily sensations, touch, and images. Individuals who suffer from sensorimotor flashbacks often feel that they have no cortical control over the occurrences or their sympathetic autonomic nervous system responses to them. Frequently, these responses are just as fragmented as the stimuli which produces them. More often than not, there is an inability of higher levels to modulate and modify these stimuli-response reactions. Thus, purely cognitive cortical interventions may not be able to touch these lower circular sensorimotor level responses.

EXTERNAL STIMULI	INTERNAL STIMULI: THOUGHTS, FEELINGS, IMAGININGS	INTERNAL STIMULI: PHYSICAL SENSATIONS
Real external threats: physical, biological, economic	Imagined threats in the present or future	Pain
Social threat: defense of social standing, attack on internal belief systems	Primitive longings for attention, love, specialiness, acceptance	Illness or disease
Present environmental stimuli which triggers past stress and past stress responses	Any self-expression which does not fit the outer persona	Lack of homeostaces
	Invasion of the ego/mind of complexes which override the capacity to be in the present	

STRESS REACTION

HYPOTHALAMUS (SEAT OF EMOTIONS)	HYPOTHALAMUS (SEAT OF EMOTIONS)	PITUITARY GLAND
Triggers sympathetic response in the autonomic nervouc system	Secretion of hormones	Secretion of hormones
Produces	Produces	Produces
Fight-flight-freeze-and/or faint responses	Secretion from glands such as epinephrine from the adrenal medula resulting in a "rush"	Neuropeptides travel to cell groups and tissues
Corresponding muscle tension increase	Secretion from nerve cells called neuropeptides	Responses from organ such as adrenal cortex (cortisol)
Nerve cells connect to all organs	Neuropeptides travel to cell groups and tissues which bind to receptor molecules in the cells	
Produces	Produces	
Restricted upper GI, volatile lower GI	Sensations and emotions such as butterflies in the stomach	
Decreased immune system response		
↑ heart rate and cholesterol		

CHRONIC STRESS RESPONSE

MALADAPTIVE COPING	STRESS HARDY
Blocking of expression through the use of childhood survival mechanisms	Coping strategies
Produces	Ability to change relationship to chronic illness or stress producing stimuli
Denial and somatic disconnection	Able to generate the relaxation response
Addictive behavior: work, retail, love, sex addiction Substance abuse: food, drugs, alcohol	producing
Decreased immune system response	Increased immune system response for health and recovery
Feeling of tension, depression, and/or anxiety	Feelings of optimism, calm, solution focused
Attachment to suffering and stress	Detachment from stress and suffering
Chronic physiological somatic complaints	Relaxed muscle tone, spontaneity, normal digestive and circulatory functioning
Inner criticism, need to control, isolation, insulation, minimization, needless and wantless	Mindfulness, full present consciousness, acceptance of the here and now

Figure 2-3. The stress-stimulus response.

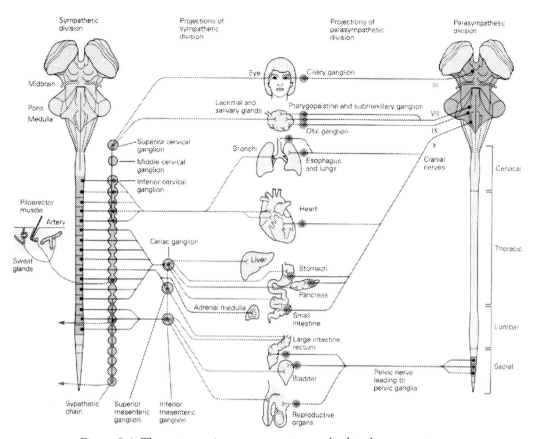

Figure 2-4. The autonomic nervous system and related organ systems.

Mindbody approaches that tap into sensorimotor processing and experience are effective in altering and regulating the responses of individuals who have suffered physical trauma (Lewis, 1993; Caldwell, 2000; Ogden & Minton, 2001). Individuals who are caught in hyperarousal, responding with hypervigilance and hyperreactivity–within the fight/flight response–frequently experience being overwhelmed, flooded and chaotically disorganized. Others who respond in hypoarousal within the freeze/faint response can feel a numbing or dulling of both inner and outer experience producing an inability to discriminate and protect themselves in their present life. These individuals use isolation, insulation and wall-like boundaries that diminish their capacity to receive any response appropriately. Body-oriented psychotherapies have been able, through an awareness of the significance of sensorimotor level held memory, traumatic flashbacks and primitive responses to danger, to facilitate the client's ability to have choice regarding their responses; thereby helping them to alter their previous sensorimotor responses (Lewis, 2000).

THE CHEMICAL NERVOUS SYSTEM: THE NEUROPHYSIOLOGIC MOLECULES OF EMOTION

"My research has shown me that the body can and must be healed through the mind, and the mind can and must be healed through the body" (Pert, 1999, p. 274).

Psychoneuroimmunology has put a magnifying glass up to the mindbody immune system relationship. There they found molecules–the tiniest element of the body that can still be considered a substance. Molecules make up every cell of the body. Certain molecules are specifically located on cell walls for the purpose of scanning for the right chemicals that will bind to the receptor and be received into the cell in a process known as binding. Once the receptor receives the message, it can result in the cell changing through the productions of new proteins, cell division or a number of other possibilities resulting, when many cells are engaged in the process, in changes in physical activity and mood.

Among the molecules that bind to these receptors are:
- Acetylcholine
- Norepinephrine
- Dopamine
- Serotonin
- Steroids such as testosterone, progesterone and estrogen, and cortisol
- And peptides which constitute 95 percent of these molecules; such as:
  - Endorphins
  - Proteins which are equal to the brain's own morphine
  - Gut cell substances which produce "gut feelings" and insulin

It is these peptides which Pert refers to as "the molecules of emotion" (1999). What has long considered to be the classical seat of the emotions: the limbic system in the sub cortex of the brain composed of the amygdala, hippocampus, and limbic cortex contains 95 percent of the various neuropeptide receptors. But there are also other anatomical locations where high concentrations of these emotion-producing peptides exist; such as: the dorsal horns of the spinal cord and all the way along neural pathways to internal organs as well as to the skin. Additionally, it has been discovered that immune cells produced in the bone marrow and thymus also store and disseminate neuropeptides themselves. Immune cells are making the very same chemicals that are considered to control the emotions in the brain. Pert (1999) writes, "The decision about what becomes thought rising into consciousness and what remains buried at a deeper level in the body is mediated by these peptides and their receptors" (p. 141). Thus, it is these molecules and their receptors which decide what is worth attending to.

And further: "if we accept the idea that peptides and other informational substances are the biochemicals of emotion, their distribution in the body's nerves has all kinds of significance which Sigmund Freud, were he alive today, would gleefully point out as the molecular confirmation of his theories. The body is the unconscious mind! Repressed traumas caused by overwhelming emotion can be stored in a body part, thereafter affecting our ability to feel that part or even move it. The new work suggests there are almost infinite pathways for the conscious mind to access and modify the unconscious mind and body" (p. 141).

Kendall at Columbia University has proven that these peptides and their receptors are the bimolecular origin of memory occurring in the body. The significance for integrated holistic health is obvious. Pert writes, "the unconscious mind of the body seems all-knowing and all-powerful and in some therapies can be harnessed for healing or change without the conscious mind ever figuring out what happened. Hypnosis, yogic breathing, many of the energy base therapies and psychotherapies centered on body work to chiropractics, massage and therapeutic touch are all examples of techniques that can be used to affect change on a level beneath consciousness" (p. 147).

THE NEUROPHYSIOLOGY OF PSYCHOLOGICAL DYSFUNCTION

It is well-known that anxiety and depression decrease the strength of the immune system. Of the two, chronic depression can be more injurious as it increases cortisol that many feel "poisons" the immune system. Chemically, depression is correlated with a diminished amount of the neural chemical serotonin secreted by the brain cells. Antidepressant drugs are used to block the reuptake mechanism allowing the serotonin to flood the receptors thereby supposedly correcting the imbalance. With new research, however, it is understood that excess serotonin can also flood the intestine producing gastrointestinal disorders.

Antipsychotic drugs can have similar disruptive effects upon the natural functioning of neurophysiology of the brain by blocking the receptors for dopamine. Researchers are concerned that drugs–legal and illegal–are further interrupting the many feedback loops that allow the psychosomatic network to function in a natural balanced way.

Research at the National Institute of Mental Health has found that depression in early childhood trauma results in chronic alteration of brain functioning. Simply, the hypothalamus, a part of the emotional limbic system of the brain identified by some as a virtual drug factory, messages the pituitary gland to secrete cortical releasing factor (C. R. F.) which, in turn, stimulates the secretion of ACTH that travels to the adrenal glands messaging them to begin to produce steroids (Hafen et al., 1996). Thus, depressed people are in a chronic state of adrenal activation because of a disruptive feedback loop that fails to signal when there's a sufficient level of steroids in the blood. Pert calls C. R. F. the "peptides of negative expectations." The plethora of C. R. F. curtails other peptides resulting in fewer possibilities in the range of emotional expression and behavior.

Body-oriented therapies that entail touching and holding can, according to Pert, break the steroids feedback loop. Pert writes, "From my research with the endorphins, I know the power of touch to stimulate and regulate our natural chemicals, the ones that are tailored to act at precisely the right times in exactly the appropriate dosages to maximize our feelings of health and well-being" (p. 272).

THE NEUROPHYSIOLOGY OF PHYSICAL HEALTH AND HEALING

Regarding physical health, it is important to note that viruses use the same receptor as neuropeptides to enter a cell. Whether or not a virus enters a cell depends upon how much a peptide for a particular receptor is available to bind. Thus, the state of the emotions will affect whether or not an individual contracts a viral infection. Simply, when a person is elated, a virus is less likely to enter the cell because the norepinephrine blocks all the potential virus receptors. Additionally, research has currently correlated the lack of expression of anger with a slower recovery rate from long-term disease processes such as cancer. These more passive cancer patients also seemed statistically unaware of their own basic emotional needs. With these individuals, the immune system was weaker and the tumors larger than for those who were not in touch with their emotions.

THE INFLUENCE OF THOUGHT AND EMOTIONAL STATES ON MINDBODY HEALTH AND HEALING

"Your body cannot tell the difference between what you are imagining through thought and emotion and reality" (Boresyenko, 2000).

Driven by the tested hypotheses that psychological distress decreases the immune system which results in increased risk of illness and reduced rate of recovery, and that holistic mindbody approaches have been proven to increase resistance to disease, the 90s culminated in a huge surge in scientific effort to begin to uncover the physiological, biomolecular mechanisms that are involved in the interconnectedness of the mindbody. Body system after body system was seen to be influenced by thoughts and feelings: the circulatory, digestive, muscular-skeletal, excretory, respiratory, reproductive and endocrine as well as central nervous system functioning and development.

Imagination and Reality

The body physiology, including the autonomic nervous system, responds the same way to imagined or reremembered danger as it does to an actual physical danger. Conversely, individuals using self-hypnosis can place themselves in a relaxation response or one which increases their endorphins resulting in suppression of pain and increase of ecstatic states even though their body might be undergoing what would be considered physical pain and therefore stressful. When the mind is calm, opiate-like molecules are created which are sent throughout the body calming every cell. Conversely, when the mind is filled with negative imaginings, anxiety and depression producing neuropeptides are created. Additionally, the limbic system gets caught in a continuous negative feedback loop resulting in the amygdala affecting the sympathetic response from the autonomic nervous system affecting bodily changes reminding the individual of past trauma thus producing more anxiety and imaginings which reaffect the amygdala, etc. In these situations, the cortex is bypassed, so rationality often cannot influence the crisis spiraling process.

Healthy Boundaries

It is vital to not only comprehend the difference between fantasy and negative thinking and reality, but individuals must also know the difference between another's thoughts and their own. An amazing number of individuals take in what others think about them without differentiating what is true from what is inaccurate. Most people tend to unconsciously project a part of themselves or transfer a former relationship they had with a significant other such as a mother into another person. If recipients of transferences do not have adequate boundaries, they may buy into all the associated thinking about themselves. They then carry others thoughts and feelings rather than connect with their own truth. This can occur collectively as well such as when, for example, a nondominant societal or cultural group believes a negative projection by the dominant group. This phenomenon can result in self-hate, increased stress and reduced life force to stay healthy.

Thoughts as Energy

"Everything you believe has an energy. What you fear controls you. You are energy before matter." If you have 100 percent energy to start, this can be diminished by bringing the past into the present and reliving it or by fearing or obsessing about the future. If 60 percent of an individual's energy is taken up with thoughts and feelings of the past or future, then there is only 40 percent of the available energy left for the present. This affects the life force available to the immune system as well as for moment-to-moment experiencing. These negative cognitions, fears, obsessive ruminations, and self-judgments all pull energy away from healthy cellular functioning (Myss, 1996).

Simply, if the mind is filled with unawareness (the lack of being fully present) and dissatisfaction (that the past happened or what is wished did not or will not occur), it is difficult to feel calm or relaxed.

Research has demonstrated that negative thoughts such as a sense of helplessness and hopelessness produce stress responses that result in adrenal exhaustion and in the lack of the body to absorb needed antioxidants such as vitamin C (Cousins, Hafen, et al., 1999).

Afflicting thoughts and feelings such as anxiety and fear, Boresyenko (2000) relates, can cause a sense of pessimism and helplessness which, in turn, produces stress and reduces the immune system's capacity to heal and maintain a person's health. Researchers have documented that the natural killer T-cells are decreased when an individual consistently feels helpless. Apathy and stoicism also point to a poor prognosis.

Many in holistic health whether they be energy healers, nutritionists, or mindbody counselors understand that unless core or limited beliefs are healed, cleared, or replaced with positive affirmations, the individual will most typically revert back to their existing symptoms and be unable to sustain health. Cognitive behavioral approaches have infused much of the holistic health field. Thoughts that limit a person's capacity to heal need to be explored and traced back to their fundamental essence. For example, a client may say that they have tried everything but nothing will ever work. The holistic health practitioner/counselor/consultant may ask what underlies this belief. The individual might say, "Because nothing works for me." Delving further could result in: "Because I am excluded from health and good things happening to me." This may become "because I am isolated, unworthy, rejected by God, fundamentally unacceptable, and/or shamefully barred from life's abundance and good will." This may reveal the core issue of abandonment that originated from lack of appropriate attunement and emotional care by the primary caregivers. The final result of this core belief which began at infancy is that "if I, an infant, am abandoned, I will die as I am too young to

care for myself." Survival and the fear of death are always underlying roots.

Nonafflicting thoughts such as peace, humor, insight, faith and a sense of personal control over one's health can produce optimism and a hearty immune system. Participating in a holistic health program or going to a practitioner often brings back a sense of control and hope which, in and of itself, can strengthen the body's capacity to fight disease and stay healthy.

In addition to a sense of control, researchers have found other cognitive constructs as having a positive correlation to maintaining health. Perceiving life's difficulties as a challenge to overcome rather than a threat to respond to defensively and experiencing meaning in something one is committed to are both positive influences upon well-being (Goleman & Gurin, 1996).

Mindfulness

Perceiving Versus Judging

Research suggests that a nonjudging but rather perceiving attitude to life may promote health and well-being. It goes without saying that if an individual is continuously filtering themselves, others and external events through an inner critic, they are less apt to find contentment nor a sense of expansiveness. A perceiving person seeks to understand and make meaning of situations and personal thoughts and feelings.

Acceptance and Self-Connection Versus Avoidance and Disconnection

Zinn (1990) writes, "We may be so busy denying and forcing and struggling that we have little energy left for healing and growing" (p. 38). This attitude is not the same as passivity. Zinn's mindfulness approach suggests the cultivation of a nonattached mind that lets go of feelings rather than holding on to them. The serenity prayer of addicts comes to mind here, imploring the Higher

Power to help the entreator to change what can be changed, let go of what cannot and the wisdom to know the difference. Here trust and connection to individual's own deepest knowing provides a foundation for health and well-being.

Important to note here is that there is no ultimate cognitive or emotional formula that practitioners can promise their clients. Life and the susceptibility to emotional and physical illness is a complex constellation of genetics, environment, nutrition, as well as elements that have as yet to be discovered. Happy centered people can get sick too.

THE INFLUENCE OF SOCIAL AND ANIMAL SUPPORT ON MINDBODY HEALTH AND HEALING

A sense of loneliness or disconnection from other living creatures also influences the amount of disease fighting T-cells. Studies show that interpersonal networks reverse the adverse effects of stress. The positive effects of social relationships correlates with the findings from breast cancer supports groups. People who have several support networks of friends as well as family have been identified as having better health in general. A sense of intimacy with at least one confidant with whom an individual can express thoughts and feelings akin to confession also increases the potency of the immune system. Studies have shown that individuals with these social networks live longer than their isolated counterparts whether they typically are in good health or not. Studies document over a 20 percent difference in mortality rates (Hafen, Karren, et al., 1996). Longitudinal studies also document these findings.

Not unsurprisingly, it is the heart which is most affected by a caring social support. As long as individuals are not held in hopelessness, if they are able to express themselves and are empathicly heard and reflected, they can often reduce their level of stress. The influxes of support groups are a direct result of these findings.

The Power of Touch

History has shown that infants in orphanages died of marasmus because they weren't being touched held or caressed except for feeding and rudimentary diaper changing. The famous Harlow monkey studies showed that primates develop attachment disorders and show abnormal relationship skills when raised in isolation. Touch has been shown to regulate heart rate and reduce depression and anxiety. The rise of touch-related complimentary heath modalities such as massage and the gentle touch in some forms of energy healing such as craniosacral, polarity, and Reiki may also be a result of a computerized society where friends and family are some distance away.

The Blessing of Pets

Studies have shown that those with pets live longer. Dogs and other pets that are being trained as pet therapy is on the rise in nursing homes and other facilities with severe organic dysfunction. Again, the heart and heart-related diseases are shown to be reduced and alleviated.

Some pets have been known to bond so deeply that they take on the disease of their beloved pet owner or the family stress in order to bring well-being back into the "pack."

HEALING VERSUS CURING

Most all holistic health centers will make sure that their clients understand the difference between curing or the entire relief of all symptoms and the concept of healing. Healing means to make whole. Wholeness is associated to connection and relationship.

Often individuals disconnect from their diseased bodies, from the part of their body that is in pain or is no longer functioning in the way in which they would choose. People, at times, have a tendency to refer to their body as an inanimate object—something that is not really a part of who they are. Reconnecting a person to their entire being requires individuals to be sensitive to the profound influence that their thoughts, feelings, attitude, life-style, and world view can often have on how they view and can remediate their illness, the process of aging, or overwrought neurophysiology.

Additionally, not only is intrapersonal phenomena interrelated in each individual, but we can also influence each other interpersonally. Social support from friends, family, groups, pets, as well as clinicians who are holistic health practitioners enhance healing and health.

Studies have also shown that individuals who are mindfully present are also positively inclined to healing, health, and well-being. The capacity for nonattached, nonjudgmental conscious acceptance allows individuals to experience themselves as pure, being present, conscious, still and infinite.

SUMMARY

In summary, the mindbody and soul/spirit are interrelated and can affect and influence both positively and negatively the health and well-being of an individual. The mind can influence the body. Negativism, hopelessness and helplessness have a destructive influence on the health and well-being of an individual. Chronic stress and depression compromises individuals' immune systems and their capacity to stay healthy and live longer. Recent studies have developed the new field of psychoneuroimmunology that further chemically connects the relationship among emotions, stress and the many aspects of the immune system.

The body influences the mind. For example, inactivity and specifically, the lack of endorphins produced in exercise, as well as the lack of touch can influence the person's attitudes toward life.

REFERENCES

Goleman & Gurin. (1993). *Mindbody medicine.* Yonkers, NY: Consumer Reports Books.

Hafen, B., Karren, K., Frandsen, K., and Smith, N. (1996). *Mind/body health: The effects of attitudes, emotions and relationships.* Boston: Allyn and Bacon.

Diagnostic Criteria from DSM-IV-TR. (2000). Washington, DC: American Psychiatric Association.

Myss, C. (2000). *Anatomy of the Spirit.* Tapes.

Ogden, P. & Minton,K. (2001). Sensorimotor processing: The role of the body in trauma. In Somatics Forum, winter, vol 5, #1 pp. 10–12.

Pert, C. (1999). *Molecules of emotion: The science behind mind-body medicine.* New York: Touchtone Books.

Shore, A. (1994). *Affective regulation and the origin of the self: The neurobiology of emotion and development.* Hillsdale, NJ: Lawrence Erlbaum Assoc.

Kabat-Zinn, J .(1990). *Full Catastrophe Living.* New York, NY: Dell Publishing.

Chapter 3

THE BIOLOGY OF OUR PSYCHOLOGY: UNDERSTANDING HOW STRUCTURE AND BEHAVIOR RELATE

CHRISTINE CALDWELL

ABSTRACT

THIS CHAPTER ATTEMPTS TO ARTICULATE some of the subjects neuroscientists and biopsychologists are investigating that have relevance to those who work with the interwoven nature of the body/psyche/mind. It does not attempt to cover treatment issues, but looks instead at theory building from the vantage point of modern Western scientific method. In particular, this chapter touches on emotion, learning, memory, and expressive movement as important elements of general body psychology theory.

The roots of science lie in biology. We can gain wisdom about psychological processes by studying the organization of the physical processes they are embedded in. Another view on this might be that biology is sloweddown psychology–that physical matter (the body) simply moves and changes more slowly than energy (the psyche), and that this stability of form protects and enhances individuals, just as "quick-wittedness" does. Similarly to physics, which sees matter and energy on a continuum rather than as separate entities, so individuals may see their bodies and psyches as existing on a continuum that on one side favors stability, pattern, and continuity (our more biological natures), and at the other end organizes around the ability to fluctuate on a more moment-to-moment basis (psychological natures).

Specifically, this chapter attends to the issue of biological and psychological influence. How individuals move expressively influences biochemistry, as well as biochemistry influencing their movement. How individuals feel emotionally, not only affects posture and motion, but hormone, enzyme, and peptide levels. The biological substrates of emotion, learning and memory highly influence what individuals think is true, and how we behave. By studying this juicy continuum, we can better articulate what it is we believe, how it relates to the dominant culture, and how this informs our clinical work.

Introduction

Advances in understanding of the nervous system may top the list of exciting scientific progress in recent years. Historically, because visible structures tended to be easier to study, the various structural components of nervous system tissues were examined first. Neurons, those electrical wizards of the brain and spinal cord have been long understood. Later, the understanding of the chemical components of the nervous system, the neurotransmitters came. Individuals could then see that, in a manner of speaking, all possess a solid nervous system with neurons and glial cells (glial cells provide a protective and supportive function, but are not well understood, and perhaps represent a frontier in this area of study). Developmentally, science has discovered that early experience, especially in utero and just beyond, strongly influences how, where and to what extent neurons grow. The emerging wisdom is that "neurons that fire together wire together" (Cowan, 1990). What individuals experience grows in certain directions that affect how humans continue to experience.

Individuals also possess a kind of liquid nervous system, made up of various chemicals that enhance or inhibit the transmission of impulses from one neuron to another. These chemicals are critical to psychological functioning via modulating our level of arousal, our mood, how our attention is focused, etc. It is here where psychopharmacology largely operates.

Another view to the nervous system lies in an understudied aspect of this structure, that of pheromones, a class of neurochemicals. Since pheromones are conveyed from one person's nervous system to another via air, it could be said that this represents a gaseous nervous system whose intent is to influence the nervous systems of other species, most notably affecting sexual and reproductive behavior (Wilson, 1980). It may be possible that pheromones influence other socially mediated behaviors, but this remains to be investigated. If this turns out to be so, this could have impressive repercussions for our understanding of the biopsychology of the therapeutic relationship, and body-centered relationship therapy as a whole.

Figure 3-1 illustrates this new way of looking at our nervous systems. The solid nervous system sits tight, always in place except when growing new connections or withering old ones via experience and chemical action. The liquid nervous system concentrates in the brain and spinal cord, but effectively circulates throughout the body, touching and influencing other structures, especially those of the gut and the endocrine and immune systems (more on that later). The gaseous nervous system is exuded via breath and sweat, to reach the nostrils of those around us and turn them towards or away from us in a dance of attraction and repulsion.

Next on the list of views of the nervous system peers into the brain itself. With its penchant for dividing things up, neuroscience has apportioned the nervous system from left to right, and from back to front. Those interested in the right brain/left brain material should consult Gazzaniga's work (2000). This split of the hemispheres relates to types of thought as well as language. However, the back to front view, pioneered by MacLean's *The Triune Brain* (1990), may be a hot area of exploration the field is cur-

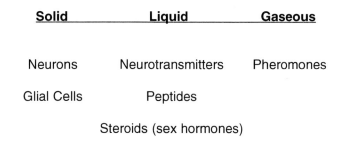

Solid	**Liquid**	**Gaseous**
Neurons	Neurotransmitters	Pheromones
Glial Cells	Peptides	
	Steroids (sex hormones)	

Figure 3-1. Types of Nervous System.

rently attending to, because it illuminates one of the holy grails of therapy, the regulation of emotion via the limbic system. Simplistically put, the hind brain and brain stem structures regulate much of human metabolism, such as breathing, heartbeat, and motor planning. MacLean dubbed this the Reptilian Brain. The midbrain, which he labels the Mammalian Brain, consists largely of the limbic system, and regulates such important psychological arenas as sensory integration, emotion, memory, and learning. Up in the front, in all its large-foreheaded glory, lies the neocortex, that which purportedly makes individuals uniquely human (or at least primate). Here is where humans reason, think, plan, reflect, and imagine.

This may be an overly neurocentric view of function and behavior. For now, we can say that these functions seem to require these brain structures, but it is also the case that they are not sufficient, and need the operations of many other tissues in the rest of the body to come about. With this overview of the nervous system in hand, we can begin to play with the biology/psychology interface in more detail.

THE BIOPSYCHOLOGY OF SOLID EMOTION

With the evolutionary advent of the mid or emotional brain, organisms were able to more quickly respond to changing environmental demands rather than operate with more fixed programs and responses. In his now famous book *Emotional Intelligence* (1995), Daniel Goleman reiterated that humans possess two minds, one that thinks and one that feels. We could add that the feeling mind also remembers and learns. Individuals may have two minds, but from a solid nervous system perspective those minds are so interlinked with bidirectional neural pathways that the limbic centers have a tremendous capacity to influence thought, as thought also influences emotion.

One of the most significant recent findings in this area of study is the fact that the solid nervous system is wired so that incoming signals from the senses are filtered first through the amygdala in the limbic system before this data ever reaches the neocortex (LeDoux, 1996). Before individuals ever form a conscious thought about an event, they have already imbued it with personal meaning and significance, because they have sifted it through stored emotional memory. Before they ever recognize an event, they have already decided whether this is something hated or feared, whether it is dangerous or pleasurable. The limbic system (more specifically the amygdala) imprints memories with an emotional context to them. The stronger the arousal was historically, the more intense the emotional imprint will be. However, this circuitry is sloppy—the memory is imprinted through association, so if one element of an old situation is present, the new situation may be perceived as a match.

This finding bears a tremendous significance for our understanding of illnesses such as impulsivity, PTSD, phobias, and affective disorders. The limbic circuitry allows it, during a crisis, to capture and drive much of the brain, including the rational mind. The popular term for this is "emotional hijacking." LeDoux feels that this wiring of the brain points to the physical existence of a cognitive unconscious, arising from emotional memories, and driven mostly by perceptions of danger. This research also lends credence to the idea that individuals are not in control of whether or not an emotion arises, but are only (potentially) in control of what is done with that emotion.

Another area of emotions' research holistic health practitioners could find usable is the realization that the amygdala is fully functioning at birth, and that the more classic, solid nervous system centers for memory (specifically the hippocampus) take as much as two years to fully come on line. Most individuals state that they cannot remember anything before the age of two or three, and this is because the hippocampus is not yet fully functional. But memory tracks are laid down in the limbic system even in utero, and are stored not as movie-like scenes, but as emotional arousals. When individuals feel emotionally reactive in a way that is out of proportion to a current stimulus, it may be that they are actually remembering a memory of a much earlier imprinted event. Rather than pushing clients to recover hippocampally-based memories, in some cases it may be more powerful to help them remember through emotional processing, to trust their feelings and relax about the details of what did or didn't happen, with whom, way back when.

Aside from providing fantasy and imagination, the prefrontal cortex also functions as the limbic systems' damper switch. When an emotion arises, the prefrontal lobes then tend to analyze the risks and benefits of various reactions, and then "choose" which behavior is in the perceived best interests of the individual, and thus keep emotional responses in balance. Emotional hijacking in this sense involves two processes: a stimulus triggering the amygdala first, and the subsequent failure of the prefrontal cortex to activate the brakes on an unhealthy response. This can be demonstrated using PET scanning and MRI's, where brain metabolism can be measured and located. In PTSD sufferers, the prefrontal cortex remains cool, while the amygdala lights up like a firecracker.

Clinically, researchers in Post Traumatic Stress Disorder believe that learning relaxation techniques, coupled with retelling the traumatic story in a harbor of safety, with as much sensory detail as possible, helps to reactivate the prefrontal lobes (Charney, 1993).

Another casualty in instances of imprinted trauma is what neuroscientists call working memory. The prefrontal cortex also organizes attention that holds the facts necessary for completing a task. If the limbic brain lights up and the prefrontal cortex fails

to come to bear, individuals' capacity to remember and learn new input can become crippled. This can be especially tragic for children in chronic emotional stress. It can literally create deficits in a child's capacity to learn and to make good decisions. It can also interfere with emotional learning and a memory, causing the child to grow up not knowing what he or she feels or wants.

As a clinical side bar, Freud's concept of evenly hovering attention begins to take on a new significance, as retraining the ability to pay attention to the right stimuli in the present moment, especially sensation itself, becomes the treatment of choice in trauma recovery.

Beginning to take the nervous system out of the strict confines of the brain, we can look at the work of Antonio Damasio (1994, 1999). One of his fascinating contributions is his concept of the "somatic marker," a term for gut feelings. He feels that what is called intuition may actually be mediated by limbic-driven surges from the viscera, and he further notes that without these visceral churnings individuals are unable to assign value to one thing over another. Humans literally have no basis for choosing, because they have no sense of what they like or don't like.

The guts seem to have a mind of their own. They certainly produce all of the same classes of chemicals responsible for liquid nervous system function (over 95% of serotonin is manufactured in the bowel, for instance) (Gershon, 1998). In the absence of input from the brain or spinal cord, the enteric or gut nervous system can mediate reflexes and perform many actions by itself. It can even have its own forms of "mental illness," which show up as ulcers, colitis, and irritable bowel syndrome. When we look at stress and its effects, we also need to look at the gut, yet traditional talk-oriented psychotherapy has been largely ineffective with this second emotional center. As Gershon states: "Malfunction of the enteric nervous system may be resistant to therapies aimed at the head, but therapies aimed at the gut just might work" (1998, xiv). Body-oriented holistic health practitioners and clinicians with their emphasis on sensory tracking, somatic awareness and expressive movement, may address this issue.

THE BIOPSYCHOLOGY OF LIQUID EMOTION

New science really comes alive for us when we look at the work of Candace Pert (1997). This former NIH, now Georgetown University neuroscientist, was largely responsible for the discovery of endorphins, the body's' natural opiates. She believes there is a biochemical link between the body and the mind, and that this link operates through chemical keys called ligands2 that act on individual cell receptors. Ligands are manufactured by the endocrine glands, and form what she calls the "molecules of emotion." She sees ligands as a separate and more ancient nervous system than the solid one we spoke of; here we begin to reframe a view towards a fully circulatory liquid nervous system, swimming in both the blood and the lymphatic system.

Seeing emotion as governed by activity in parts of the brain seems largely inaccurate to Pert, who notes that less than 2 percent of communication occurs across neural synapses. Peptide communication (peptides being a type of ligand) throughout the body especially influences the somatosensory area of the brain, and the limbic system in general. In this liquid view, we can see that emotions and body sensations are intricately intertwined in a bi-directional network where each can alter the other, resulting in changes of behavior and mood. Pert even believes that there may be specific peptides related to specific emotions.

Her work also unifies the nervous, endocrine, and immune systems. Her holistic approach sees the immune system as a floating endocrine system and that both these systems are in constant communication with the nervous system via peptides. Called "the body's brain," the immune system may help define individuals' sense of self (evolutionary biologists often call the immune system our "kinship recognition system," helping us define who they are by who they aren't, and responding accordingly). The key here is that emotions have a powerful effect on all these liquid operations, altering such powerful processes such as insulin levels, blood pressure, what cells the immune system chooses to attack or let be, etc., (Pert, 1998).

Pert validates mindbody unity by asserting that the mind is a flow of information as it moves through the tissues of the body; that it is immaterial, but has a physical substrate that is both the body and the brain, and that it has a nonphysical substrate that is information flowing. Mind becomes body, and what is called body is the outward manifestation in physical space of the mind. Emotions are the information messengers that link the systems of the body into one unit. Emotions are cellular signals that translate information into physical reality–mind into matter. Emotions exist as a back and forth flow between matter and information, influencing both.

In this view, stress-related disease in the liquid nervous system can be seen as an information overload–the mindbody becomes so overloaded with unprocessed sensory input in the form of suppressed trauma or undigested emotion that it bogs down and cannot flow freely. Stress prevents the molecules of emotion from flowing freely where they are needed, and breathing, blood flow, digestion, and elimination, collapse and cannot function well. Pert concludes that meditation and movement let peptides flow again, resulting in emotional and "mental" health.

A SECOND LOOK AT THE COMMUNAL NERVOUS SYSTEM

We do not yet know if pheromones do more than drive sexual attraction to others and other reproductive factors such as the timing of ovulation. There is some evidence that plants prime each other's immune systems via the transmission to other plants of airborne molecules of aspirin when one plant is attacked by a pathogen. If we can find these same influences in humans, we could begin to appreciate in a very physical way the presence of "healers." What if the very molecules a healthy person exudes could be healing?

Until this area is investigated, we must be content with more observable forms of human interaction, that of awareness of each other through the senses. Here again the importance of body level emotional acuity is beginning to be appreciated. Researchers who study emotional states such as empathy and compassion find that they build on self-awareness (Goleman, 1995). In other words, the more that is known about one's own feelings, the better an individual is at reading others, which is of course what is termed emotional attunement. The key to intuiting others feelings lies in reading nonverbal cues–tone of voice, gesture, facial expression–and the ability to read these cues also makes us better adjusted emotionally, more popular, outgoing, and more sensitive. It is said that 90 percent of emotional meaning is conveyed nonverbally, through body language, voice tone and facial expression. Interestingly, empathy's roots lie in motor mimicry; if an individual moves with another person, it is possible to feel something of what the other feels. Developmental psychologist Daniel Stern's (1985) concept of attunement comes directly from this observation–that microlevel nonverbal exchanges between the parent and child helps the child know his or her own emotions will be met with empathy and acceptance. These attuning movements are different than imitation. Imitation tells another that the person knows what they did, not how they feel. With a lack of attunement, the child simply begins avoiding expressing or even feeling these emotions.

In physiological readings of couples, those whose bodies were in synch (i.e., if he sweats, I sweat, if her heart races, so does mine) experienced the most empathy with each other. Emotional rapport also occurs through unconscious movement synchrony, which for many of us occurs out of our awareness. High levels of this synchrony translate to people liking each other, which helps to construct an adult-based attunement. The ability to train ourselves as conscious movers becomes crucial when we realize movement's implication in relational healing.

MEMORY AND MOVEMENT

Previously this chapter noted that emotional stress or trauma could interfere with memory formation, particularly the ability to transfer short-term memory into long-term memory. It was also mentioned that memory could be seen in two ways: like videotape being replayed with images and sound (more hippocampal), or like an emotion welling up, at times out of context (more amygdala). Some neuroscientists state that these two types of memory could be called Limbic and Forebrain.

In the limbic memory system, memories originate as sensory impressions. These sense impressions route first to the amygdala and hippocampus. Repetition or strong emotional states function to lock in this route, and transform perception into durable memory. The memory gets stimulated when the same or similar sensory events occur. Interestingly, the emotional amygdala mediates the association of memories formed through the different senses. The amygdala not only enables sensory events to develop emotional associations, but it also enables emotions to shape perception and the storage of memory. This could be the structural basis of selective attention–an important filter that limits learning to stimuli with emotional significance. This finding, that emotions influence what is perceived and learned, helps us as holistic health practitioners and therapists to continue developing our emphasis on emotional expression and expressive movement.

Addiction

This limbically-mediated memory system has gotten a lot of attention of late, because it so strongly explains PTSD and trauma. But there is also a second memory system, and it behooves clinicians to keep their attention on it as well, because it illuminates an area of work that has as much or perhaps even greater social significance–that of addiction. This noncognitive memory system exists independently of limbic circuits, and has to do with stimulus/response repetition, or habit. It lives in the area of the brain called the striatum, in the forebrain. It receives input from many parts of the cortex, and sends fibers to the parts of the brain that control movement.

This ancient area of the brain that helps individuals to form habits develops quite early. Infants do quite well in habit formation tests, for instance, but poorly in memory formation tests. So it can be seen that habit and emotional imprinting exist quite early, and that classic memory comes later. This habit-oriented memory system first works to store movement habits (called motor plans), which points to the clinical significance of therapists understanding early movement patterning as a way to understand how individuals "repeat" themselves as adults. It is my belief that the roots of adult addiction lie in this system, and in early need deprivation that affects individual's ability to motor plan (Caldwell, 2000).

Because the striatum-based memory system so connects with movement centers, it is important to take a more detailed look at what is known about the biological bases of movement to begin to more deeply understand the significance of working with the body.

A Look at Movement

One of the fast-moving areas of research in the field of movement has to do with how complex motion is learned. Previously, it was thought that individuals only learned movement via a combination of enlisting reflexes in the service of motor planning and practice. This still remains quite true, but it has recently been discovered that there exists a powerful visual and social component to motoric learning as well. What are now called mirror neurons have been found in area F5 of the premotor cortex. This is the area of the brain where neurons specialize in grasping movements. Area F5 also comprises part of a circuit that translates the three dimensional features of an object into the motor programs required to take possession of that object. The breakthrough occurred when it was demonstrated that these neurons can be triggered both when humans execute the grasping action and *also* when they observe the same action performed by another individual (Gallese, 1996; Rizzolatti, 1996). These neurons are called mirror neurons because their visual properties mirror or replicate their motor properties. Mirror neurons discharge during specific goal-related motor acts. This implies a new mechanism for social learning among mammals. Humans see an action and they replicate it in their own bodies without thinking. This has far-reaching implications for a possible imprinting mechanism in individual's viewing of such things as violent acts (whether real or on TV) or loving acts, physical problem solving, movement empathy, and a host of nonverbally mediated communicative behaviors.

Movement and intelligence now appear to be intimately intertwined. The two areas of the brain that were previously thought to be associated solely with the control of muscle movement–the basal ganglia and the cerebellum–are now found to be important in coordinating thought (Hannaford, 1995). These areas are connected to the frontal lobe area where planning the order and timing of future behavior occurs. Hannaford states that "to pin down a thought, there must be movement. A person may sit quietly to think, but to remember a thought an action must be used to anchor it" (p. 98–99). She also notes that a coordinated series of movements produces increased neurotrophins (natural neural growth factors) and a greater number of connections among neurons. This gains importance when it is combined with research that shows it is not so much how many neurons a human possesses, but the amount of connectedness or networking between them that factors greatly in IQ and other measures of intellectual ability (Calvin, 1999). As holistic health practitioners and therapists who use somatic and expressive movement approaches in combination with tracking sensation and verbalization, we can feel more confident that the efficacy of what we do enjoys a scientific underpinning.

Evolutionary biologists as well as physiologists have championed this bridging of intelligence with movement. Researchers such as Calvin (1999) hold that intelligence evolved primarily through the refinement of a brain specialization that involves quickness, versatility (the ability to move appropriately towards many different food sources), social complexity, and the ability to plan ahead. Behavior emerges, says Calvin, through the matching of sensory templates to responsive movements. Interestingly, he believes that play behavior may be a free opportunity to try new combinations of sensory templates with movement (Ibid.).

The ability to sequence things one after the other develops an ability to plan ahead. Evolutionarily, this behavioral sequencing ability came from the development of movement sequencing, especially ballistic movement (hammering, throwing, and clubbing), and may have promoted language, music, and intelligence. Ballistic movement requires a surprising amount of planning; slow movements leave time for improvisation and course corrections. On the other hand in ballistic movement, which requires ordering the sequencing of dozens of muscles to move quite rapidly, no during-the-movement corrections are possible, so it has to be planned ahead of time in the brain, perhaps with the aid of mirror neurons. This coordination of movement occurs at the sub cortical level in the basal ganglia or cerebellum. Novel movements tend to depend on the premotor and prefrontal cortex. This realization led Calvin to state that "Thoughts are combinations of sensations and memories–in a way, they are movements that have not happened yet (and maybe never will)" (1999, p. 66). This hearkens back to the famous line from Humerto Maturana, the biologist who has so heavily influenced family therapy. He once quipped that the mind is not in the head; the mind is in the behavior.

Biologist Isaac Golani has been investigating movement processes in many different life forms, and concentrates on mammals. He studies the effect of different psychotropic drugs, both endogenous (made in the body) and exogenous (administered from outside the body). He now asserts that movement occurs along a continuum. "Behavior progresses along a mobility gradient from immobility to increasing complexity and unpredictability. A progression in the opposite direction, with decreasing spatial complexity and increased stereotypy, occurs under the influence of dopamine-like drugs" (1992: 263). Most addictive drugs, as well as many prescribed medications for "mental" illnesses influence dopamine circuitry. What this may point to is a connection between movement stereotypy and addiction, first pointed out in the popular literature by the author (Caldwell, 1996).

An emerging view of movement processes can be organized along a continuum of highly patterned to highly impulsive, as illustrated in Figure 3-2 below. It is the authors contention that health can be seen as an ability to oscillate responsively along this entire continuum.

By using biologically organized movement processes as a relevant feature in body-centered diagnosis, we can form even more intelligent treatment practices for our clients, ones that compliment and share language with other disciplines such as occupational therapy and physical therapy. Another way to view our field's organizing principles is by articulating sensorimotor processing from a biological perspective. Figure 3-2 attempts to take a phylogenetic view of how we develop via the loop of sensation and movement, tying together much of the previously discussed material.

In this view, individuals exist along a continuum of pure biological purpose to highly conscious behavior, culminating in the finest expression, that of play. Perhaps from here

those in the field of holistic health can more precisely articulate what it is we do, and why. This chapter does not represent an exhaustive articulation of what science has investigated in the body/mind area in the past decade. Hope blossoms that in the future we can incorporate a deeper understanding of other body systems as well, especially the immune, endocrine, and integument (skin). Connective tissue seems to bear another look, as it now is known to possess and influence electromagnetic fields. We are becoming capable of not being so neurocentric in our views, which may be a holdover from a Cartesian-based mind/body dualism. By extending our hand out to science, we may find a companionable dialogue ensues, one that enriches us, our clients, and the society at large.

REFERENCES

Caldwell, C. (1996). *Getting our bodies back.* Boston, MA: Shambhala Press.

Calvin, W. (1999). The Emergence of intelli-

Pattern				Impulse
Forced ____ __Motor Plans __ __Attuning __ __Nonverbal _____ Play				
Forced Movement	Motor Plans	Attuning Movement	Nonverbal Communication	Play Movement
Fixed Action Patterns	Locomotion (walk/fly/swim)	Shape Flow	Posture/ Gesture/Tone	Exploring Curiosity Experimentation
Orienting Responses	Drives (push, reach, yield)	Tension Flow	Pacing/ Facing/Spacing	Reflexes/Tropisms

Notes:
* Forced Movements are species-specific and require no practicing—they are hard wired and inherited
* Motor plans are also species-specific, but require practice
* Attuning Movements are species driven but require practice and begin to be influenced by culture
* Nonverbal Communication Movements are largely learned culturally
* Play Movements oscillate between inner impulse & culture

Figure 3-2. Movement Processes.

| Sensation | | | | | Reflex Action |
| (6 senses) | | | | | (knee jerk, etc) |

Sensation _____	Emotional _____				Defense Reaction
	Designation				(the 4 F's)
	(limbic & ligands)				

| Sensation _____ | Emotional _____ | Perception _____ | | Reaction |
| | Designation | (attention + tone) | | (habit) |

| Sensation ___ | Emotional ___ | Perception ___ | Reflection __ | Responsive |
| | Designation | (aware/own/apprec) | | Action |

Notes:
* The sixth sense = proprioception
* We are aware of reflexes only after they occur
* Limbic structures include the amygdala, hippocampus, cingate gyrus, hypothalamus
* Ligands is a general term that can cover hormones, neurotransmitters, and peptides
* The 4 F's are: fight, flight, freeze, and faint
* Awareness, Owning, and Appreciation are three of the phases in Caldwell's Moving Cycle (1996)
* All actions are movements that create influences towards incoming sensation and emotional designation—a feedback loop

Figure 3-3. Levels of Sensorimotor Processing, from simple and primitive to complex.

gence. *Scientific American Quarterly, 9*(4), 126–135.

Charney, D., et al. (1993). Psychobiologic mechanisms of posttraumatic stress disorder. *Archives of General Psychiatry, April 50,* 294–305.

Cowan, W. M. (1990). The Development of the brain. In Lyons, R. (Ed.), *The Workings of the brain: development, memory, and perception,* 39–57, New York: W.H. Freeman and Company.

Damasio, A. (1994). *Descartes' error: Emotion, reason, and the human brain.* New York: Avon Books.

Damasio, A. (1999). *The feeling of what happens: Body and emotion in the making of consciousness.* New York: Harcourt, Brace, and Company.

Gallese, V., Fadiga, L., & Rizzolatti, G. (1996). Action recognition in the premotor cortex. *Brain, 119,* 593–609.

Rizzolatti, G., Fadiga, L., & Fugues, L. (1996). Premotor cortex and the recognition of motor actions. *Cognitive Brain Research, 3,* 131–141.

Guessing, A. (Ed.). (2000). *Cognitive neuroscience: A reader.* New York: Bleakly Publica-

tions.

Gershon, M. (1998). *The Second brain.* New York: Harper Perennial.

Golani, I. (1992). A Mobility gradient in the organization of vertebrate movement: The perception of movement through symbolic language. *Brain and Behavioral Sciences,* Cambridge University Press. *15,* 249–308.

Goleman, D. (1995). *Emotional intelligence.* New York: Bantam.

Hannaford, C. (1995). *Smart moves: Why learning is not all in your head.* Arlington, VA: Great Ocean Publishers.

LeDoux, J. (1996). *The Emotional brain: The mysterious underpinnings of emotional life.* New York: Simon & Schuster.

Lob, J. (1973). *Forced movements, tropisms, and animal conduct.* New York: Dover Publications.

MacLean, P. (1990). *The Triune brain in evolution.* New York: Plenum Publications.

Mishkin, M., Appenzeller, T. (1987). The Anatomy of memory. *Scientific American.* June.

Pert, C. (1998). The Psychosomatic network: Foundations of mind-body medicine. *Alternative Therapies, July 4*(4), 31–40.

Pert, C. (1997). *The Molecules of emotion.* New York: Simon & Schuster.

Routtenberg, A. (1978). The Reward system of the brain. November. *Scientific American.*

Shore, A. (1994). *Affect regulation and the origins of the self: The neurobiology of emotional development.* Hillsdale, NJ: Lawrence Erlbaum Associates.

Sheets-Johnstone, M. (1999). *The Primacy of movement.* Philadelphia, PA: John Benjamin.

Stern, D. (1985). *The Interpersonal world of the infant: A view from psychoanalysis and developmental psychology.* New York: Basic Books.

Wilson, E.O. (1980). *Sociobiology: The abridged edition.* Cambridge, MA: Harvard University Press.

For further information and training:

Christine Caldwell, Ph.D., LPC, ADTR
Director, Somatic Psychology Department
Naropa University and the Moving Cycle Institute
P.O. Box 19892
Boulder, CO, 80308

Chapter 4

THE OBSERVABLE BODY: UNDERSTANDING BODY POSTURE AND MOVEMENT AS A WAY OF KNOWING HEALTH AND HEALING

EXERCISE AND MOVEMENT

DOCUMENTED RESEARCH HAS identified that exercise and movement decreases stress and helps prevent some diseases; including coronary heart disease, osteoporosis, arthritis, hypertension, vestibular dysfunction, diabetes, as well as other diseases of aging, and depression. Active exercise influences the production of endorphins, the body's natural mood elevator. Softer forms of exercise such as the Eastern approaches of tai chi and yoga influences the calming parasympathetic relaxation response which can elevate the body's natural immune system and promote healing. Expressive movement found in dance movement therapy allows for a full range of individually prescribed active and calming movement experiences which serve to reinforce the mind-body emotional spiritual interconnection, releasing body blocks, clearing of past trauma and repetitive outmoded survival behaviors, enhancing body image, interpersonal relatedness, and reconnection with moment-to-moment embodiment.

HUMAN DEVELOPMENT

Body movement is the most primary means of communication of the infant. The mother through the observation of the baby's movement begins to attune to the needs and wants of her child. If the attunement is successful the infant will experience the world as safe and need satisfying rather than depriving or abusive. The movement ministrations of the primary caregiver are crucial to the development of the child. Caldwell sites that the brain grows through the interactions with the caregiver. Deprived baby's brains are 20 to 30 percent smaller (Caldwell, 2000). The dyadic movement interaction (the tension flow and shape flow) between the mother and the child actually grows the limbic system of the infant if the mother is empathetically attuned. The mother is seen as the "neurological programmer of the infant." The amygdala is the locus of feeling-toned memories that are inextricably interconnected with bodily memories on a cellular level. Holding gives an infant a sense of existence and a comfort in inhabiting his/her body. Handling, caressing in an attuned manner, gives a sense of personhood, identity and uniqueness. The effects of early parenting both positive and negative remain on a body level and can be observed in an individual's posture and movement interaction with the nonhuman and human environment.

Development is seen as a progression of various stages. Within each are key relational elements that are needed in order for the infant to grow into a healthy child and adult. If, for whatever reason, a stage is unsuccessfully integrated, it will result in that particular developmental building block becoming weak. When stress arises in an individual's life, the developmental milestones which rest upon this unsuccessful stage can tumble, resulting in an individual regressing into thoughts, survival mechanisms and actions of childhood. This phenomenon has been called "a fixation," that is, the individuals are "fixed" in a particular developmental phase. In recovery theory, these individuals have been identified as "adult children." Because of the dominance of phase-related issues and behavior, individuals capacity to adapt to the moment and utilize other more appropriate behaviors is curtailed. Although the particular pattern may be appropriate in some instances, it will undoubtedly be inappropriate all the time.

Within each phase of development, key movement qualities dominate to help support the learning on a sensorimotor level. For example, biting and chewing is a required movement when a teething toddler is learning to consume food. If the needed developmentally-based relationship with the primary caregiver is not present during the teething or differentiation phase, this will effect the adaptive use of the biting/chewing rhythm. Later in life, individuals may show a dominance of this rhythm in their movement personality or a lack of adaptive usage. Thus, the presence or absence of these physiologically phased movements will identify when an individual is fixated at a particular

phase of related psychoemotional development. Mindbody interrelationship is confirmed when individuals repeatedly move a certain way or omit needed movements from their vocabulary that were naturally dominant when the associated emotional or relational issues were developmentally figural to be integrated.

All the elements described below need to be present in individuals' emotional-movement mindbody repertoire. The concern of the holistic health practitioner is dictated by the adaptive use of the movements and postures; that is, are individuals employing the appropriate body movements for their moment-to-moment needs, expression and adaptation to the environment? If not, the phase at which the individual was to integrate that behavior was compromised. Barring the presence of severe physical trauma either due to congenital or inherited dysfunction, illness or externally induced crises, much childhood failure to develop has been due to unsuccessful relationships with primary caregivers. Thus, by observing the body movement and posturing of an individual, much can be understood regarding their psychological development, mindbody health and potential to heal.

THE KMP PARADIGM OF OBSERVABLE HUMAN MOVEMENT IN MINDBODY HEALTH AND HEALING

Of all the methods of ways of knowing and assessing body posture and movement which incorporates neurophysiology, healthy development, psychodynamic and recovery psychotherapy theories, the Kestenberg Movement Profile appears to be the most inclusive. Dr. Judith Kestenberg, a Viennese psychiatrist, child psychoanalyst and protégé of Anna Freud and Margaret Mahler, developed a method of observing, notating, and assessing observable posture and body movement utilizing Rudolph Laban and Warren Lamb's concepts of Effort-Shape (Amaghi, Loman, Lewis, & Sossin, 1999). The Kestenberg Movement Profile (KMP) identifies the emotional-behavioral development of the individual, intrapsychic conflict and primitive (sympathetic nervous system) responses to real or imagined chronic stress. Additionally, a person's capacity to respond spontaneously to every moment adapting their body to the present rather than reacting as if it were the past or the future is observable from a KMP trained eye.

"The unconscious lies in the body" was and is a realization that emerged from the father of psychotherapy. Much of human movement is purposeful, conscious and rationally, ego-based. Even habitual movement responses such as driving a car come from a cortical source within the brain. But within all movement there is a hidden unconscious body posturing and movement which addresses primitive physiologic needs and their psychological derivatives. These include affective responses and indicators of a sense of self and other. These movement elements in the KMP are called "flow." They can be observed in both tension flow addressing the dynamics of movement and shape flow addressing the actual physical structure of body attitude and movement.

TENSION FLOW: TENSION FLOW RHYTHMS IN DEVELOPMENT

Tension flow is the alternation between agonist and antagonist muscle systems. This flow of muscle tension is intrinsic in all movement. Kestenberg noticed in her longitudinal studies that there were patterns or rhythms of tension flow changes. These rhythms parallel key physiological needs in early stages of development. All these rhythms and various combinations are needed in order for an individual to meet their needs and express them motorically for the purpose of satisfaction. Using this observable paradigm, holistic health practitioners can identify if an individual is stuck in an earlier developmental phase thereby inhibiting their capacity to meet more complex needs that dominate higher levels of development. This repetition of earlier phases of development is due to the lack of the presence of the needed stimulation and interpersonal and environmental factors that are required for growth. Conversely, individuals may also demonstrate a lack of adaptive use of a particular rhythm where the presence of that rhythm would be appropriate to facilitate satisfaction of primitive and emotionally derivative needs. An example of this might be if an individual is seeking to be nurtured or to self-soothe, the presence of an oral level sucking rhythm mixed with the nurturing swaying movement of the of the primary caregiver produces the mixed rhythm of rocking. An individual may be unable to self-rock or receive this form of comfort from another if they are stuck in another developmental phase. This might be the case if they were fixated at the rapprochement phase of development characterized by power and control behaviors. Here the presence of the anal straining high tension holding of the torso seen in the rigid posturing of the anal character would curtail the rocking behavior.

These unconscious motoric expressions of needs and drives are identified based upon their functional psychophysiological purpose (see Figure 4-1, Tension flow rhythms).

With adults and age-appropriate children, all rhythms need to be present in pure form in order for the drive to be sufficiently differentiated. If a rhythm is absent, it may be due to the fact that they have not developmentally arrived at a phase or it may be that the drive has been repressed because it is culturally gender specific or considered unacceptable or too dangerous to express in the family or culture. For example, classic

Mexican culture reinforced the anal straining rhythm in macho men and the coquettish anal libidinal twisting in the Marianissma quality in women. Barring cultural markers, a fixated dominant rhythm identifies the age of the child within or "inner child" coined in recovery theory.

Oral Sucking Rhythm Symbiotic Dependence Dominance

Oral libidinal sucking rhythm dominance occurs during the symbiotic phase of object relations development described by Margaret Mahler (1968). It is the initial rela-

Age	Psycho-Physiologic function	Movement Description
0-6 mons	incorporating sucking	alteration of free & bound flow
6-9 mons	separating and discriminating biting and chewing	sharp transitions between free & bound flow short holding transitions in chewing
9-18 mons	ambivalent playful twisting passive defecation	low intensity flow adjustments
18-24 mons	asserting power and control straining in controlled defecation	high intensity bound flow and release
2-2.5 yrs	uncontrolled flowing out passive urination	gradual decrease of muscle tension
2.5-3 yrs	runs stopped go flight response; starting & stopping in bladder control	abrupt changes into bound flow at various intervals of free flow
3-3.5 yrs	creativity and imagination Inner genital contractions; nurturing	wave-like contractions of gradual increase & decrease between free & bound flow
3.5-4 yrs	birthing and surging	high intensity gradual bound flow of long duration followed by release into free flow
4-5 yrs	externalized exuberant excitement outer genital surges; sexual excitement	abrupt high intensity with smooth transitions
5-6 yrs	penetrating spurting, intrusive ramming, sexual penetration outer genital ballistic fighting response	abrupt high intensity with sharp transitions
Adult	androgynous expression; orgasm	Adult integration of inner & outer genital rhythms

Figure 4-1. Tension flow rhythms.

tional stage between the mother (object) and infant. When good enough attunement of the sucking rhythm occurs, the infant's primary narcissistic experience of being at one with a loving need satisfying environment occurs. The self-object dual unity promotes several phenomena: basic trust and a sense of safety in the environment, a sense that the self-environment matrix can satisfy needs, a positive body image, and a developing sense of wholeness of self. The latter develops from an enteroceptive belly sense of wholeness that comes from an ease or satiation through being nourished. In recovery theory, this process addresses the development of an inner child (corroborative evidence can be seen with patients that are asked to imaginally enter their bodies and locate their inner child). Invariably they put their hands on their stomach denoting where the child within resides. This is further corroborated in Pert's (1996) research that substantiates that the gut or belly itself is a source of emotional molecular chemical expression.

If the mother is not able to attune to the infant's sucking rhythm, the infant will not be able to successfully feel empathy or feel that the fundamental needs and wants can ever be met. Hopelessness and helplessness follows. In other instances due to organic problems such as: severe developmental delay, attention deficit hyperactive disorder, autism, or congenital anomalies, clef pallet, colic, allergies etc.; the infant himself may have difficulty achieving or sustaining the oral sucking rhythm. Under these circumstances the organization of the rhythm may need greater encouragement over a longer period of time. Individuals who have an overabundance of oral libidinal indulging rhythms in their movement are said to be orally fixated. Oral rhythms may appear in different parts of the body, manifested in constant rocking, hand-to-face gestures like hair twirling, head nodding and soothing foot movements; or in addictive behavior as with compulsive thumb-sucking, eating dairy and sweets, cigarette smoking or con-

stant drinking. These patterns are associated with the oral character described later in the section on body attitude. Often these individuals demonstrate a desire for merger through longing eye-to-eye contact, reflection of others' tension flow as seen with codependent individuals and a general disinterest in engaging in anything which involves standing or ambulating for long periods of time.

When other rhythms are present in primarily mixed form (in combination with) oral rhythms, these rhythms and their associated drives and object-related derivations are not sufficiently differentiated. In addition, since the oral libidinal indulging rhythm reduces aggression, the consistently merging oral rhythm could inhibit needed aggression, resulting in a diminished capacity to discriminate through the expression of the oral biting rhythm or stand up and assert oneself through the expression of the anal straining rhythm.

Some individuals will demonstrate dysfunction through a profound diminished use of the oral rhythm entirely. Since the presence of this and any other pure rhythms are needed in order to meet basic needs, it can be assumed that although they may be able to consume food, derivatively, such individuals may be fundamentally incapable of soothing themselves. This may result in their inability to receive narcissistic supplies, to maintain sustenance for a full and realistically positive sense of self, and to feel that they are capable of trusting that the environment is safe and can satisfy their needs.

Oral Biting and Chewing Differentiating Rhythm Dominance

The oral biting and chewing rhythms are crucial in Mahler's first phase of separation and individuation i.e., the differentiation of the infant from the primary object. The same biting rhythm is used in patting and tapping the infant's self and the environment. Self-patting helps establish the needed body boundary. Tapping the environment establishes its material presence and "otherness."

This same rhythm intrapsychically aids in the formation of the ego boundary thereby enhancing the individual's capacity to distinguish their inner experience, thoughts, feelings and imaginings from outer reality. Ego boundaries assist ego formation by promoting a holding container for its developing mediational functions.

Some individuals are seen to have an overabundance of the oral sadistic fighting rhythm. When this fixation is present individuals can be seen incessantly tapping their hands and feet, talking with a quickened, sharply enunciated tone, along with a heightened tension in the jaw. They may constantly chew gum or food, bite their nails and suffer from TMJ and nocturnal teeth grinding. Their eyes are frequently glaring. They tend to be critical and hold onto ideas or relationships unable to let go. These individuals have a biting or snapping personality. They are not "cuddlers," and when hugged, are quick to give a differentiating pat or tap to the other persons back indicating that they are uncomfortable and want to separate. Relationally, it is always safer for them to speak on how they or their ideas are different from the other persons. These individuals are typically the ones who suffer from childhood abuse of omnipresent undifferentiated mothering or the boundaryless invading mother. They may have mothers who were themselves fixated at the oral sadistic fighting stage and therefore, demanded heightened boundaries. Whenever people stay in close physical or emotional proximity with one of these individuals they eventually receive the negative mother transference and a heightened separation dance occurs.

If the mother is unable to separate from the infant, dysfunctional survival patterns develop. This could occur if the mother had an insufficient sense of self—either through improper parenting by her mother or through cultural or gender devaluing of her worth. She may unconsciously project her undeveloped self during the in utero and neonatal merged phase and then not support normal separation. This phenomena produces the smothering, enmeshed or engulfing mother who unconsciously through tone and movement gives the message to the baby that it isn't OK to separate. The image of the devouring witch mother who wishes to consume the child's nascent sense of self can be present here. This form of abuse of aborted development can be seen with the mother who wants the infant "in her lap" all the time or fills the child with anxiety about the environment when they begin to separate.

Other mothers utilize their children as narcissistic extensions of themselves. They therefore only mirror their children's primary narcissism and maintain children's view that they are the center of the universe and everything must reference them and their well-being. This would result in the maintenance of a grandiose sense of self and in the demand for perfect undifferentiated mirroring and continuous nurturance in the form of narcissistic supplies. These children become narcissistic personalities.

In contrast, some mothers may demand mirroring from their children and do not allow them to separate. They can be given the message that to act on one's own needs and wants is to be selfish and that one must care about the other first. This is particularly taught to females in our culture and is typical in many Asian and ethnic Catholic families. This frequently results in mirroring and caretaking, resulting in the presence of more libidinal indulging rhythms and few sadistic fighting ones. Oral aggressive responses are unheard of. In its extreme form, some females are taught never to hold onto anything and to continuously let the other take it. Many of these women will come to holistic health practitioners and therapists complaining of physical ailments, as expression of emotional distress is considered an act of selfishness.

In other cases, the infant may be abandoned by the primary object and thus never be able to sufficiently separate because there was no one there from whom to choreograph differentiation. In these situations, the derivative use of oral biting as well as all other separating (i.e., sadistic fighting) rhythms may not be present as the individual struggles to receive enough primary parenting. Without the derivative use of oral sadistic rhythms, individuals will have difficulty maintaining protection of themselves. Due to their lack of body boundaries, they may find themselves repeated victims of physical abuse. In addition, the intrapsychic lack of ego boundaries may result in the ego being flooded with unconscious material or bombarded by inner constellations such as the inner shamer, critic or judge. They will frequently swallow what other persons say about them through projection as they will be without the capacity to discriminate i.e., to spit out what doesn't apply and internalize what does.

Anal Twisting Ambivalence/Practicing Independence Dominance

Developmentally, twisting movements dominate the second year of life. Their presence addresses Mahler's second sub-phase of separation and individuation: practicing. During this phase toddlers practice leaving Mommy and returning for "refueling" (loving reassuring hugs) and "customs inspection" (exploring clothing and body parts) of the primary caregiver to reassure themselves that she's still there. The parents need to respect and value toddlers' attachment to their anal products and emphasize that it is the toddlers' own creation and not produced for them. This reinforces in toddlers the sense that they can produce something of value and can identify and feel pride in it–vital foundation for the capacity to work.

Mothers who either leave the toddler when the toddler practices moving away or withhold their positive regard when the child explores separation will often bring forth a fixation or excessive presence of the anal twisting rhythm. In these situations toddlers feel they can't leave and become more self-sufficient because with the former, mother won't be there if needed; and with the latter, mother will emotionally abandon them if they engage in this natural ambivalence phase.

Individuals who have an anal libidinal twisting dominance don't know whether they should hold off or let go, be in a relationship or leave it. They can neither commit nor sustain a relationship. If they become intimate, the negative engulfing mother transference typically gets constellated, and they move away and diminish contact. When the hopeful partner finally gives up, they then place the abandoning mother transference in them and begin moving closer again through phone calls, dating or resumption of sexual intimacy. They will be unable to stand on their own two feet for any long periods of time. They will shift back and forth in a twisting movement. Assertion is unavailable and they may, at times, have a whining ambivalent tone to questions requiring self-statements.

The holistic health practitioner may expect that this individual will be unable to commit to alternative or complimentary practices and to the continuity of appointments with the practitioner or with others to whom the practitioner might refer them. It is vital that the individual be able to explore the ambivalence within the setting with the holistic health practitioner. Canceling appointments and distancing outside of the healing relationship only repeats ambivalent child-like patterns and does not allow for the client to begin to heal.

Anal Straining Defecatory Power and Control Assertion Dominance

When there is a dominance of anal straining exhibited and expressed constantly even when such an assertive stance is inappropriate, an individual could be said to be anally fixated. In terms of object relations this parallels the third sub-phase of separation and individuation: rapprochement. Relationally, toddlers have internalized enough of a sense of self that they feel ready to stand up and test the authority. This period has been called the "terrible two's." In adulthood, they can then stand up for themselves and assert what they believe in. In terms of recovery theory, they have healthy external boundaries that are neither wall-like nor "leaky." They are able to ensure that no one violates their personal space and consequently give off the nonverbal message that they are not potential victims. Parents who give the message that it is not "OK" to have personal needs and wants or to stand up for oneself will frequently deny their children the right to integrate the anal straining defecatory rhythm. Here can be found an absence of the derivative use of the rhythm, or even its presence mixed with other more indulging rhythms used to "tone down" the intensity. These individuals are unable to stand up for themselves and are pushovers for others.

Conversely, some individuals decide to identify with their rageful or otherwise over-controlling authoritative parents and develop anal maso-sadistic characters described in the body attitude section under "vertical plane." These are individuals who always make sure they are in positions of power and control. The anal straining rhythm is held in their body like a time bomb waiting to explode. Instead of straining and releasing downward, they strain and hold upward producing clenched gluteals and external rotator buttock's muscles. Their second chakra and the flow of energy from their first chakra—all the power of the kundalini is held in the lower back. Metaphorically or literally, their bowels are retained symbolizing unexpressed childhood anger. They explode periodically in rage attacks at spouses, children, and other vulnerable individuals. Chronic low back pain is common.

Urethral Limitless Flowing Rhythm Dominance

The boundaryless flowing of movement into neutral gives the appearance of adults that flow everywhere without a responsible sense of time. Body boundaries become liquid; their gentle flowing nature may put them in harms way or result in their obliviously pouring into another person's personal space.

If families' messages are that children must do something in order to be loved or that indulging in free floating, revitalizing reverie is a sign of sloth and laziness, then this rhythm may not be derivatively present in individuals' repertoires. Conversely if there is a predominance of this limitless flowing rhythm, individuals may have difficulty doing anything. Complete oblivion regarding time and task completion may result in an individual's inability to maintain a job or get anywhere on time. They may have a dazed look about them and be identified as "space shots," "zoned out," "New Agey" or "not on this planet."

Fixation in the urethral phase is often a result of the unwillingness to be fully present in the world. Potential child abuse will need to be focused upon with the additional goal of their feeling safe enough to let go of a survival pattern that keeps them at least two inches off the ground.

Urethral Bladder Control Run-Stop-Go Operational Dominance

With the beginning of an internalized sense of self and other, toddlers can gain pleasure in the movements that are required for bladder control. Here toddlers run everywhere stopping and starting the flow of their own movement. The toddler can leave their mommy's side and mentally feel they have taken her with them. With the integration of the capacity to operate and get things done comes the vital development of the ability to work.

Parents who want to keep their children tied to them frequently instill anxiety or judgment in them regarding the act of doing. For example, "Oh, don't run too fast–you might fall" or "Are you sure you are capable of doing that?" Other mothers will literally take everything the child does and claim it as theirs so that children get the message that nothing they do is for themselves. In these instances, this operational rhythm is curtailed and absent in their repertoire. They will come to therapy complaining that they can't ever complete a task or feel good about what they are doing. They often become passive-aggressive when asked to carry out tasks resulting in others becoming frustrated. Those individuals who have requested something from the (elimination [anal and urethrally] fixated) adult-child unwittingly become the recipient of the person's negative transference of their dominant mother or father.

Parents who produce narcissistically disordered children can also curtail the joy in doing with the message that "unless you are the best or do the greatest things immediately, you will not be the wonder person I have told you you are." These persons, fearful of being "just like everyone else" and loosing the grandiosity their parents inflated them with, do nothing.

Positive fixation is the result of work-addicted families who convey the message that people are not worth anything unless they "do something." Others have a predominance of urethral run-stop-go rhythms as an adaptation in order to attract attention and win the love they never got. Their view is, "well, if I keep doing things, maybe then I'll be acceptable and cherished." These individuals are always running with many tasks to do at once and never have time for refueling or real relationships. Culturally, the Protestant work ethic has produced many fixated worked addicts who even "work at play" and have a diminished ability to employ the urethral flowing rhythm which might allow them to indulge in time, relax and just be. These individuals are frequently Type A personalities and, require techniques, which helps them become fully present in the moment. Meditation, yoga, authentic movement, tai chi and other alternative and complementary approaches can be beneficial to these individuals.

Inner Genital Indulging/Maternal and Fighting (Birthing) Rhythms Dominance

The swaying rocking movement that mothers naturally engage in to soothe their infants is a very same movement that occurs internally during uterine contractions and the shifting of the *tunica dartos* in male genitalia. These inner sensations are more subject to primary process thinking. They are more present in creative reverie or nurturing self or others utilizing the right hemisphere and the more primitive instinctive systems of the brain rather than with left brain rational analytic reasoning. In terms of object relations, mothers are identified with by both sexes for her capacity to create. This is vital if individuals are to experience themselves as creative in adult life.

This inner genital rhythm with its graceful caressing, swaying, lyrical movements is society's stereotype for the female gender thereby curtailing the full androgynous instinctual expression in both males and females. Males may feel uncomfortable being tender if they were shamed for playing with dolls and doing things identified as feminine during this developmental phase.

The deep high intensity of the inner genital sadistic birthing rhythm may be present when an individual, during an authentic or improvisational movement experience, is giving birth to themselves. It is unlikely that this rhythm would be seen dominating a person's movement repertoire suggestive of fixation.

Outer Genital Thrusting, Penetrating and Ballistic Rhythm Dominance

In the same way that the graceful inner genital rhythm has been stereotypically assigned to females, the outer genital ballistic rhythms have, in the past, been assigned to males. Feminist outrage has now expanded sports and military duty to include women who utilize these rhythms. Aggressive women are still discouraged in business where competition and hierarchical ranking requires outer genital rhythms.

Males or females who have an over abundance of inner or outer genital rhythms need to claim the drive and its movement expression that they deny within themselves. This appears in their gender-based attraction or repulsion of others via a projection onto an individual or a prejudice against a group. Frequently these instinctually-based tension flow rhythms appear in day and night dreams and various art expressions such as writing, visual arts images or improvisational drama or dance characterizations. They can symbolically be represented as animals, children, and/or possibly volatile characters. Snakes and cats (domestic and wild) can house the inner genital rhythms and mobsters, rapists and grizzly creatures can express the outer genital waiting to be confronted, embodied and claimed. In this process they are humanized, civilized and transformed as the ego mediates the genital drives. When they appear imagistically as children, they can grow and develop through active imagination embodiment. The union of contrasexual sides and their associated body movements can occur via creative improvisation, energy work, and visualization producing adult gentility and a balanced inner feminine and masculine side.

Adult Genital Rhythm Dominance

The combination of the inner and outer genital rhythms results in the experience of medium to high intensity rhythms gradually rising in falling in tension. These rhythms dominate adult life and are utilized in sexual gratification in movement during coitus and the powerful contractions during orgasm. Interpersonally the presence of this rhythm demonstrates the capacity of the individual to be vulnerable with protection, to creatively bring forth their ideas and put them out into the world, to network with others and to join together in consensus.

TENSION FLOW: TENSION FLOW ATTRIBUTES: HYPOTHALAMIC RESPONSES TO SAFETY AND DANGER

Six elements and their combinations characterize the flow of muscular tension. They are: low intensity, high intensity, gradual increase or decrease of tension, abrupt increase or decrease in tension, adjustments of tension and even flow of tension. These attributes can either be present in free flow in which only the agonist muscle system is activated producing an uninhibited relaxed flowing movement or bound flow in which both the agonist and antagonist muscle systems are activated producing stabilizing or inhibiting tense movements. Kestenberg referred to tension flow attributes as "affective potentials" (1971) stimulated by the autonomic nervous system and the limbic system's hypothalamus (see Figure 4-2, The hypothalamus).

The hypothalamus is the coordinating center for the autonomic nervous system that "integrates various inputs to ensure a well-organized coherent and appropriate set of autonomic and somatic responses including the peripheral motoric expression of emotional states." This definition of the functioning of the hypothalamus has been documented by lesion studies that have corresponded to expression of a vast range of emotional expression (Kandel, Schwartz, Jessell, 2000, p. 986, 1971).

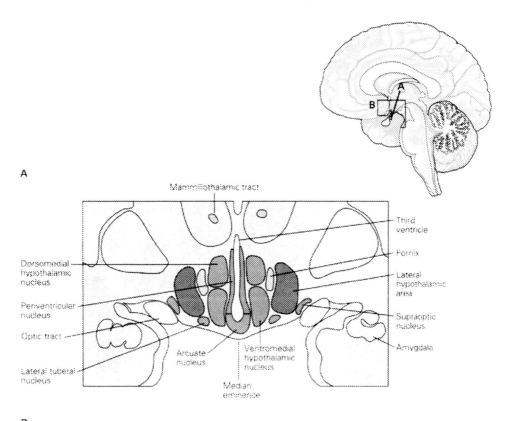

A. Frontal view of the hypothalamus (section along the plane shown in part B).
B. A medial view shows most of the main nuclei. The hypo-

thalamus is often divided analytically into three areas in a rostocaudal direction: the preoptic area, the tuberal level, and the posterior level.

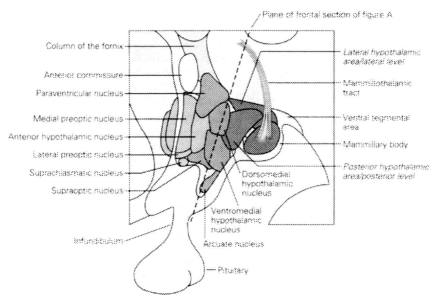

Figure 4-2. The structure of the hypothalamus.

This affective center of the primitive brain addresses motor inhibition and discharge. With regards to inhibition: stopping, delaying, diminishing, or reversing movement becomes the basis for fear responses for such hypoarousal defensive patterns as freeze and faint and psychological survival behaviors such as denial, minimization, repression, isolation, insulation and splitting. With regards to motor discharge: the continuity of movement becomes the basis for hyperarousal responses of fight or flight and the foundation for displacement, acting out, identification with the aggressor, manic flight and projection. The motor discharge in free flow is also employed in the parasympathetic response of ease in coping with the environment found in the relaxation response.

Tension flow attributes (TFA) function as affective need regulatory mechanisms. If free or bound flow is brought to the extremes, the former can result in unrestrained behavior while the latter can result in body blocks and rigidity. If there is a lack of range between free and bound flow, the individual may be said to have lost elasticity and be in neutral flow which results in flat affect denoting depressive or numbing features that can be seen in the sympathetic response of hypoarousal. Very low intensity: neutral free flow creates a rag doll-like flaccidly seen in suicidal patients. High bound neutral flow produces brittle nonadaptive personalities as seen in the sympathetic response of "freeze." If neutral flow is predominant, the individual appears to be uninhabited as in the response of "faint." If the family of origin environment is repeatedly abusive TFA flight or flight childhood movement responses will develop and become habitual survival patterns that continue into adulthood. Although these sensorimotor survival modes were useful in childhood, a time when there is frequently no way out of abusive situations, they become detrimental in later life. These archaic affective responses which were once used for protection now keep the person from being fully present in the moment and appropriately responding to the situation.

Free Flow

An overuse of free flow could indicate a lack of boundaries. Healthy boundaries exist at three levels: ego boundaries, body boundaries, and external boundaries or personal space.

EGO BOUNDARIES. In psychodynamic and humanistic psychotherapy, the ego is considered the psychological construct which maintains an individual's sense of reality, mediates between various intrapsychic thoughts, feelings, imaginings, and unconscious material and external reality. With the absence of or faulty ego boundaries; the psyche could be flooded with unconscious, intrapsychic schema or complex material, traumatic responses of hyper or hypoarousal from the sensorimotor level of the brain, or psychologically possessed by addictions, unmediated drives or negative internalized objects.

BODY BOUNDARIES. Without body boundaries the individual may not be able to discern what feelings, thoughts, and imaginings originate from themselves from what belongs to another. The individual may project or transfer onto another or group split-off parts of themselves or their history with another significant person in their lives. Conversely, individuals may not be able to discriminate when other people accuse them of behavior, traits or motivations that are not their own. Additionally, the individual may be unable to say "no" to being touched or handled in ways that are undesirable and be subject to physical violation.

EXTERNAL BOUNDARIES. Without external boundaries, the individual can give off the message that his personal space can be approached thereby setting himself up as the perfect victim.

The adaptive presence of the rhythms of biting and chewing are indicative of the individual's capacity for ego boundaries and body boundaries. The adaptive presence of the straining bowel control rhythm is indicative of an individual's capacity for external boundaries and the ability to stand up and say, "no" to personal space violation. By avoiding bound flow, the individual is basically expressing that everyone in everything is safe to be with.

Bound Flow

EGO BOUNDARIES. Within an overuse of bound flow, wall-like boundaries develop blocking on an ego level the individual's access to her own feelings, wants and needs.

BODY BOUNDARY. On body boundary level she is unable to express her feelings or receive any affective responses of others.

EXTERNAL BOUNDARY. With rigid external boundaries she sends out the message, "Don't approach me" thereby isolating herself from the possibility of experiencing a more benign relationship.

Even Flow Dominance

Even flow occurs when individuals move in a held level of tension. If individuals move utilizing even tension flow they may be seen to be even-tempered. However, if they persist in utilizing this monotoned movement even though it is adaptively not called for, a more primitive survival mechanism may be manifesting. These individuals may have utilized the role of the "smoother over" in their family attempting to calm a volatile labile environment. When even flow is bound in tense movement expression, a wary caution occurs when individuals bind their tension to "keep the lid on" spontaneous expression perhaps stemming from potentially explosive parental responses. When even tension flow is combined in neutral, individuals are seen to deanimate or exhibit the "faint" sympathetic response. Individuals who sustain this behavior are living in continuous shock and functioning out of the sensorimotor level due to physical abuse through beatings, sexual assaults, major surgery or physical accidents.

Flow Adjustment Dominance

Individuals who have a habitual abundance of flow adjustments are continuously initiating micromovements. It looks as if they can't feel comfortable in any given position or are responding to internal discomfort. This may be a real, present phenomenon with chronic pain or in may be a result of chronic traumatic sensorimotor response. If the latter is the case, these individuals may have needed to continuously adjust their own feelings as they may have been trained to read other individual's moods and needs before addressing their own. If this is the case, these individuals are identified as codependent and in severe cases, they may not even know what they feel or need. When flow fluctuation is combined with bound flow, these adjustments and temperament are influenced by caution. Clinically, these individuals have a form of hypervigilance, looking around feeling uneasy about the environment no matter whether the present environment is actually safe or not. They are repeating their sensorimotor response that developed in the initial traumatic environment. Their family of origin may have abusively violated spatial boundaries through physical abuse, overprotection, controlling or smothering. These individuals often describe a "yucky, queasy feeling in their stomachs." Their constantly unsettling movements deliver uneasiness to those who observe them. If high intensity is added to flow adjustments these individuals become prone to emotional disorganization. Adding the time factor of abrupt changes in flow, personality fragmentation will occur. When combined with neutral flow, their affective responses become loose-jointed. They may give in to expressing deeper levels of unconsciousness. Bizarre twisting gestures such as tics and autistic-like features develop.

High Intensity Dominance

When the majority of muscle fibers contract, individuals can be said to be moving in high intensity tension flow. These people are able to express strong needs and drives and feel deeply about life. They also can feel elated, exuberant, passionate, deeply upset or ragefully angry in temper tantrums. When high intensity is combined with free flow, they tend to be easily excited and can derail and lose control. Clinically these individuals may not have the needed boundaries to contain the extremes of their emotions. Co-dependents and rage or love addicts describe being on an emotional roller coaster ride. Without the needed bound flow for boundaries these individuals exhibit poor impulse control. Individuals with narcissistic components also exhibit this attribute combination in their grandiosity and rages at not being perfectly mirrored. When combined with bound flow, the intense feelings are held and restrained producing a "time bomb" feeling around these potentially explosive individuals. Frequently, it is anger that is stored in the body, as the "uptight" individual tends to be negative and furious. Clinically these are the classic anal-retentive personalities who hold their rage and then burst forth in abusive ways. The childhood pattern of identifying with the aggressor creates little bullies and later, child and work-related abusers and wife beaters. Because their rage is retroflexed, that is, turned back inward on themselves, they are frequently masochistic with shame-producing inner critics.

When neutral flow is added, the core of their inner child is surrounded by deadness. Here the adult ego remains split off from the child self or from the split bad self that occurs during rapprochement (Lewis, 1994). When the adult ego continues to banish the child self located in the third chakra or solar plexus into a neutral dead zone, the inner child remains held in a frustrated deanimated state until the individual accesses his split

part of the self through body-felt awareness. These individuals have been described as wooden, heavy, inert "like molasses" and can be passive-aggressive.

Low Intensity Dominance

Individuals, who use low intensity as a survival expression, are seen to respond with little feeling to trauma that may have befallen them. Instead of being hurt or angry, they can often be seen smiling. These individuals who are afraid of their anger or the anger of a parent may neutralize and minimize their feelings. Their voice is often in high register with minimal amplification moving away from lower chakras that might support assertive expression. Clinically, when low intensity is combined with bound flow, individuals may be afraid to feel too deeply; but when deep feelings come close to the surface, they may need to bind up though muscle contraction in bound flow and avoid the flow of expression lest any enters ego consciousness. When individuals combine neutral flow with low intensity, they have drifted so far away from their real feelings that they no longer care about anything. Their bodies are fluid but weak. They have given up feeling that what they want and need can matter in the world. The world may be abundant but not for them.

Abruptness Dominance

Users of the predominance of abruptness can be volatile in life while inner survival expressions remain alert. When combining abruptness with free flow, these individuals tend to be impulsive about their feelings and quick to uninhibitedly be filled with feelings or collapse in relief. Clinically, these individuals have poor impulse control and cannot sustain attention. They can frequently be seen in anxious manic flight looking to utilize the "flight" sympathetic response as if the present environment were as abusive as their childhood. Frequently combined with flow fluctuations, they are literally all over the place emotionally and otherwise. When abrupt change is combined with bound flow, these individuals can move quickly into restraining their expression or its reverse, decreasing in caution. Clinically, these individuals are jumpy, often having come from a family of origin in which they never knew where or when the attack would come. This form of hypervigilance would also allow them to quickly utilize the "freeze" sympathetic response so as not to draw attention to themselves as potential victims.

Organically-based attention deficit hyperactive disorder (ADHD) is also slotted here. These individuals describe not being able to feel deeply or pick up effective cues from others as they cannot sustain time long enough to sensitize themselves. With a lack of control, they often violate others boundaries without being aware. Coordination becomes difficult and they leave a wake of chaos in their path.

Graduality Dominance

With the preponderance of graduality, clinical concerns develop when individuals need faster transitions in situations when flight and fight responses may be required. These individuals are said to have "slow reflexes." This may result from a dysfunctional family in which any abrupt changes might have effectively set someone off into abusive behavior. When combining graduality with bound flow, individuals are cautious and become less intense in a restrained manner or conversely become more and more an affectively charged. Like someone who has a slow fuse, they gradually begin to boil with anger or effervesce excitement. Clinically speaking, these slow-fused individuals are often difficult to calm down especially when even high intensity flow is added. They stay adamantly locked into the intensity of their feelings and in impressing their concerns on whomever is around, unable to adjust and adapt to others effective expressions. When combined with neutral flow, a gradual disassociative spacing out occurs as these individuals leave their bodies during flashbacks of severe physical abuse.

SHAPE FLOW: THE UNCONSCIOUS MANIFESTATION OF A SENSE OF SELF AND OBJECT INTERNALIZATION

Shape flow is seen when the body grows during inhalation and shrinks bodily dimensions in exhalation. Shape flow gives structure and form to the motoric expression of needs and emotions in tension flow. Bilateral shape flow (simultaneous movement of opposite sides of the body horizontally, vertically or sagittally) is seen in individuals responses to the environment. Although there is a natural growing and shrinking during the breathing process, individuals can be seen to maintain more of an opened body position supported by growing shape flow or a closed body position foundationally reflected in shrinking shape flow. Growing in shape flow is associated with feelings of comfort, safety, and trust. Individuals expand extending their body into space when the environment feels supportive. Shrinking in shape flow is associated with feelings of discomfort, protection and mistrust. Individuals contact and close off their bodies to the surround if it feels deleterious or not supportive of comfort and well-being. During diaphragmatic inhalation, individuals widen bilaterally from side to side, lengthen upward and downward, and bulge forward and backward. During exhalation, individuals narrow bilaterally, shorten downward and upward, and hollow forward and backward all toward the midline of the body. The body grows and shrinks in relationship to the internal and external environment. The body grows when it takes in food and other content that it feels to be appropriate to receive and shrinks when it wants to excrete internal waste as well as disengage from a potentially noxious external environment. The body opens and feels relaxed in environments that are supportive of life and shrinks and contracts in environments that are uncomfortable. These environments may be atmospheric such as warm or frigid weather. They may be emotional environments that are caring and nurturing or hostile and abusive, and/or they may be energetic environments that are positive and filled with conscious light or negative filled with unconscious darkness. The more sensitive an individual, the more sensitive the shape flow response to the immediate surrounds.

Individuals' self-in-relation to others is expressed in shape flow. Shape flow thus provides for the motor apparatus for the flow of pleasure and protection between self and other. Through this structure body boundaries are aided along with the internalizations of self and other as described in the theories of object relations and self-psychology (Lewis, 1993). Bipolar shape flow gives three-dimensionality to individuals' sense of wholeness of self and serves healthy narcissism or the capacity to feel that one is worthy, lovable, and has a right to be considered.

Held shape flow in body postures and attitudes tell the observing holistic health practitioner about individuals' sense of self and their initial relationship to the primary caregiver or primary object. This shape flow body attitude indicator identifies the type of early nurturing or abuse the individual received and the resultant sense of self. The individual has only to walk into your consulting room and sit down. Often if primary caregivers were not attentive to the health and well-being of clients, then they too may be unaware of how to care for themselves. Recommendations will fall on deaf ears. Clients may want you to "fix" it without any appreciation for the power and influence of their own mindbodysoulful capacity to heal.

Because the office of the holistic health practitioner and the furniture chosen sym-bolically translates to the client your capacity to hold them appropriately, it is vital to attend and be aware of the nonhuman environment as symbolic projections of you. By the same token, the individual who is seated in front of you will tell you through his/her shape flow, the effects of early parenting on the mindbody. Observing the client's posture, the therapist/practitioner/consultant can imaginally create what type of early nurturing and parenting the individual had by designing in your mind an image of the individual's parent held in their energetic field. For example, if an individual is in a shrunken closed position in front of you sitting in an awkward position, and you know yourself to be a caring attuned supportive human being in a warm comfortable environment, it is clear that the individual is not responding to the present. Imagine in your mind a holographic image of the client's parent(s) in physical relationship to your client's held body position or attitude. This will give you added information in order to support and make recommendations for integrative holistic health interventions.

This holographic image will also serve you in terms of any possible transference. Whether working on a table, in a studio or sitting in relationship to the client, the person may at any time transfer that very image of that parent held in their energetic field into you. Being aware before hand of any possible transference allows you to discuss this with the client first, and establish strategies with the client before the primitive sensorimotor defensive response is triggered and you are responded to as a potential predator instead of who you genuinely are.

Widening Dominance

A dominance of bilateral widening in individuals' body attitude seen in expansion of both sides of the rib cage with the possibility of arms extended in abduction on the side of a chair, demonstrates an object-seeking response which suggests that the initial relationship with the primary caregiver was one in which there was a physical availability and affection. It is expected that with a healthy amount of widening in an individual's repertoire, the individual would be able to receive. With a sustained dominance of widening, however, a narcissistic sense of importence may be present. These individuals typically take up a great deal of personal body, verbally expressive and energetic space. In this case the individual would require perfect mirroring from the environment. This phenomenon is present due to the fact that widening in the horizontal is associated with the first developmental phase of symbiosis. In this oral sucking phase the relationship to the environment is a merged one as self-object or the infant-mother dual unity is seen as encompassing the entire surroundings. Those who have a dominance of widening often feel that unconsciously everyone is "mother" and therefore should dote on their every word and wish. Without the balance of shrinking in the horizontal (narrowing), their grandiosity is not relativised in reality. This typically occurs with one of two mother-child scenarios: The mother, empty of a sense of worth and a connection to her own inner child or self, sustains the symbiotic phase of undifferentiation with the infant and places all her unmet compensatory monumental fantasies in the child. An alternate origin stems from the client compensating for feelings of inferiority due to devaluing from the primary caregivers through acting like they are better than. In either case, you may feel the countertransference of being energetically squished.

Widening is associated with free flow and the tension flow attribute of flow fluctuation. When mismatched with bound flow, the individual may be manifesting a fear of falling apart, resulting in outer manifestations of the inner split or fragmented self.

Narrowing Dominance

A dominance of bilateral narrowing is seen when the rib cage contracts and moves toward the body center drawing the arms back in adduction to the torso. This gives the message that in childhood it wasn't "OK" to expand oneself, to reach out to another, or to take what one needed. These self-contained individuals don't know how to get what they need or be sensitive to the needs of significant others. Their arms are drawn tightly to the sides of their body or are frequently crossed over their solar plexus disconnecting them from their sense of self and or barring access to their core self and their own vulnerability in relationship to others. They constrict their interactions with the environment and give the message that it wasn't safe for them in their childhood. They tend to shy away from social interaction. They can feel defeated, powerless and helpless to reach out for anything they need. If their arms are also showing neutral or limp levels of tension flow, it could be assumed that they might have been more severely abused or abandoned by the primary object during infancy.

If high intensity bound flow is present in their arms, they can be seen as being in conflict between wanting to extend and reach out and fearing abuse or the lack of satisfaction. Kinesthetically, the agonist muscles contract in forward outward movements and the antagonist muscles contracts holding them back and down. This might indicate a volatile or abusive object in which case the individual may also be turning his or her own aggression back on the self.

Narrowing is matched with even flow of tension and the oral biting and snapping rhythms associated with the differentiation subphase of separation and individuation in object relations theory. A natural balance between widening in narrowing reflects the individual's capacity to experience trust and mistrust appropriately—a vital developmental foundation for life. Without this balance, these individuals are unable to sustain intimate relations or have faith in themselves and their capacity to get what they need in life.

Lengthening Dominance

Dominance of bilateral lengthening upward and downward gives individuals an experience of being tall, becoming bigger hierarchically in stature and status in relation to others. Our culture has reinforced bipolar lengthening due to its patriarchal competitiveness, where being the "alpha" or "top dog" is associated with one's own sense of well-being. This world view differs from the horizontal more self-in-relation feminist networking model. Bound lengthening suggests someone who is filled with an anal level rage and/or someone who is compensating for feeling less than by a false persona of being "bigger than."

Persons who lengthen upward but not downward are not grounded. For these individuals, being present in the world in this reality is to be avoided at all costs due to previous trauma. They shy away from lower chakras along with the associated power of kundalini energy, the depth of emotional expression and the connection to the self and will. They often seek holistic health practitioners incorrectly believing that New Age practitioners support this body splitting. These individuals are seen to deny their own instinctual physical reality and seek to utilize transcendence as a defense against embodied presence. They confuse detachment with the desired nonattachment. This detachment supports a disconnection of self from the undifferentiated wholeness that connects all of existence. These individuals are seen to metaphorically flow into the holistic health practitioner's consulting room almost as if they had no contact with the floor. Their tension flow of low intensity matches their disengagement with the deeper more passionate feelings or life force.

Shortening Dominance

The dominance of shortening in shape flow is seen with individuals who shrink in stature, frequently feeling inferior to others due to low self-esteem, and/or living with a core of shame surrounding them from an abusive childhood. Culturally, certain groups of repressed individuals can be seen shortening their height in order to suggest submission. There was pressure on African-Americans in the South prior to World War II to adopt this pose.

In terms of object relations and recovery theory, if individuals without cultural precedence, frequently present themselves in a shortening position, it gives the impression that they are waiting for someone to dominate them and/or take care of them. These individuals may be codependent, dependent personalities or raised to be victims of another's control and potential abuse. Counter-transferentially, the holistic health practitioner might be aware of growing taller and/or feeling a demand to fix their problem, mother them or even be controlling.

If bound flow combines with sustained shortening, individuals may figuratively be all tied up inside. When both lengthening and shortening are utilized appropriately, individuals can be said to have stability, balance and self-control.

Bulging Dominance

The dominance of bulging growing in shape front and back is associated with feelings of wholeness, satiation and gratification. In terms of object relations, if bulging is present at a healthy level, the individual may be said to have a strong sense of self. Exaggerated bulging or bound flow bulging can give the appearance of someone bursting with feelings. This body shape flow occurs in food and alcohol addiction when individuals strive to fill an empty relational void with oral cravings.

Hollowing Dominance

The dominance of hollowing: the drawing into the body center front and back, is suggestive of a lack of an internalized sense of self in object relations and a lack of the connection with the inner child in recovery theory. Since the sense of self is experienced as an enteroceptive or belly self experience (Spitz in Lewis, 1994), it is understandable that the lack of sense of self is reflected in the hollowing of the solar plexus or third chakra area of the body. This posturing is further described in the body attitude of the oral character delineated below. These individuals frequently feel rejected and unlovable. They often do not know what they need and want, deferring to others or cultural stereotypes to tell them what they should want. These individuals can secretly hunger for relationships but feel so depleted they have no idea how to get what they need.

A natural balance between bulging and hollowing provides a healthy sense of confidence that is associated with object constancy, an ongoing sense that one is not alone but has an internalized caring parental figure, and a realistic sense of self.

BODY ATTITUDE: FIXED UNCONSCIOUS HABITUAL RESPONSE

Comprising what Irmgard Bartenieff (1980) conceptualized as the body attitude is a gestalt of factors such as a person's characteristic standing and sitting body position, use of body parts, carried body shape and readiness for certain patterns to emerge. These generalized factors may reflect body image, self-feelings, object relations, collective culture, gender and socioeconomic factors as well as individuals' present reaction to the environment and events which are occurring. It is the somatic core of individuals' presentation of the body that changes

with each developmental phase. Basically, the body attitude represents that which the KMP observing holistic health practitioner can see without having to suggest any movements or interventions. Often the practitioner therapist will make hypotheses regarding earlier childhood and caregiving. Fixed survival patterns may be frozen in the body or in readiness to be reactivated at a moment's notice. Gender and cultural preferences of body planes, shape and alignment, the available use of the whole body or restrictions to potential movement of certain body parts or certain relationships to space, gravity and time can be gleaned as well from this paradigm.

Body Action Attitude: Tension Flow Tension

Since the writings of Wilhelm Reich (1949) therapists have been aware of tension spots. These so-called dead spots indicate previously emotionally charged areas in an individual's body. These areas store childhood memories of abuse and affect-laden split off parts of the self. Frequently, there are also constellations of held bound flow in various parts of the body which have an interrelationship to one another such as with the anal statistic masochistic character. These individuals tense their arches, gastrocnemius, quadriceps and hamstrings in their legs. Their external rotators and pectoral muscles are overdeveloped along with the muscles in the lumbar and cervical areas in their torso. Triceps are also held and are in contracted conflict with the antagonist biceps.

LOCALIZED TENSION. Various areas frequently carry specific clinical meaning. For example, if individual's lower torso is frozen, this may indicate cultural influences regarding diminished outward expression of sexuality such as Puritan-based Euro-American and northern European heritages. If their torso is truly locked into a one-unit torso, sexual abuse or the fear of any lower chakra expression may be involved. Because women's power resides in their hips and thighs, held tension may indicate cultural or family of origin messages that full expression of strength and assertion is not permitted in women.

Low back pain frequently addresses blocked anger, sexuality and/or assertion. Men frequently complain of low back pain because of held tension in the lumbar area. When stress occurs and the burden to shoulder is too intense, the lower back is easily injured with simple torquing or bending movements.

Tension in the third chakra belly area is easily assessed by a lack of shape flow alteration. This factor indicates that the internalized sense of self or inner child is split off, damaged or not developed. Tension in the forth chakra chest area is also detected by a lack of shape flow changes in breathing. This phenomena is typical of white males in the West who have been given the message that vulnerable heart-related feelings such as hurt, pain, loss, longing for love and sadness are "unmanly" to have. Upper back tension is quite common in the West as it is a favorite storage place for perfectionism, inner taskmasters or inner critics. Neck tension results in a split between instincts and feelings stored in the body and cognitive logos rationality. This fifth chakra tension also can inhibit vocal expression. Temporomandibular joint tension (T.M.J.) and nocturnal teeth grinding are also body blocks to speaking out, emotively expressing as well as orally receiving.

Tension in the agonist and antagonist muscles systems in the legs and arms indicates individuals somatic conflict between the desire to stamp their feet, kick out or move forward or reach out, bar access, or aggressively punch out respectively.

Body Posture: Shape Flow Held Position

Healthy posturing adapts from moment-to-moment. Individuals tend to research,

explore possibilities and communicate in the horizontal plane (the plane of the horizon). They tend to present, represent, have intention and sell in the vertical plane (the door plane), and operate, move on a decision and proceed in the sagittal plane (the cartwheel plane). If individuals are stuck utilizing only one plane to the adaptive exclusion of others, then their body alignment can be said to be held delineating a fixation in a personality or characterolgical body attitude.

Developmentally speaking infants begin their life with only the ability to lie on the horizontal plane. They then are able to sit up and finally stand unattended in the vertical plane, and finally are able to ambulate in the sagittal plane. Indicators of fixation at the first three years of life may be etched into individual's body attitude.

HORIZONTAL PLANE DOMINANCE. Individuals who function primarily out of the horizontal plane tend to lean to the side while sitting (e.g., tilting the head or leaning on either arm). This is the plane of listening, exploring and communication. Individuals fixed in his plane literally collapse out of the vertical as if pulled downward toward the horizontal. Standing, the classic S-shape curve can be detected: the weight of the body is on the heels, the back is swayed back with the pelvis forward and the belly emptied or hollowing back. The jaw is tilted forward and movement is generally initiated by the head. These sagittal plane adjustments are due to an inability to achieve vertically due to being clinically fixated or stuck in the earlier developmental horizontal plane. This posture gives the impression that individuals "can't" do what needs to be done in order to be proactive and move forward in life. They appear lifeless and frequently the muscles and dynamic expression is underdeveloped. This S-shape form may be slight or severe.

Clinically speaking since developmentally humans are first in the horizontal i.e. the lying down plane, the holistic health practitioner can posit that this individual may have unresolved issues from the first year of life. These issues may stem from lack of appropriate primary care giving typically either due to emotional or relational abandonment (denoting psychodynamically a negative fixation) or smothering and enmeshment (denoting a positive fixation) or both. These individuals can be identified as oral characters. Those drawn to the horizontal plane or issues in the first few months of life may prefer holistic health practices which have the individual lying on a table such as with massage, acupuncture, Rubenfeld synergy or energy healing. These individuals may expect the holistic health practitioner to "fix" the problem and become dissatisfied if asked to consciously participate.

VERTICAL PLANE DOMINANCE. Individuals who function primarily in the vertical (up down, door) plane tend to sit upright in an unsupported or self-supported manner. They typically exhibit a bipolar shaping of their body in the vertical. This is true in the standing position as well. This is the plane of presenting, assertion, power and control. Developmentally this dominates during the toddler phase of the "terrible two's" of rapprochement which begins about 18 months. Clinically speaking, if an individual remains in this position no matter what the adaptive context we may notice tightly contracted arches, overdeveloped calf muscles, quadriceps, and hamstrings. The pelvis is tilted forward frequently with contracted external rotators buttock's muscles resulting in a widened second position (ballet) or duck-like stance. There is often a strong muscular development with an expansive chest and low back tension frequently resulting in chronic pain. The message of the vertical personality shifts to "I won't." This posture can be typically seen in the classic state troopers stance or salesman presenting persistently without communicating or listening. This anal character frequently has anger stored in the lower back area which can be held down for periods of time followed by rage explosions not unlike the temper tantrums of a two-year-old. These clients come into the holistic practitioner's consulting room with chronic back pain, type A hypertense personalities at risk for cardiac arrest and coronary ailments. They tend to have a chronic fight sympathetic response and can have a difficult time letting go into anything that entails their imagination such as visualization, guided imagery or improvisational creative play.

SAGITTAL PLANE DOMINANCE. Individuals who function primarily in the sagittal (forward backward) plane tend to sit forward or retreat backward. They typically narrow bipolarly so that the body has an arrow-like penetrating appearance. If forward in the sagittal, they often have to keep busy doing to avoid feeling deeply. They may appear officious, impatient and work addicted. They may also demonstrate a held upper torso shift forward or backward. Clinically, this plane can be detected in the histrionic personality and incested or molested posttraumatic stress individuals both moving forward in the upper torso and holding back in the pelvic area. Along with this stance can be seen frightened eyes and elevated shoulders as seen in the flight or freeze sympathetic responses. Their behavior can include sexualization of relationships, occasionally with a coquettish flirtation.

These individuals come to holistic health often seeking stress reduction. They have particular difficulty letting go of the busy mind which interferes with meditation, yoga, and other techniques which attempt to still the person bringing them into presence from moment-to-moment as these individuals are caught re-doing the past or obsessing about the future.

SUMMARY

Holistic health practitioners and consultants understand the mindbody connection. Comprehension of a rich developmentally-based window into the identification of early sensorimotor development and primitive limbic and sympathetic system responses to safety and danger through the Kestenberg Movement Repertoire can offer an understanding of key elements which are crucial in recovery, health and the maintenance of well-being.

REFERENCES

Amaghi, J., Loman, S., Lewis, P., Sossin, M., Eds. (1999). *The meaning of movement: Developmental and clinical perspectives as seen through the Kestenberg Movement Profile.* Newark: NJ: Gordon & Breach Pub.

Lewis, P. (1993). *Creative transformation: The healing power of the arts.* Willmette, IL: Chiron Publishing.

Lewis, P. (1984). *Theoretical approaches in dance-movement therapy* Vol 2. Dubuque, IA: Kendall/Hunt Pub.

Lewis, P. (1986). *Theoretical approaches in dance-movement therapy* Vol 1. Dubuque, IA: Kendall/Hunt Pub.

Lewis, P. and Singer, D. Eds. (1983). *The Choreography of object relations.* Keene, NH: Antioch-New England Graduate School.

Lewis, P. and Loman, S. (1990). *The KMP: Its Past Present and Future Applications.* Keene, NH: Antioch-New England Graduate School.

Chapter 5

IMAGINATION, INTUITION AND THE PERSONAL & COLLECTIVE UNCONSCIOUS IN HOLISTIC HEALTH, HEALING AND TRANSFORMATION

And when we see our own identity and our destiny in relation to the unseen world-God or dharma or the Tao or Nirvana-then myth as myth is given an added impulse, for we imagine the invisible through the visible and give life to our faith through symbols. (Smart, 2000, pp. 85–86)

ORIGINS OF THE CONCEPT OF THE UNCONSCIOUS

THE UNCONSCIOUS CAN BE simply defined as that which individuals are not consciously aware but is, nonetheless, within their mindbody experience. This phenomenon was first conceptualized in the early twentieth century when the inner workings of the psyche were explored. Freud, Jung and Adler are considered the founding fathers of bringing the focus of the unconscious into a new field called psychoanalysis and later psychotherapy.

Freud, in addressing the question of the dynamics of the unconscious, formulated the concept of libido and expanded his view to include a developmental perspective of psychosexual stages. The libido is seen as the pleasure-based driving life force of the personality at the disposal of Eros–the instinct of love. This life force, serving connection and growth, modifies and revises at each stage of early development focusing upon specific sources of pleasure and learning.

This developmental orientation, in turn, was broadened through the work of ego psychologists such as Anna Freud, (1966) and Eric Erikson, (1963) who expanded the range of human development to include stages throughout the life span. Adler, too, attended to this phenomenon from a child development perspective within what is now identified as a family system's orientation.

C.G. Jung (1948) wrote "Depth psychology is a term deriving from medical psychology, coined by Eugen Bleuler to denote that branch of psychological science which is concerned with the phenomenon of the unconscious" (XVIII, par. 1142). Jung felt the driving force of the unconscious came from the Self–an archetypal organizing principle of wholeness that moves persons through an individuating process. Humanistic psychologists espoused Jung's concept. Maslow, Perls, and others felt that the motivational force of the unconscious is a propensity toward personal evolution called self-actualization, an innate human tendency toward growth and the greater fulfillment of individuals' potentials.

Jung's findings resulted in his view that the unconscious consisted of "two layers: a superficial layer, representing the personal unconscious, and a deeper layer representing the collective unconscious" (Jung, 1948, C.W. XVIII, par. 1159). The personal unconscious, like Freud's view, was comprised of repressed childhood trauma, split off parts of the personality and internalized significant objects in the individual's early life. The collective unconscious is the domain of universal eternal images, themes, sounds and gestures called archetypes.

One of the original theorists of the mindbody relationship to the unconscious was Willhelm Reich, a member of Freud's elite Vienna Psychoanalytic Society. Reich conceptualized the libido as functioning at a physical level rather than at a mental level as Freud suggested. He translated the concept of "psychic energy" into "physical energy." Reich, like Freud, focused on sexual drive and its expression as key. Like the ego psychologists and object relations theorists who followed Freud, other's, most notably, Lowen expanded Reich's ideas into bioenergetics and developed one of the original body-oriented psychotherapies. (Looking from an Era II medicine: mindbody interrelationship perspective, the argument as to whether the unconscious lies in the mind or body is now a moot point.)

All of these originators valued the importance of accessing the unconscious not only to unlock the mystery of the disease but also to aid in the individuation (Jung), self-actualization (Humanistic) and working through (Freud) with such techniques as transforming the transference, expression of blocked early childhood movements, metaphoric embodied enactments, free association and active imagination. This value of the unconscious and its symbolic world has continued to have a profound and integral influence in mindbody understanding and healing.

THE ANATOMY OF THE UNCONSCIOUS AND THE IMAGINATION

The left hemisphere of the cerebral cortex is typically thought of to provide rational analytic assessments. Time is seen as quantitative, linear. Most events have a cause and effect relationship to one another. This portion of the brain basically ascribes to two tenants: "what you see is what there is," and "if it cannot fit into an existing logical scientific model, it doesn't exist." This is the realm of reductive thinking and interpretation.

Juxtaposed to the left hemisphere is the right hemisphere. This is the realm of imagination, creativity, the mysterious, the intuitive, synchronicity and qualitative time. The language of this realm is symbol and metaphor. In this realm is the threshold to the unconscious filled with the unacceptable, the horrible, and all the potential of who one could be waiting for the right time to come forward. These painful events along with childhood survival patterns and toxic aspects of significant others organize themselves into autonomous feeling toned complexes or schema. These so-called complexes become anthropromorphized or theriomorphized into human-like or animal–like symbolic entities in the psyche.

The sensorimotor foundation for the unconscious lies in the more primitive limbic system and the body. Even in Freud's and Jung's time it was clear that the unconscious had a somatic source. "The unconscious lies in the body," Jung proclaimed early on. Thus, the mindbody interrelationship was understood well before neurophysiologic documentation. Repressed trauma and split off parts of the self can be located in the body covered over by the "frozen" tension spots described in the former chapter. These corresponding dead spots are also seen in energy medicine as well, and will be discussed in Chapter 7. Reclaiming preverbal memories that lie in the body and bodily sensations allow both the client and therapist the ability to reconstruct, recover from and/or clear early trauma. Winnicott has stated that many memories are "pre-verbal, nonverbal and unverbalizable" (1971, p. 130). Since many memories of abuse occur prior to language, they are often held in unconscious somatic schemata that can only be recalled by kinesthetic, energetic and/or movement reconstruction. For example, many patients report feeling nauseous often suggesting early trauma in what Freud called the oral phase, object relations called the symbiotic phase, ego psychologists called the stage of trust verses mistrust and behaviorists called the sensorimotor phase. Thus mindbody techniques such as found in the process orientation of body-oriented psychotherapies can allow individuals the vehicle to fully experience, claim, and transform. Through embodiment, prior trauma can be healed and as yet undeveloped parts of the self-claimed and integrated.

THE PERSONAL UNCONSCIOUS

The unconscious has been likened to the metaphor of the ocean into which unacceptable or unsafe parts of the personality, traumatic experience too painful to remember, and other discarded occurrences are thrown into like some vast receptacle for unwanted or unusable material. This so-called "personal unconscious" also contains those sub-personalities which individuals are to integrate into their existing psyche as they progress through their life span. These self-parts are developmentally waiting to be washed onto the shores of consciousness when the time and health of individuals are right.

If the family does not provide the needed environment for healthy development but does not get identified by social service as too dangerous for the children to remain, the children are typically caught "imprisoned" until they are old enough to leave. Children develop behaviors to survive these painful years that become habitual automatic unconscious blocked ways of responding long after they are needed. For example, an individual may have a judging survival mechanism which was created in childhood based upon the premise that if the child could judge his or herself more severely than the parent or other criticizing individuals, than she/he would be protected from further shameful pain. This inner judge complex frequently becomes personified as a relentless voice criticizing the person. Rationality would say that, of course, there isn't a little nasty figure of a judge inside; but the imagination, where it resides, knows very well that it exists.

The self or inner child(ren) complex(es) also exist and are frequently stuck imprisoned and disconnected from the adult self in the body unconscious of the third chakra. Pert's research regarding gut feelings confirms that there is more occurring in the solar plexus than "digestion."

THE COLLECTIVE UNCONSCIOUS

Complexes reside in what Jung called the personal unconscious, but at their core is always an archetype from the deeper layer or collective unconscious (Jung, XVI). In this realm, time is relative. Past, present, and future all reside in the now. Access to the collective unconscious typically shakes loose any rigidities which have kept individuals from the "bigger picture" and their relationship within it. Jung (1948) writes, "These experiences usually concern individuals in the second half of life, when it not infrequently happens that didactic changes of outlook are thrust upon them by the unconscious" (C.W. XVIII, par. 1161). Jung goes on to say, "The relating influences of the collective unconscious can be seen at work in the psychic development of the individual, or the individuation process" (par. 1162). Access to this archetypal unconscious allows individuals a window into the spiritual realm. It is understood that faith and a connection to the spiritual or mystical is not a rational empirical left hemisphere experience but rather addresses the capacity to connect to the collective or archetypal universal Holy Other (Spiritual belief) or Undifferentiated Light (Mystical belief). The right brain experience of this universal realm is conversely called the capacity for Consciousness in Buddhist and other Eastern traditions. It is said that newborns bring this consciousness with them, lose it through the reinforcement of the unconsciousness of others and then, if they are sentient beings, rediscover or remember this truth after a long spiritual journey. The journey can be described as circular evolving as described in Figure 5-1.

HEALTH, HEALING, AND GROWTH THROUGH THE IMAGINATION

The shores of the unconscious can be seen as the imagination. Whatever washes ashore onto the imagination utilizes the language of symbol and metaphor. D.W. Winnicott (1971) identified the imagination as a transitional space. Winnicott's transitional space in analysis and the liminal phase in shamanic healing have a common experiential link. In both cases, the individual is experiencing the moment in an area that lies between reality and deep unconsciousness. It is a combination of both utilizing conscious empirical awareness and the symbolic language of the unconscious. It is a liminal realm in which children play in order to learn and grow and adults artistically create and explore in order to reveal the universality of the human condition, evolve and heal.

As children, most individuals have engaged in fantasy and pretended to be any number of characters. During this time, they knew that they weren't really this character or that–not to know would mean they were paranoid or suffering from a disassociative reaction. But they nonetheless had a rich experience of being these characters in every inch of their bodies, so that their movements emerged naturally from this imaginal core. Needless to say, this playing has a profound effect in shaping individuals' adaptation to life. Various techniques have been developed in rites of passage, ritual, and therapeutic processes to re-invite adults into this transformational imaginal realm.

Accessing the Imagination through the Arts

Jung, as did Freud, understood that dreams came from the unconscious, but Jung also utilized the arts knowing that they came from the same symbolic source. Thus painting, drawing, sand play, story writing, stream of consciousness journaling, visualization, poetry, improvisational sound, movement and drama all come from and access the imaginal realm. It is vital when employing the arts in health, healing and individuation not to switch over to the left brain and interpret. Interpretation kills. Rather it is vital to enter into the imaginal realm with the artist-client where healing and transformation can occur.

Because the abuse, inner core child selves, childhood survival patterns, all of the shadow aspects of who one could be, as well as access to the spiritual realm all lie within the unconscious, it makes sense that here is one avenue into healing and transformation. Although it may be possible to understand what happened and why a person is the way they are in the left rational hemisphere, this knowing often changes nothing. A transformational experience cannot be had by teaching, either. This naive reductionistic view supposes that one behavior pattern can be

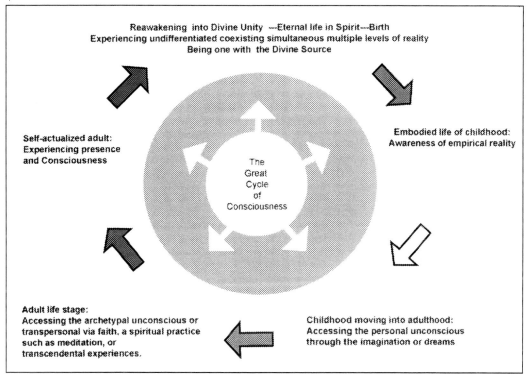

Figure 5-1. Circular journey to Consciousness.

superimposed on or replaced by another. Rather individuals can access and enter the imagination–"the royal road to the unconscious" (Jung)–where their history and future potential lie, and can recover, heal, and transform. The embodied arts of drama and dance-movement are most powerful as the person is experiencing the healing process as it is happening within the mind-body experience.

This often requires not only the client, but the therapist as well to enter into the bipersonal imaginal realm (Lewis, 1985, 1987, 1988b, 1992, 1993). Therapists join in the play, improvisation, visualization, guided meditations, body scans, or ritual allowing their interventions to be within the symbolic-metaphoric language of the imagination (Turner, 1969). Holistic health practitioners know, as did ancient shaman counterparts, that through experience within the unconscious symbolic imaginal realm, there is a possibility for healing and transformation (Lewis-Bernstein, 1982, 1985; Johnson, 1982; Lewis, 1989, 1993, Kabat-Zinn, 2001).

When the holistic health practitioner values this liminal unconscious transitional space within the imaginal realm, it facilitates the patients' doing so themselves within the many containers for this experience. In this imaginal realm, clay shapes, drawings and sand play figures are embodied and their symbolic power infused by their creator. In this imaginal realm, the patient's body, like that of the shaman's, may feel as if it is being pulled apart, turned to mush, or archetypally filled with golden, penetrating rays (Lewis, 1986a, 1988a). In this realm the individuals may allow a dream, or an aspect of their psyche to fully manifest in their bodies and an invoked spirit; angry monster, divine guide, or a tender infant self may emerge.

But when childhood abuse violated physical boundaries, embodiment may be too powerful and literally send individuals out of their bodies triggering the childhood survival pattern of dissociation. In these instances, arts media, which externalize trauma-based complexes may be far more appropriate. Through art, poetry, story writing, and journaling, the individual can distance themselves from the events; then personifying different aspects, they can interview them and can begin to put the pieces together in a way that doesn't tear them apart in the process. Visualization, meditation on themes within a non-doing peaceful practice, and guided present-oriented sensory awareness which reduces the excitation of the triggered amygdala and sympathetic response may begin to unravel the chronic re-traumatization whether the pain is emotional-relational or physical in origin. It also has been shown that meditation and the hearing of archetypal poetry during mindfulness can stimulate the left prefrontal lobes of the cortex thus assisting in the reconnection and subduing of the overactive amygdala (Kabat-Zinn & Santorelli, 2001).

Accessing the Imagination through Visualization

It continues to be clear that the imagination plays a profound role in heath, healing and well-being. Readers have only to recall the importance of double blind studies in drug testing due to the documented placebo effect to realize that just imagining taking a drug can often produce the same restorative physiologic responses as the actual drug itself. The successful use of visualization to reduce phobias, anxiety, depression, and to increase T-cell assaults on cancer cells has been documented. Simply, positive imaginings encourage growth; negative imaginings limit it. These imaginings trigger biochemical responses (Pert et al.) which can reduce stress and its bodily repercussions.

Accessing the Body Unconscious Through the Somatic Countertransference/ Somatic Intuition

Carl Jung was the first in the field of psychotherapy to point out that analysands and their analysts communicate on several different levels. First, there is the explicit conscious-to-conscious communication between the clinical two in which reality-based information is discussed. The patient also shares unconscious information with the therapist typically in the form of free association or dream material. Additionally, neo-Jungians began to address other vectors of unconscious information. Nonverbal communication such as discussed in the former chapter on body movement also conveys unconscious phenomena to the clinical practitioner. In these two instances, the clinician receives the unconscious material into her consciousness. Jung (1997), however, talked about an unconscious-to-unconscious connection in which the patient's unconscious communicates directly to the unconscious of the therapist. When the therapist does not bring this material into consciousness, personal countertransference may occur. Here the unaware therapist begins to act upon or react to the unconscious material given to him or her. For example, this can occur if the client idealizes the holistic health practitioner and the practitioner starts believing the idealization and becomes inflated with the client's projection. In this instance the clinician holds on to a belief that he or she is an "omniscient healer" instead of giving the pedestaling regard back to the patient through empowering statements.

This third unconscious-to-unconscious phenomenon has been given much exploration in Freudian as well as Jungian depth work and has been called projective identification (Schwartz-Salant, 1983-1984; Stein,

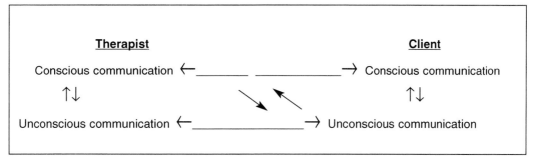

Figure 5-2. Types of communication between client and therapist.

1984; Grostein, 1981) and the somatic countertransference (Lewis, 1981, 1986b, 1986c, 1988a, 1988b, 1993a).

Many practitioners have described this receipt of the client's unconscious material as having a key somatic component. The material is received into the third chakra of the therapist producing a gut feeling or sensation (Motoyama). Typically, whatever is not integrated into the consciousness of the client remains split off in the unconscious and can be projected unconsciously into the therapist. The therapist (or any individual for that matter) may receive for example: sensations of queasiness, nausea, sexual excitement, aching pain or frantic fragments bouncing off the wall of the stomach; feelings of rage, sadness, fear, joy, or love; or in the mind images such as wounded inner children, toxic parents or metaphors. Some practitioners predominately receive feelings, others kinesthetic sensations, others images which can be either symbolic or literal, others auditorily receive ideas, still others a combination of the above.

Practitioners need to be able to distinguish between their own feelings and responses and that of the clients. A sure indication that the phenomena belongs to the client is that if the client begins to claim the sensations, feelings, or images they will immediately disappear from the body unconscious of the practitioner. Additionally, when clients leave, these phenomena will leave with them. If practitioners find themselves with lingering sensations, feelings, images or ideas, then the material is either theirs or has triggered a personal countertransferential response. This occurs when the clinician has not completely dealt with or healed a related issue with which the client is struggling.

It is important when utilizing the technique of the somatic countertransference to create a centered meditational inner state. Some imagine an inner sacred vessel within the belly or third chakra to receive any material from the client. Important to note is that not all practitioners are receptive to these phenomena. If, for example, they had their own boundaries energetically violated in childhood, strong energetically-based survival mechanisms may have developed to ward away anyone else is unconscious material.

This body unconscious to body unconscious connection is a two-way street. Holistic health practitioners can imaginally heal or transform, hold, and/or send back to the client split off feelings or recovered held inner core selves. In this realm, attending to the somatic countertransference it is possible; for example, to imaginally transform projected split off aspects of a person's psychology through remembering, and neutralize and detoxify transferred negative primary caregivers. The therapist may receive the patient's negative judgmental or engulfing parent from the patient's somatic unconscious. And, like the shamans who receive the poisonous or negative "spirits" that sought to rid their patients of their sense of self, the therapist heals and transforms these feeling-charged images while still in the therapist's body vessel. With others, their infant self may be imaginally received for love and healthy gestation to be retransferred when the patient is ready.

When working with post traumatic stress disordered individuals, it may be important to hold some of the trauma such as sensations, images or feelings. To send these back might overload the client sending them out of their body, into a sympathetic nervous system response and/or overfiring the amygdala creating emotional hijacking disconnecting these primitive reactions from the calming effect of the prefrontal lobe.

Motoyama (1990) sights a similar phenomenon in his work as a Shinto Priest doing "therapeutic counseling" with his parishioners. He states, "I intentionally attempt to activate my manipura (3rd chakra) in order to gain paranormal knowledge about deeper causes of people's physical and emotional problems" (p. 102). When he sends healing or otherwise split-off material back to the client to be reclaimed, he moves the material up to the heart chakra to be imbued with compassion and then out. Utilizing the AMI machine (apparatus for measuring the function of the Meridians and their corresponding internal organs) which successfully and accurately measures Ki (chi) energy, he has been able to monitor healers use of the manipura and anahata (4th heart chakra) during the receipt and transmission of client material on behalf of the client. The pilot study showed statistically significant differences in the meridian systems as they were passing the Ki energy.

The use of the technique of the somatic countertransference (Lewis, 1993) allows for practitioners to not only receive transferred objects or projected split-off effect, self and shadow aspects, sensations, and images from the client's personal unconscious but grace

and numinosum from the transpersonal archetypal unconscious on his/her behalf. Individuals, who are identified as psychics or medical intuitives such as the well known and documented Edgar Casey, access material from the client and on behalf of the client. Those who utilize this high intuitive ability have been able to look into another's body at varying depths. These medical intuitives report being able to receive an inner picture of the diseased or traumatized area (see Chapter 9).

INTUITION

The capacity for intuition comes from an access to the archetypal unconscious. Chakra-based models see this as an open functioning 6th chakra or third eye. Many in energy medicine identify this phenomenon as high sense perception (Brennon, 1987). It is fundamentally a way of perceiving things beyond the normal ranges of human senses (p. 5). The images that are perceived in the mind's occipital cortex do not originate from empirical reality.

This phenomenon has been called clairvoyance or psychic reading and is seen as the capacity to tune into the universal hologram and to read information that exists out of linear time. Operationally Brennon describes this process as light entering her third eye and natural eyes and flowing along the optic nerve circumnavigating the pituitary, then bifurcating entering the occipital lobes and the thalamus and ending in the pineal gland which serves as a "detector" for internal vision (p. 163). This so-called central brain scanner can also receive information from other sources beyond that of the client. Receiving on behalf of the client has been called channeling. Information can be received as a thought or image. Recommendations on behalf of the health and healing of the individual can be gleaned.

THE TEMENOS

Whether or not information is received via the somatic countertransference, from the client or from the supraconsciousness via the archetypal unconsciousness on behalf of the client, practitioners need to create a series of sacred spaces starting with their own body as a temple, followed by a larger temenos which includes the bipersonal field between the holistic health practitioner and the client, and a larger third which encompasses the entire consulting room. The practitioner's body must become a sacred vessel to receive on behalf of the client. Formal practices which can include a sacred or religious discipline, meditation, yoga, breathing, diet, prayer and periodic cleansing of energy fields as well as personal mindbody work aid in creating and maintaining a clear field. The inner vessel described earlier aids in this process.

Practitioners are also aware of the energetic field that exists between the two of them or surrounding a group that allows for intimacy, confidentiality, boundaries and sacred space. Through prayer, ritual, or meditation some create an energy field within which healing can occur. Material received from the body unconscious of the client and sent back must remain within this bipersonal field.

The consulting room itself must also be a temenos–a sacred temple in service to the healing and well-being of all those who enter. Practitioners, depending upon their spiritual or mystical beliefs, create and maintain their space through a variety of methods from indigenous saging to Christian prayer. Regardless, the space must be a *vas bene clausum*–a well-sealed vessel allowing the alchemical process of healing and transformation to take place in an uncontaminated space, metaphorically in much the same way a surgeon requires a sterile operating room. The intent and energy must be for the greater good of the client(s) with the practitioner's detached objectivity and open compassion present from moment-to-moment.

THE PERSONAL AND ARCHETYPAL UNCONSCIOUS IN HEALING AND TRANSFORMATION

Healing and transformation work is seen in two distinct although occasionally overlapping phases that were delineated in Jung's view of working with the personal unconscious followed by the archetypal collective unconscious. The first phase entails healing from childhood and other previous physical and/or emotional trauma along with the transformation of any addiction(s) and dysfunctional patterns. The second phase addresses the individuation process that facilitates the integrating of as yet undeveloped aspects of the psyche and an individual's unique unfolding of their personal journey which culminates in greater spiritual consciousness or wakefulness. The goal of the work is to be fully present with a spontaneous mindbody, have healthy boundaries and a capacity for intimacy with oneself, others, and the transpersonal through a spiritual or mystical connection.

The Personal Unconscious: Healing Previous Trauma

In the first phase, individuals enter therapy because their lives are not working for them. For example, they cannot sustain relationships and/or jobs, or they have begun to move from denial into accountability regarding their addictions, or they are beginning to have flashbacks of abuse, or all the implicit promises of their childhood survival patterns such as, "if I am a perfect giver, then I will get what I need," are not panning out.

In the nineties, the concept of trauma and child abuse has expanded from physical beatings and sexual perpetrations to include all forms of emotional, verbal, and spiritual assaults. Symptoms of these forms of abuse have been hidden in our culture for some time. For example, Western society has considered it appropriate for white males to feel better than, invulnerable, perfectionistic, angry, antidependent and hierarchically competitive (Mellody, 1989, p. 27); while women were to feel less than, have no boundaries, be co-dependent caregivers and carry the more vulnerable feelings of hurt, fear and sadness for the male.

Addictions go hand-in-hand with improper parenting. Like the definition of child abuse, the concept of addictions has expanded as well. The list enlarges from alcohol and substance abuse to include eating disorders such as bulimia, anorexia and obesity, smoking, gambling, retail shopping, sex, love, money, power, work, etc. These dysfunctional patterns are learned from families, peer cultures or represent personal intrapsychic adaptations whose motivation is based on childhood survival. These patterns continue into adulthood and outlive their appropriateness. Individuals experience present reality as if it was a carbon copy of their past. They act and react in significant relationships based upon their abusive relationships with their primary caregivers, and they respond in social and work settings as if it were their family or prior peer culture.

Because they may have had nonnurturing and devaluing parents, they were unable to experience a realistic sense of self. This lack of self-esteem results in a person feeling empty, less than or reactively better than others. These abusive primary caregivers are then internalized and become inner critics and shamers, abandoning or traumatizing the inner self (sometimes referred to as the inner child). Occasionally, the abusive parent wants to live off the child's greatness and so never relativizes their natural grandiosity. When internalized, this inner object never allows the ego-self to live a regular, normal life. Their capacity to work is atrophied because they are somehow supposed to reach the pinnacle of greatness without ever having to exert any time or attention to it.

If separation and independence is trau-

matized through personal space violation, as with physical abuse or denial of privacy, individuals will have inadequate boundaries. For example, they may have no boundaries and be perpetual victims to others' perpetrations. They may have wall-like boundaries and isolate themselves; or have faulty boundaries in certain areas and continue to receive the type of abuse they incurred in childhood.

If too much separation is given through abandonment or overstressed as with males in our culture, they may become "needless and wantless" and employ additions as false mothers to avoid the reality of having needs. If individuals are encouraged to remain dependent, as many women are, or those whose parents cannot separate, they may become overly dependent or codependent resulting in their not being able to meet their own needs.

If the home environment is unstable, children will not have the needed, consistent, emotionally present parenting. This results in immature, emotionally labile adults. If children become parentified or spousified within the nuclear family, they will tend to continue to be overcontrolling and hyperresponsible as adults.

Health and Goal of Therapy

Health and thus the goal in the recovery process is to have the capacity for intimacy with oneself, others, and the transpersonal. Additionally health is seen as the capacity to be fully present in the moment. That means that individuals are no longer reacting to the present as if it were the past dramas and no longer allowing childhood survival patterns to keep them from experiencing their whole self in relation to the world in a spontaneous manner. Health also requires strong ego boundaries ensuring that individuals' consciousness does not become possessed by fantasy, the past or future thoughts or by early survival behaviors. Working body boundaries ensue a distinction between what comes from the inside as versus what is projected or transferred from or onto the outside; and resilient and adaptive external boundaries ensure that individuals' personal space is not violated nor are wall-like boundaries constructed inhibiting appropriate intimacy with another.

Dysfunction

Dysfunction occurs from abuse, less than good enough parenting, cultural oppression, and the repeated ineffectual use of survival patterns that were created in childhood in the place of healthy boundaries. Dysfunctional families are unable to instill in a child a healthy realistic sense of self with an intact functioning ego, body, and personal space boundaries. This results in fragmented or split-off parts of the self, faulty boundaries, and habitual survival mechanisms created in order to endure what could not be escaped. Addictions are seen as one category of survival patterns. These are called "false mothers" as they frequently try to convince the addict that they can take care of them: fill the inner emptiness or stop the pain and that the addict does not need anyone else. Addictions whether they are alcohol, drugs, food, retail shopping, sex, love, money, power, or work use the same strategy as other survival mechanisms such as isolation, shutting down, people-pleasing, or judging oneself and/or others. They all attack intimacy on three levels: with the inner core self or what recovery therapists call the inner child (ren), with other individuals and with the spiritual transpersonal realm (see Figure 5-3).

Method of Identifying the Health-Dysfunction Continuum

The method of identifying and evaluating health and dysfunction is carried out by interviewing regarding the individual's distorted core beliefs, limiting thoughts and behaviors as well as presenting problem.

Additionally, the use of the embodied psyche technique, sand play, dreamwork, art, mindfulness practices and other venues into the imagination that reveal the functioning of their psyche aid in assessment.

Recovery Stage Therapeutic Process

The therapeutic process of the phase of recovery entails the therapist identifying the presenting problems and goals of the client through initial client interview. The therapist then assesses ego strength and explores within the imaginal mindbody process, the presence, accessibility and connection to the core self or inner child. Through the use of techniques such as the embodied psyche technique, the personality and intrapsychic structure is revealed, including those survival mechanisms, addictions, trauma, and/or parental and societal introjects which conflict with health.

In the second phase, that which inhibits a connection to the self, others and the transpersonal is transformed utilizing techniques which employ the imagination such as visualization, the embodied psyche technique and recovery and healing of the inner child(ren) from trauma. The former technique entails the personification through art and/or role playing of various complexes or habitual thinking or feeling so that individuals can become more aware through externalizing and gaining distance, be fully present and mindful, and connect to their core self (Lewis, 2000). One method of healing child abuse requires individuals to return imaginally to each abuse setting and occasion; take their inner child to a safe place; and if they choose, as an adult, return imaginally and confront the perpetrator(s). When addictions are used as false mothers in attempts to fill the void of the absence of self and object, they, too, need to be confronted as the abusers they really are. Once the inner child is freed from the abuse, re or co-parenting can occur in the choreography of object relations (Lewis-Bernstein, 1983;

Lewis, 1986, 1987, 1990a, 1993a) or indirectly though other holistic approaches which entail caring touch such as massage therapy. With a healed loved inner child and a supportive positive internalized parent who ensures and encourages healthy boundaries and expression of needs and wants, the individual is freed to respond appropriately in the moment and continue to unfold in their life.

The Embodied Psyche

Because self-formation and the internalization of the object is accomplished in and with the body, mindbody techniques, which employ the imaginal-transitional play space, are utilized (Lewis, 2000). Whether working individually, with groups, or couples therapy, it is vital to know "all the players." The first cast of characters is always in the head of each individual present. Within the initial interview the therapist can assess the level of health of the individual based upon the presence, relationship, and the amount of power or psychic energy distribution of the various inner voices. These inner characters are called complexes by Jungians, schemata by cognitive therapists or subpersonalities by those who utilize psychosynthesis. The following complexes are looked for in a person's psyche and can be role-played:

EGO OR INNER ADULT: CHAIRPERSON OF THE PSYCHE. A healthy psyche has a functioning ego which acts as the "chairperson of a board of directors" listening to what different subpersonalities have to say. The ego, referred to as the inner adult (transactional analysis), is the mediator and reality tester. The ego deciphers inner reality from outer reality; it assesses what belongs to the person and what does not. If healthy, the ego will know what projections and transferences are being sent out by the psyche, or being received from another person. In order to execute this filtering process the ego needs healthy ego boundaries that differentiate what is part of the individual's psyche from

what is someone else's.

The boundaries must also be secure so that toxic intrapsychic complexes do not invade the ego and "possess it." The person is often unaware when this happens and operates from a false belief that it is the inner adult that is speaking. This occurs, for example; when an addiction invades the ego and individuals "think" they should reabuse a substance, when a rage possesses the ego and individuals batter another, or when an inner critic complex enters and clients misperceive the voice to be their rational ego who is self-trashing.

SELF OR INNER CHILD: SOURCE OF FEELINGS, NEEDS AND WANTS. The ego is expected to have a good connection to the core self (object relations and self-psychology) also referred to as the inner child (recovery theory and transactional analysis). This connection means that the chairperson of the psyche always knows what the person feels, needs and wants. Without access to the self, the person will not be able to give the self what it needs nor fill the self with realistic positive love and regard. Without this connection, self-esteem and an experience of being seen and understood is impossible. This disconnection begins in the first few years of life with a parent that does not provide the ego with a role model of a healthy parent-child relationship. The parent or primary caregiver either emotionally or physically abandons, attempts to control, or violates the developing child. The self, instead of feeling full of love and realistic positive regard, remains depleted and in pain and fear.

CHILDHOOD SURVIVAL BEHAVIORS: DEFENSES AGAINST INNER PAIN, SURVIVAL FEAR, AND EXTERNAL OTHERS. The child then soon develops behaviors to disengage from any ongoing pain, loses, emptiness and/or survival fear. These survival behaviors are designed to disconnect the ego both from the inner core pained self and from external others. Initially they are needed in childhood as children cannot "fire" their parents and so must somehow endure growing up in the family. However, these survival patterns do not leave in adulthood, but stay, keeping the ego forever disconnected from the self and caring others. The following are some examples of these survival complexes:

- *The denier*–"I have no pain; no needs and wants; I had a happy childhood."
- *The insulator*–"It's not safe to be vulnerable, I'll hide the child self so no one not even you (the ego) can find it."
- *The inner critic*–"Do not say or do anything spontaneously, someone might find out that you are unacceptable and abandon you or judge you adversely."
- *The controller*–"Remember it was not safe having our parents be in control; or it was not safe having needs in that chaos. I'll just protect you by controlling others and by controlling your vulnerable feelings."
- *The abuser*–"You know what it felt like to be the victim; it's much better to be the one on top. Get that needy self away from me! I'm the bully now and I won't have that vulnerable self messing this up. So let's find someone to project onto and attack."
- *The victim/martyr/people pleaser*–"If we just focus on other peoples needs than sooner or later someone will focus on us and heal the child. Besides it's selfish to focus on your own needs."
- *The forgotten one/isolator*–"If we do not say anything then no one will notice us and no harm will come to us."
- *The ambivolator*–"If we never take a stand or never make a decision then we won't get anything wrong and end up alone, shamed or abused."
- *The scapegoat*–"If we agree to be the bad one then it will please the family and draw attention away from the real problem: mom and/or dad."
- *The perfect one*–"I can't control what is going on outside, but I can control myself." Or "Maybe if I am perfect; then I can fix my family."

ADDICTIONS: THE INNER COMPELLING VOICE OF THE ADDICTION. Like survival behaviors, addictions too split the inner adult ego off from the core child self and from the possibility for intimacy with others. These "false mothers" tell the ego that they'll take care of the child, stop the pain, or fill the void. They demand total obedience and control over the addict's life.

INNER OBJECTS: MOTHER OR FATHER COMPLEXES: THE INTERNALIZATIONS OF THE CHILD'S PARENTS. Early in childhood, the many experiences with individuals' mother, father, and any primary caregivers are internalized. If a parent was absent there will not be the constant inner parent who offers advice to the ego to support and care for the inner child or encourage the adult to develop. If any parent was verbally abusive, individuals will internalize an inner abusive judge and will feel "less than." If the parent lived off the greatness of the child, individuals will internalize a complex that views the ego as "better than" and entitled to all their needs and wants being met. Negative parental complexes continue to treat the child self in the same unhealthy way their actual parents treated them and advise the adult ego to do the same. They, too, can disconnect the ego from a functioning connection to the core self.

Often when parents and other authority figures are toxic, individuals disconnect from access to a Higher Power especially if their parents acted like gods. Other individuals feel that if there were a higher consciousness then it would be like a human parent and hold their view on what an appropriate family of origin would be. Since their family was hurtful, they surmise that there is either no God or that they are being punished in some way. This can result in a disconnection from the transpersonal.

DEVALUING NEGATIVE COLLECTIVE: THE INTERNALIZATIONS OF SOCIETY'S DISTORTED WORLD VIEWS. Dysfunctional families are not always the only source of disconnections of the ego from the core self or external others. Minorities, whether they be people of ethnic diversity, socioeconomic stigma, or do not fit the ideal stereotype due to physical appearance, psychological or physical health, or intellectual ability, often internalize negative devaluations of themselves and so disconnect as a result of the painful assaults on the core self. Additionally, they feel ashamed and/or feel that God has punished them in some way and thus disconnect from external others and the transpersonal.

ANIMUS AND ANIMA: INNER MASCULINE AND FEMININE ASPECTS. When an individual has successfully connected to the self and healed their pain, access to their contra sexual inner masculine or animus in women or inner feminine or anima in men becomes more available. Frequently the same sex parent can occlude a relationship to this contrasexual complex. For example, if a man has a controlling mother complex, he frequently sees all women as potentially controlling. His *anima* may render him moody and depressed, but if freed, she is often a beautifully wise hierophant. Likewise, if a woman had a judgmental or unprotective father, she may not trust men and have a piercing derisive inner *animus* that attacks her and castrates other men. There are an infinite variety of *animi* and *animae* that can organically emerge from the unconscious to be claimed. They often make excellent advisors to the ego particularly if they are not projected out of the psyche and onto someone else.

The collective world view and family scripts often hinder individuals from claiming their androgyny through a relationship to his anima or her animus. The collective voice might say, "Men shouldn't take care of the children" or "Women shouldn't be powerful."

Within these personal contra-sexual aspects, lie archetypal cores. A woman's animus might have an inner rational Apollo or protective Mars; a man's anima might have a wise Sophia or romantically loving Aphrodite (see Figures 5-4 and 5-5).

SHADOW ASPECTS: INNER SAME SEX ASPECTS WAITING TO BE CLAIMED BY THE EGO. Likewise, same sex aspects or shadow complexes wait to emerge to be integrated into the ego or remain as advisors when the need arises. These aspects may initially appear in dreams as highly instinctual and uncivilized, but, with embodiment and intrapsychic dialogue with the ego, frequently become more civilized. They then are invited on to the inner board of directors.

Just as family roles and the collective can negatively influence the integration of animi/ae, so can they curtail the ego's relationship to the same sex shadow complexes. For example, a sibling may already have been identified as the smart one or the artist or athlete, leaving a younger sibling to be given another role.

As with *animi/animae*, shadow aspects also have archetypal cores to be discussed later in the chapter (see Figures 5-4 and 5-5).

SOUL: THE ETERNAL SELF. The soul, an individual's eternal being, lies within the core self or inner child. If individuals do not connect to the self, they will never be in relation to their soul. Thus they will never be able to connect to whom they truly are and what it is they are meant to do in this lifetime. Figure 3-1 represents the disconnected psyche.

The Technique Itself with Groups, Individuals, and Couples

Basically, individuals' psyches are externalized, thereby gaining conscious distance through art, sand play or role-play. If they are part of a group, various group members can take on the different roles and may be arranged in an initial tableau not unlike Satir's family sculpture. Each personified complex is given a characteristic phrase and movement. The person can observe and is then asked, "Is this the way you want your psyche to be?" If the answer is no, then the drama therapy process commences with the person role-playing parts of their psyche with whom they want to connect to, such as their inner core self, soul, animus/animae or

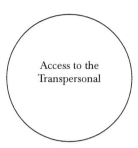

Disconnection from the transpersonal due to:

Internalized Toxic Parent	Any Addictions	Childhood Survival Behaviors	Devaluing Negative Collective

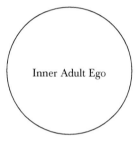

Disconnection from the core self/inner child due to:

Internalized Toxic ParentParent	Any Addictions	Childhood Survival Behaviors	Devaluing Negative Collective

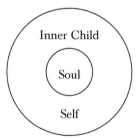

Disconnection from external others due to:

Internalized Toxic Parent	Any Addictions	Childhood Survival Behaviors	Devaluing Negative Collective

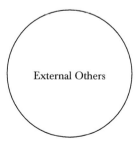

Figure 5-3. Dysfunctional disconnected psyche.

shadow aspect and have the therapist or others personify complexes that need to be externalized and depotentiated: survival mechanisms, addictions, and toxic introjects. Role reversal by the client is encouraged with complexes to be empowered and drawn into closer relationship to the ego (Lewis, 2000). This technique has proven helpful to increase mindfulness both during formal and informal practices, and has substantially reduced anxiety and stress.

The Archetypal Collective Unconscious: Individuation and Expanding Consciousness

The second phase of the work addresses the process of claiming more of who one is whether it be a shadow aspect or a contra-sexual animus or anima to employ Jung's terminology. Once this integration occurs, an individual's life direction becomes more clear to them. Eventually the individual comes to enlarge their awareness to grasp an ever-expanding relationship to community, humanity, the planet, and the many levels of spiritual connection. This connection to the spiritual or mystical aids in the healing process which needs to occur in chronic physical illness, pain or life-threatening injury or disease.

Jung, (1955) found that this journey often began during midlife and entails an assault on much of what came before, he writes,

> The Self in its efforts at self-realization reaches out beyond the ego personality on all sides; because of its all-encompassing nature it is brighter and darker than the ego, and accordingly confronts it with problems that it would like to avoid. Either one's moral courage fails, or one's insight, or both, until in the end fate decides.

> The ego never lacks moral and rational counterarguments which one cannot and should not set aside so long as it is possible to hold on to them. For you only feel yourself on the right road when the conflicts of duty seem to have resolved themselves, and you have become the victim of a decision made over your head in defiance of the heart. From this we can see the numinous power of the Self, which can hardly be experienced in any other way. For this reason *The experience of the Self is always a defeat for the ego.* (1955-1956, par. 778)

The Self that Jung spoke of is the archetypal organizing self-actualizing principle of wholeness. This defeat or death of the ego often results in a disintegration of life as it was known followed by a descent into a hellish darkness—like an arctic winter, in which much of who one is, is let go. It is an experience that is often precipitated by a crisis e.g., a life threatening disease, a loss of a job or relationship, or a physical injury. The resolution of this cycle comes like the spring—the individual experiences a rebirth of a new more authentic expanded self.

Health

Health is seen as the capacity for self-actualization. This ability supports the process of individuals to become freely and spontaneously more fully who they are. Shadow aspects that have been waiting in the wings can now enter the stage and be integrated into a person's life. Once this begins to occur, individuals have a better sense of what their personal myth is, i.e., what they are meant to do. This journey occurs after individuals have gone through recovery. Once freed from habitual patterns, everything is "up for grabs": relationships, livelihoods, old survival patterns. Everything must reflect and resonate with the goal of becoming who they truly are (see section on Alchemy in Chapter 8).

Once this occurs, there are gradual shifts from self-focus to an ever-expanding one in which the community, the earth, and the many realms of spiritual reality engage their interest and investment. Thus, the individuation process inevitably brings individuals toward an evolving spiritual consciousness.

The capacity for mindfulness, spontaneously responding from moment-to-moment without expectation or attachment can expand and deepen an experience of the interconnected undifferentiated whole of which humanity and all life is a part.

Dysfunction

Dysfunction is viewed when individuals remain focused upon themselves and their problems and are not fully free to be present. Dysfunction is also seen with individuals who limit their view of existence to the empirical realm of physical reality. Thus the "bigger picture" is obstructed from their awareness and interest. Their capacity to expand their consciousness and be in relation to the sacred either from a spiritual Judeo-Christian-Islamic I-Thou perspective or from a mystical Hindu-Buddhist-Taoist: "we are all one with the Light" is blocked.

Method of Identifying the Health-Dysfunction Continuum

Method of identifying and evaluating health and dysfunction is through tracking what genuinely gets individuals' attention. There are those who have utilized spiritual practices as a defense and escape from doing their own work. These individuals are often characterized as being *Puers* or *Puellae*–eternal youth, inspirational, charismatic, with high flying ideas without the groundedness that comes from claiming its polar opposite– the *senex* or wise woman. These individuals eventually crash for they tend to soar too high and think they do not need to abide by human rules such as committing to a job or relationship or, if they have power, to abuse it through inappropriate monetary gains, status, fame or sexual acting out. Assessing through access to the archetypal and its balance in the psyche both from the inner masculine and inner feminine perspectives is useful through the embodied archetype technique and other accesses to the transpersonal in sand play, dreams, guided shamanic and psychosynthesis journeys, and other connections to the collective archetypal unconscious (see Figures 5-4 and 5-5 to view masculine and feminine archetypes). Like the Taoists, balance is vital as each archetype also has a shadow side if the opposite archetype is not constellated in a person's psyche.

Individuation Stage Therapeutic Process

The therapeutic process within the individuation phase entails interviewing of clients regarding what their goals are as well as gleaning any information regarding the outcome of any past recovery therapy. In the second phase, the unconscious is sourced for the direction of the work through such techniques as dreamwork as theater, authentic sound movement and drama, shamanic journeying, visualization, embodied sand play, and archetypal poetry read during mindfulness meditation. The transformative process occurs within these techniques. As clients become more of who they are and are impacted with the experience of transpersonal grace, their presence becomes more soul-directed and their relationship to what guides and influences them shifts profoundly. These are individuals who experience nonattachment, healing, and loving compassion for themselves and others.

CONCLUSION

The concept of the unconscious is an integral phenomenon in holistic health. Although the transformative power of the use of the imagination can only be truly understood through experience, this chapter attempts to demonstrate that entering into the unconscious imaginal realm through mindbody and soulspirit allows for healing from childhood trauma and addictions and the unfolding of the individuation process toward Spiritual Consciousness.

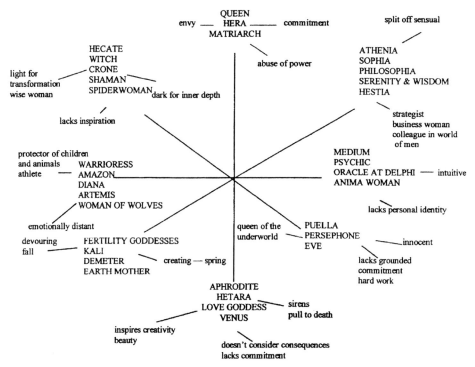

Figure 5-4. Archetypal inner feminine.

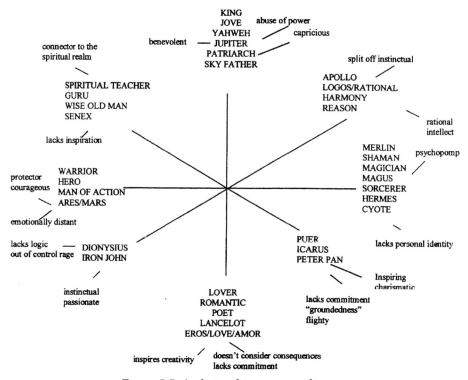

Figure 5-5. Archetypal inner masculine.

REFERENCES

Erikson, E. (1963). *Childhood and society*. New York: W.W. Norton.

Freud, A. (1966). *Normality and pathology in childhood*. New York: International Universities Press.

Grotstein, J. (1981). *Splitting and projective identification*. New York: Jason Aronson.

Johnson, D.R. (1982). Developmental approaches in drama therapy. *The Arts in Psychotherapy, 9*, 172–181.

Jung, C.G. (1977). *The collected works of C.G. Jung* (Vols. XII, XIII, XIV, XVI, XVIII). New York: Bollingen Foundation. (Original work 1953).

Lewis-Bernstein, P. (1972). *Theory and methods of dance-movement therapy*. Dubuque: Kendall/Hunt.

Lewis-Bernstein, P. and Bernstein, L. (1973-1974). A conceptualization of group dance movement therapy as a ritual process. In *Writings on body movement and communication* (Vol. III). Columbia: American Dance Therapy Association.

Lewis-Bernstein, P. (1982). Authentic movement as active imagination. In Jusuf Hariman (Ed.), *The compendium of psychotherapeutic techniques*. Springfield, IL: Charles C Thomas.

Lewis-Bernstein, P., & Singer, D. (Eds.). (1983). *Choreography of object relations*. Keene, NH: Antioch University.

Lewis-Bernstein, P. (1985). Embodied transformational images in dance-movement therapy. *Journal of Mental Imagery, 9*(4).

Lewis, P. (1981). The somatic unconscious and its relation to the embodied feminine in dance-movement therapy process. Paper presented at the American Dance Therapy Association Conference, Madison, Wisconsin.

Lewis, P. (1986a). *Theoretical approaches in dance-movement therapy*, Vol. 1. revised. Dubuque: Kendall/Hunt.

Lewis, P. (1987). The expressive arts therapies in the choreography of object relations. *The Arts in Psychotherapy, 14*, 321–331.

Lewis, P. (1988). The transformative process in the imaginal realm. *The Arts in Psychotherapy Journal, 15*:309–316.

Lewis, P. (1988a). *Theoretical approaches in dance-movement therapy*, Vol. II. Dubuque: Kendall/Hunt.

Lewis, P. (1988b). The unconscious as choreographer: The use of tension flow rhythms in the transference relationship. In Cheryl Planert Geffen (Ed.), *Moving in mealth (Monograph No. 4)*. Columbia, MD: American Dance Therapy Association.

Lewis, P., & Loman, S., Eds. (1990b). *The Kestenberg Movement Profile: Its past, present applications and future directions*. Keene, NH: Antioch University.

Lewis, P. (1992). The creative arts in transference/countertransference relationships. In *Arts in Psychotherapy, 19*, 317–323.

Lewis, P. (1993a). *Creative transformation: The healing power of the arts*. Wilmette: Chiron Pub.

Lewis, P. (1993b). The use of Chace Techniques in the depth dance therapy process of recovery, healing and spiritual consciousness. In *Foundation of dance/movement therapy: The life and work of Marian Chace*. Sandel, A. et al, Eds. Columbia: The Marian Chace Memorial Fund.

Lewis, P. (1993c). Following one's dreams: Dance therapy as transformation. In *Following Our Dreams Dynamics of Motivation*. 28th ADTA Conference proceedings. Columbia: American Dance Therapy Association.

Lewis, P. (1994). *The clinical interpretation of the Kestenberg Movement Profile*. Keene, NH: Antioch University.

Lewis, P. & Johnson, D. Eds. (2000). *Current approaches in drama therapy*. Springfield, IL: Charles C Thomas Pub.

Mahler, M. (1968). *On human symbiosis and the vicissitudes of individuation*. New York: International Universities Press.

Meerloo, J. (1968). *Creativity and eternalization: Essays on creative instinct*. New York: Humanities Press.

Melody, P. & Miller, A.W. (1989). *Recovery from codependency*. San Francisco: Harper and Row.

Schwartz-Salant, N. (1983-1984). Transference and Countertransference. Course presented at C.G. Jung Institute, New York City.

Smart, N. (2000). Worldview's: Cross-cultural explorations in human beliefs. Upper saddle River, NJ: Prentice-Hall, Inc.

Stein, M. (Ed.) (1984). *Chiron: Transference/countertransference*. Wilmette, IL: Chiron.

Turner, V. (1969). *The ritual process.* Chicago: Aldine.

Whitehouse, M. (1986). C.G. Jung and dance therapy: Two major principles. In *Theoretical approaches in dance therapy*, Vol. I by Penny Lewis, 61–86. Dubuque: Kendall Hunt.

Winnicott, D.W. (1971). *Playing and reality.* New York: Penguin.

Chapter 6

NUTRITION AND HEALTH

Edward Bauman

SORTING OUT FACTS AND FANTASY

THERE IS LITTLE DEBATE in the scientific community about the importance of nutrition to promote health and prevent disease. Less is known about the value of clinical nutrition to reverse previously diagnosed illness, or for the synergistic application of therapeutic diets and supplemental nutrients to improve the outcome of conventional medical therapies using surgery, drugs, hormone replacement or radiotherapy. *Biochemical individuality* is a defining concept in the field of clinical nutrition. This term begs for an operational definition, methodology and nonproduct-driven research. The study of how diet, lifestyle, medication and environment influence genetic expression in the *sequelae* of common health complaints such as fatigue, pain, obesity and mood disorder warrants in-depth investigation.

The nutrition field is in its adolescence, relatively speaking. Hyperbole rules! Health claims typically exceed research or reality. Hardly a month goes by without another revolutionary breakthrough of a diet program, herbal panacea, powerful antioxidant or oriental herbal formula to reverse aging, injury and serious illness while increasing stamina, sexual prowess while bringing both

health and financial independence. All of this is hard to swallow for a common sense health provider or confused, media-saturated consumer. Television, radio and magazines have a greater impact on health and nutrition choices than information gleaned at school, work or from one's family doctor, if they have one, HMO or alternative health practitioner.

In sorting out the facts and fantasies of the popular and scientific nutrition press, it is helpful to present a balanced and respectful position on the state of the art and science of nutrition. While there are many schools of thought in the nutrition field, as exemplified by the *Great Nutrition Food Fight*, a media event pitting the High Protein Power approach of Dr. Robert Atkins with the low fat, vegetarian, carbohydrate-laced meal plan of Dr. Dean Ornish. It is quite likely that neither edge of the food spectrum is health promoting for many if they continue to eat a limited amount of mediocre foods and fail to identify and satisfy their unique nutrient needs.

It is difficult to unequivocally state what is fact and what is fantasy in nutrition. The answer to many complex biochemical questions is "it depends." Nutritional needs depend on variables of genetics, age, ethnicity, activity level, metabolism, endocrine status, digestive competency, environmental exposures, diet history, recreational drug use, dose and duration of pharmaceutical drugs and health/disease status. What follows is a critique of some of the myths and verities of today's nutritional Wild West.

Doctors are beginning to recognize the value of using nutrition with the standard medical treatment of chronic, degenerative illness. *FACT:*

"I remember a time when I told patients that they needed no vitamins, minerals or substances other than what is found in a healthy diet. However, after using many of these natural agents in my practice of internal medicine as either adjuncts or sole therapy, and having reviewed extensive literature from this country and abroad, I certainly feel differently at this time.

"Regardless of our level of clarity or confusion surrounding natural therapeutics, our patients are taking them for a host of disorders. Because of this, we need to become as comfortable with **nutraceuticals** as we are with the pharmacologic agents that we have come to know and trust.

"It behooves us to learn the basics of this form of therapy. We need information regarding herb-drug interactions, drug-nutrient depletions, and herb-herb interactions. After all, the basis of modern pharmaceuticals is the field of natural therapeutics, the science of pharmacognosy." Leonard A. Wisneski, MD, FACP, Chief Medical Editor, *Integral Medicine Consult.* July, 2000 (2) 7 80. *www.onemedicine.com.*

Commercial food production's reliance on synthetic fertilizer, chemical pesticide and herbicides and genetically modified foods has improved the quality of our food and national health. *FANTASY:*

Before the chemical revolution of the 1950s, farmers depended upon mulching, manure and crop rotation to support the health of the soil. Early agricultural experiments found that many plants could grow on a mixture of nitrogen (N), phosphorus (P) and potassium (K). The loss of top soil due to erosion, overgrazing of grasslands by stock animals, and an ignorance of soil nutrition has depleted our soil of essential trace elements such as selenium, chromium, magnesium, calcium, iron, copper, iodine, zinc, molybdenum, boron, and vanadium (Colgan, 1994: 11).

Poor soil ecology has engendered nutrient-poor food and a generation of bugs that are resistant to many of the chemicals used to deter them. Similarly, human health, intestinal ecology and natural immunity to opportunistic viral, yeast and bacterial microorganisms and industrial chemicals have declined.

Little is known about the health effects of genetically modified foods, though the risk of increased food and environmental sensitivity is menacing for infants, children and adults with multiple food and chemical sensitivities and senior citizens in poor health.

Organic food standards and labeling is a significant issue for health and nutrition consumers. *FACT:*

The 1990 Organic Food Production Act mandated the creation of a national organic standard, but USDA's first proposal, released in 1997, was a huge failure. In the largest public response to a proposed rule in USDA history, more than 275,000 overwhelmingly negative comments from consumers, growers and industry members forced a rewrite. It was the first time an industry went back to the government and requested tighter restrictions. It was also the first time the Internet was used to both receive comments and publish them for public review. The revised proposal prohibits the most controversial aspects of the first version-use of genetically modified organisms (GMO's), irradiation, sewage sludge as fertilizer and antibiotics in animals–and largely follows the recommendations of the National Organic Standards Board.

On March 7, 2000, The USDA released its Revised Version of the proposed national organic standard, a 650-page document defining farm practices, allowable materials, certification standards with proposed labeling guidelines. One hundred percent certified organic can be labeled as such, products with 95 percent or more organic ingredients can be called *organic*, products with 50-95 percent organic ingredients can be described as *made with organic ingredients* and up to three organic ingredients can be listed. Even nonorganic ingredients in this category cannot contain GMOs, be irradiated, or be fertilized with sewage sludge. Products with less than 50 percent organic content may only use the term organic on the ingredient information panel.

Research by Bob Smith at Doctor's Data Lab (1993) demonstrated in a well controlled study that organic produce had 2-8 times the trace mineral content of commercial foods grown under similar conditions, with 50 percent less toxic metals, such as mercury, lead and cadmium.

One dietary system fits all. *FANTASY*:
This is the bane of any credible nutritional consultant's existence. It is well-demonstrated that *diets don't work*. By definition, special diets are limited in either calories, macronutrients (protein, fats and carbohydrates), micronutrients (vitamins and minerals) or phytonutrients (favorable biological response modifiers). Metabolic typing systems such as D'Adamo's Blood Typing Diet or Ayurveda's tri-doshic dispositions, kapha (earth and water), pitta (water and fire) or vatta (air and ether) attempt to correlate physical, emotional and physical tendencies with differing amounts of concentrated or diluted foods. These typing systems are a filter that helps to distinguish some food do's and don'ts, and hypothetical nutrient needs based upon self-reported metabolic tendencies. However, if taken literally they tend to become static and oppressive over time, as needs change.

The Bauman "Eating for Health Model" offers a plant-based, seasonal, organic 5-food group system of fresh fruits, vegetables,

seeds, whole grains and legumes as staple foods. Booster food condiment suggestions include algae, nutritional yeast, ocean fish, sea vegetables, herbs and culinary spices to add nutrition density and enhance the digestion and absorption. Foods to be eaten occasionally include organic, range-free poultry, eggs, dairy products, olives and avocados. A diet direction can be chosen to determine the blend of foods that is either building (more protein and fats than carbohydrates), balancing (as much protein and fats to carbohydrates) or cleansing (less proteins and fats to carbohydrates, with more fresh fruit and vegetables than grains and legumes). Herbal teas, fresh juices and purified water is preferable to caffeinated beverages, soft drinks, alcohol and tap water.

Food sensitivities can be keyed out by removing commonly overconsumed foods for 7-14 days, and reintroducing them one at a time, and charting physical, mental and emotional symptoms. Provocative foods should be removed from the diet, and a program of desensitization can be employed.

Animal protein is superior to vegetable protein. *FANTASY*:
Proteins are amino acids that are abundantly supplied by whole grains, legumes, nuts and seeds, nutritional yeast, protein powders, algae, and fruits and vegetables to a lesser extent. An intelligent vegan or vegetarian can obtain ample protein in a whole food diet. The limiting feature for nonmeat, poultry or dairy eaters is a poor digestion of legumes and glutinous grains that may reduce the actual amount of protein absorbed. It is advised to vary the sources of protein in the diet to protect against developing food sensitivity to overconsumed foods. A person in poor health may benefit from a supplement of amino acids to compensate for the inability to metabolize food proteins and make conditionally essential amino acids from essential amino acids. Goat's whey powder is a well-tolerated source of complete amino acids.

Traditional healthy foods that reflect a

person's ethnic background are often preferable to foods from foreign cultures. Examples of this are lactose intolerance by Asians and African-Americans, and soy intolerance by people from Northern European origins (Fallon, *Nourishing Traditions*, 1995).

Good quality fats are essential in the diet. *FACT:*

Both very low-fat, no-fat diets and high fat diets based upon animal, dairy fats, fried foods and margarine are damaging to health. Fats are easily used as food and provide heat and insulation for body tissues. Essential fatty acids, from plant sources, such as flax seed, pumpkin seeds, walnuts, soybeans, hemp seeds and the oil of black current seed, borage, primrose and deep ocean fish oils are important components of the membranes surrounding every cell of the body. Essential fatty acids support the health and repair of the brain, inner ear, eyes, adrenal glands, liver and reproductive system.

Animals that eat grass and algae have significant amounts of essential fatty acids. Wild fish and game and free-range poultry and beef have a favorable blend of saturated and unsaturated fatty acids. Fish raised in farms and fed soybeans and grains are sorely lacking in the omega 3 fatty acids their cold water ocean cousins make to insulate themselves from the frigid ocean waters. A grain, meat or dairy-based diet will be higher in pro-inflammatory omega 6 fatty acids than a seafood, vegetarian and seed-based diet, such as that proposed by the *Eating for Health Model* (Bauman, 2000).

Carbohydrates are the most important nutrient for blood sugar stability. *FANTASY:*

Times are changing regarding the central role of carbohydrates in the diet. In response to the heavy consumption of refined carbohydrates, such as the breads, pastries, pasta and confections made from refined flour and sugar, many people are finding that they have difficulty in balancing blood sugar. These conditions are called hypoglycemia,

hyperglycemia, and a new metabolic disorder, called Syndrome X, named by Dr. Gerald Reaven at Stanford University (Bland, 1999) describing a constellation of symptoms such as visceral weight gain, hyper-lipidemia and high cholesterol. Several researchers have found that balancing the protein and carbohydrate fractions of the diet have an insulin-sparing effect that is salutary in stabilizing blood sugar, improving metabolism, contributing to weight management and a cessation from carbohydrate cravings.

A major benefit of eating a proteins and vegetable-based diet rather than one based upon grains and fruit is a lower glycemic index (GI). GI is a comparison of insulin response to a specific food as compared to either white bread or sucrose. Lower glycemic foods do not feed unfriendly organisms in the gut, such as candida albicans and certain anaerobic bacteria. Clearly, complex carbohydrates have an important role to play in providing a slowly digested food staple with ample amounts of B vitamins, vitamin E, magnesium, zinc, soluble and insoluble fibers, all beneficial to health. It is suggested to keep one's life simple and carbohydrates complex (Fuchs, *Nutrition Detective*, 1990). Neither a high carbohydrate nor a carbohydrate diet is appropriate for most people. Minimizing refined carbohydrates and eating nutrient rich in both organic plant and free-range animal food will go a long way toward improving blood sugar stability and curbing excessive snacking and sugar craving.

Antioxidants are not adequately supplied by a standard American diet. *FACT:*

The Standard American meal has changed from a plate of meat, potatoes with gravy and a green vegetable or iceberg lettuce salad with ranch dressing, to a fast food meal of a hamburger, french fries and a coke or shake. Another version of today's Americana cuisine is a large pizza dripping with melted cheese, nitrate-laden, hormone-enhanced meats and genetically modified tomato sauce served with a pitcher of lite beer or diet soda. None of these *All-American meals* have adequate vitamin A, E, C, bioflavonoids, selenium or zinc, which will be needed in abundance to deal with the food toxins in these entrees.

All of the antioxidants are needed to protect our bodies from free radicals generated from oxidized fats, unstable oxygen molecules, ionizing radiation, electro-magnetic frequencies and industrial chemicals that bombard us daily, creating inflammation, stress and damage to sensitive nerves and body tissues. Eating 3-5 servings of vegetables and 2-4 servings of fresh fruit will provide enough antioxidants for most people to *not* have to take an antioxidant supplement. Those eating a poor diet are well advised to supplement with antioxidants to minimize their risk of cardiovascular disease, cancer and diabetes.

Water quality in the United States is excellent. *FANTASY:*

The most abundant component of our bodies is water. Seventy percent of the brain is water, 82 percent of the blood is water. Even the bones are 25 percent water. The majority of Americans still use unfiltered tap water to drink and in cooking. In 1988, the United States Department of Public Health warned that 85 percent of American drinking water is contaminated. More than 55,000 of the regulated chemical dumps in America are leaking into the water table across the country (Norman, *Science*, 1983 as cited in Colgan, 1994). Bacteria are not only a third world problem. Over 900,000 people become ill each year from drinking United States water laced with bacterial toxins (*USA Today*, 9/27/93 as cited in Colgan, 1994).

The addition of chlorine, fluoride to the water only adds to the problems. Chlorine combines with organic wastes to form trihalomethanes, which are known carcinogens that increase the risk of colon and rectal cancer. Trihalomethanes also double the risk of bladder cancer, which strikes 40,000 people

per year (*US News and World Report*, 7/29/91; Lawrence et al. *J Nat Cancer Inst.* 1984 as cited in Colgan, 1994). Adding insult to injury is the fact that people of all ages drink more caffeinated, naturally or artificially sweetened soft drinks, coffee, tea, beer, wine and imitation milks and fruit beverages than they do simple, pure water, herbal teas or diluted, fresh pressed juice.

Culinary herbs and spices play an important role in promoting health and preventing disease. *FACT:*

All over the world, people enjoy culinary herbs and spices such as garlic, ginger, cayenne, chili's, paprika, cumin, turmeric, coriander, cardamom, cinnamon, nutmeg, allspice, basil, oregano, thyme, rosemary, tarragon, sage, dill, fennel, lemon and orange zest. These tasty plants enhance digestion, improve circulation, and are supportive to the blood and immune system. Pleasant herbal teas such as mint, chamomile, lemon grass, rose hips, nettles, dandelion, burdock, licorice, gingko, gota kola, oat straw and horsetail and alfalfa, to name a few, are rich in trace elements, bioflavonoids and other phytonutrients that help the body to buffer stress, toxicity and inflammation.

The global emergence of healthy festive, therapeutic, eclectic ethnic cuisine presents an exciting possibility in combining simple plant substances in cooking in a daily soup, salad, grain pilaf or stir-fry. Adding herbs and spices to our foods encourages us to be more creative, alchemical, and low budget in satisfying to our nutritional needs. Eating for health with organic foods and booster food condiments is a viable alternative to overconsuming supplements in the form of pills, powders, and power bars. As consumers buy poor quality food, with food additives, preservatives, artificial flavors and pesticide residues, their health suffers. This *sick food* creates a need for nutritional supplementation or medication. A person without good food sense will rely on pricey supplements in hopes they will regain their lost vitality. When supplements don't produce an expected lift, then it is back to using coffee, chocolate, cookies and soft drinks to make it through the day. Once a person learns how to shop for, prepare and enjoy wholesome, chemical-free natural food, health improves gradually day-by-day. With a diversified, nutrient rich diet, therapeutic herbs, supplements and medications will also be more efficiently utilized to maximize their targeted benefits and promote deep and lasting healing.

EATING FOR HEALTH

So many people ask, "What diet is right for me? Is it the Zone? Adkins, Ornish, Weil, Pyramid, or Blood Typing? I need to lose weight, gain energy and get fit . . . in a hurry. I've tried and failed so many diets that I am ready to give up, but I can't. I feel lousy and look worse. I've turned my mirrors inside out–to no avail. I am raging about my aging. I need help!"

For the past 25 years, this author has been guiding people of all ages and stages of life with a myriad of health problems: some cosmetic, many life-threatening. I have devised a *system*, not a diet, called "Eating for Health." Each individual has unique genetic tendencies, needs, tastes, and tolerances, all of which should be factored into a customized food and nutrition plan. One size *does not fit all* with food plans.

People are different, even in the same families. As such, they need differing amounts of healthful foods and nutrients to cope with a fast-paced, stress-filled toxic world. Similarly, individual metabolism is challenged to adapt to changes in seasons, situations, climate and health challenges. What individuals ate as children, a mediocre *standard American diet*, will not nourish them as aging adults.

Change is the one constant in life. Clients need to change for the better to improve their health by supporting their metabolism, brain function and ability to self-heal. Cleaning up the diet, clearing out the debris

in their pantries, refrigerators and medicine cabinets is called for. Finding out how to shop for, prepare and enjoy the foods that are most healthy for each individual is the key that unlocks the door to their rejuvenation.

It helps to have a map to follow to find an individual's destination in the most direct way. An in-depth intake, assessment and analysis of the individual's situation is required. If they are struggling with one or more health issues, the consultant can review and evaluate the latest research and advise them on the specific therapeutic foods, herbs and nutrients that will support their healing.

The client is the co-creator in the "Eating for Health" process. They remember the healthy foods that were nourishing and healing in times past. Likewise, they alone know the foods they have been relying on for energy or emotional gratification, that tend to add to their malaise later on when the distraction wears off, pleasure fades and disease takes over.

Nutrition is a major form of health investing. It is safer than the stock market or blind dates to hedge against the inflation of illness. When individuals eat poor quality food, they are dipping into the nutrient reserves in their bones, soft tissue, organs, glands, skin and hair. They wear the results of being overdrawn nutritionally–an unhealthy appearance, and feel the warning signs of ill health– fatigue, pain and mood disorder.

Healthy diets require fresh, seasonal, chemical-free, nutrient rich, organic foods. These add nutrients back into those body parts whose reserves have been drained by nutrient robbers that many individuals have been living on.

The usual suspects, also known as *health banditos* are the stimulants, sugars, pastries, pastas, processed cheeses, nutrasweet and margarine that wind up in people's mouths as white flour-laden, over-processed, frozen, microwaved meals served in restaurants or grabbed on the run. These foods are manufactured to taste good, too good, so that individuals forget the crunch of a carrot, or the juice of a mango, or the zest of fresh, roasted garlic. While it's hard *not* to overeat nutrient-poor, sugary, salty, greasy snack foods, it's hard to overeat naturally satisfying, nutrient-rich vegetables, grains, seeds, legumes and lean proteins.

THE HEALING POWER
OF FOODS

Foods heal in many ways. Food:
- contains important, macro, micro and phytonutrients
- has energetic properties: warm, cool, moist and dry
- has tastes that influence organs, glands and tissues
  - Sweet: pancreas, sugar metabolism
  - Salty: adrenal glands, kidneys
  - Bitter: lymph, protein metabolism
  - Sour: liver detoxification, fat metabolism
  - Pungent: antiinflammatory, improved assimilation
  - Hot: blood circulation, antimicrobial
- Has chemicals that calm or excite brain and nerve cells
- that is fresh, chemical-free, nutrient-rich and enhances the healing of tissue damaged by toxicity and malnutrition.
- Has variety and flavor that optimizes nutrient diversity and density.

DIET DIRECTION

A diet direction is a way to organize the amounts and variety of foods a person chooses to eat to achieve a specific effect. Like life, diet directions change, sometimes intentionally, sometimes impulsively. The three main diet directions are Building, Balancing and Cleansing. In helping a client choose the best way to create an Eating for Health program, the benefits of their follow-

ing either a building, balancing or cleansing diet are discussed. Additionally, the length of time the person will follow a designated diet direction, or until the desired health outcome is realized is explored. It is common for a person to follow a brief cleansing diet (3-14 days) followed by a longer balancing diet (14-21 days) followed by a longer building diet (21-42 days). The building diet programs are longer in duration as the great majority of the people who need help are tired, nutrient depleted, and have been eating poor quality foods, with stimulants, not nutrients keeping them going.

Building Diet

A building diet is comprised of a higher percentage of calories from protein and fats relative to carbohydrates. The Zone Diet is a building diet, with its formula of 30 percent calories from protein, 30 percent calories from fats and 40 percent calories from carbohydrates. The Atkin's Diet, a high protein, high fat, no carbohydrate diet, in its most extreme (and unhealthy) form is another form of a building diet. Building diets are appropriate for persons who are growing rapidly, like children and teenagers, adults who are competitive athletes, doing manual labor, or recovering from illness or injury. It is crucial that a person who is on a building diet eat ample amounts of fresh vegetables (5 servings per day) and fruits (2-3 servings per day) and drink herbal tea rather than caffeinated beverages to maintain a healthy acid-alkaline, or pH balance.

Balancing Diet

A balancing diet is comprised of equal amounts of protein and fats relative to carbohydrates. A prudent application of the USDA Food Pyramid, Cancer and Heart Association diets would be examples of this approach. A balanced diet would include a wide variety of healthy foods that would typically supply 20 percent of calories from protein, 30 percent of calories from fat, and 50 percent of calories from carbohydrates. The key to this approach is that the foods be seasonal, local, and organic, whenever possible. The type of diet an Eating for Health nutritionist considers to be balanced would be quite a bit different than the so-called "balanced diet" advised by industry driven nutritionists and dietitians. Eating for Health suggests using whole, nonglutinous grains, such as rice, millet, and quinoa as staple grains in lieu of the traditionally overconsumed and more allergenic grains such as wheat, corn, oats and rye. Roughly equal amounts of fruits and vegetables may be consumed, with an emphasis on eating whole fruits rather than juice or fruit products made from concentrates, to moderate the amount of sugars the body will have to metabolize at one sitting.

Cleansing Diet

A cleansing diet consists of more calories from carbohydrates (>60%) relative to proteins (20%) and fats (<20%). As such, this is a fat sparing, adequate protein, high complex carbohydrate, and low glycemic (sugar content) diet. The Ornish, Weil, McDougall, hypoallergenic, and various cleansing diets are in this category. The emphasis is to lower the fat content, while maintaining adequate protein, and increasing the amount of fruits and vegetables, while reducing the amounts of starchy vegetables, such as potatoes, carrots and yams, and reducing breads and cereal grains almost completely. Dairy products would also be eliminated due to their mucous forming properties. Proteins from vegetable sources such as legumes, seeds and

Nutritional Preferences For Aging	Building Diet	Balancing Diet	Cleansing Diet
Young 0-28 years	x		
Middle Age 29-56 years		x	
Older Age 57-84 years			x

Preferences for Common Conditions	Building Diet	Balancing Diet	Cleansing Diet
Fatigue Injury recovery	x		
Pain Mood Stability		x	
Weight Loss Allergy			x

Preferences for Special Needs	Building Diet	Balancing Diet	Cleansing Diet
To Improve Fertility Pre & Post Natal Care	x		
Puberty and Menopause		x	
Detoxification of Drugs/Alcohol			x

Figure 6-1. Building, balancing and cleansing diets.

nuts, and marine algae would be preferred over eggs, fish or fowl. Maintaining an alkaline-forming diet with generous amounts of fruits, vegetables and their fresh juices, with the addition of chlorophyll rich foods, herbs and powders would replenish minerals that are commonly missing from a nonplant-based diet (see the following Figure 6-1).

The key to using a diet direction is to build the food plan on top-notch quality, whole foods. A commercially-oriented diet will explain how a person can choose from a menu at McDonalds or a Round Table Pizza. What it is not taken into consideration is that the food quality will be diminished in most commercial restaurants and with most packaged food items. Fresh is best. The diet direction is a reminder to eat more of certain kinds of foods, say nuts and seeds, in a building diet, and less of other foods, say bread products in a cleansing diet. Having an intention to eat well to be well helps persons know what they want to eat, and what to pass up. Cookies, candy, ice cream, sodas, and foods with artificial colors, flavors and preservatives are best left on the shelves for any of the diet directions.

As a person gets comfortable with their food choices, they become more in touch with how a certain combination of foods feel to them. At certain times of the day, when hunger hits, and hits quickly, that person knows what food to have on hand that will satisfy hunger and provide a good source of nourishing energy. Almonds and raisins are more nourishing than a Milky Way, and the energy that is produced clears the brain and mobilizes the body into action.

Eating for Health is a skill that is learned with the support of a food coach who can serve as a mentor and resource. Adding one new food per week will increase a person's repertoire by four foods per month or forty-eight foods per year. What about parties or a food craving that just won't quit? It is fine to socialize with foods and drinks. The key is to not be too hungry or tired before a big occasion, or else overeating and excessive drinking may prevail. Nutritional consultants are working to develop a strong foundation of foods that will support growth, insulate their clients from the insults of the world, and allow them to live up to their potential as dynamic, creative human beings.

REFERENCES

Bauman, E. (1997). *Nutrition and your health: A potluck of writings.* IET Publications. Cotati, CA. *www.iet.org.*

Bauman, E. (1997). *Nutrition research reports.* IET Publications. Cotati, CA. *www.iet.org.*

Bland et al. (1999). *Clinical nutrition: A functional approach.* Institute for Functional Medicine, Inc. Gig Harbor, WA.

Colgan, M. (1994). *The new nutrition: Medicine for the millennium.* CI Publication. San Diego, CA.

Fallon, S. (1995). *Nourishing traditions: The cookbook that challenges politically correct nutrition and diet dictocrats.* ProMotion Publishing. San Diego, CA.

Fuchs, N. (1990). *The nutrition detective.* Tarcher Press. San Diego.

Lipson, E. Organic Rules Again. *Lohas Journal.* May/June, 2000. Volume 1, Number 2: 52–53.

Smith, B. (1993). A comparison of organic and conventional food for trace and toxic element status. *Am. J of Clinical Nutrition, 32*(3) 87–93.

Wisneski, L. Nutrients and herbs in a new therapeutic armantarium. *Integral Medicine Consult.* July, 2000 (2) 7 80. *www.onemedicine.com.*

For more information contact:
Edward Bauman, M.Ed., Ph.D.
Director of Partners In Health clinic and the IET Nutrition Consultant Training Program: A classroom and home study professional training program with 5 campuses in Northern California. Dean and faculty
University of Natural Medicine
Santa Fe, NM.
e-mail at *iet@sonic.net.*
Dr Bauman also leads Rejuvenation Retreats in Northern California and in Mexico.

Chapter 7

ENERGY MEDICINE:
WAYS OF KNOWING THROUGH CHI,
CHAKRAS, AND THE AURIC FIELDS

INTRODUCTION
AND HISTORY

ENERGY MEDICINE REFERS to those therapies that use an energy field to screen and treat health conditions. Among these forms are electrical, magnetic, sonic, acoustic, and bioenergy. Various energy medicine practices utilize the paradigm of subtle energies. These bioenergies are defined as systems of life sustaining energy. These systems each have their own frequencies and affect the mindbody and soulspirit of an individual. Information is received, encoded, stored, and transmitted within these human fields.

In 1989, the International Society for the Study of Subtle Energies and Energy Medicine was founded. Therapeutic Touch, Reiki, External Qi Healing, Acupuncture, Brennan healing, shiatsu massage, craniosacral, T'ai C'hi, yoga, and Qigong are just a few of the alternative and complementary approaches which utilize this way of knowing. Most of the foundation for understanding these human energy fields has emerged from Eastern traditions identifying this unseen vital force energy as C'hi, Ki, Qi, prana, and Kundalini which organizes in the body via energy centers such as chakras and linear networks within the body such as meridians and nadis, as well as outside the physical body in auric and subtle body fields.

The Indian concept of prana dates back 5000 years; in China, c'hi dates at least back 3000 years; the Jewish Kabala dates nefish, an egg shaped bubble of light surrounding the human body, from 700 BC, and the Christian halo depicted on many of the paintings of Christ and saints is a visual confirmation of auric fields that dates back a millenium. In fact Krippner and White list 97 different cultures and names which identify the human energy fields (Talbot, 1991).

These subtle energies were first scientifically noted in the West on plants. In 1939, Yale University's Burr and Northrup correlated the health of plants to the measurement of what they called the plant's "life-field." Other research at Upstate Medical School in Syracuse mapped an electrical field which was shaped like the body naming it "the Direct Control System" (1979). The Russians identified a "bioplasmic energy" field composed of ions, protons and free electrons at Kazakh in the fifties. Soviet scientists from the Bioinformation Institute of Aspopv announced their findings that all living organisms emit vibrations of energy between 300–2000 nanometers. These findings were reconfirmed at the Medical Science Academy in Moscow as well as in Western European research centers.

RESEARCH AND MEASURE-MENT INSTRUMENTS

This bioenergy is generally thought to be identifiable as higher levels of vibration and has been visually tracked by Kirlian photography. Dr Valerie Hunt at UCLA recorded extremely low frequencies reliably analyzed through electromyography that corresponded to the body energy centers called chakras. These waves were consistent with the actual colors associated with human chakras (1988). Other measurement instruments were designed specifically to detect and measure the presence and quality of the human energy field. The AMI machine or apparatus for measuring the function of the meridians and their corresponding internal organs created by Dr Hiroshi Motoyama (1978, 1990) and Green's Copper Wall Project at the Menninger Clinic (1995) are two examples. The latter research measured the transfer of subtle energy by measuring the electromagnetic voltage of healers or "sensitives" as well as a control group. These findings were highly significant demonstrating surges with the energy healers that were 10,000 times greater than the heart's electrocardiogram voltages and 100 times greater than the electroencephalogram voltage detected from the brain. It is understood that subtle energy itself is not electromagnetic in origin but nonetheless stimulates the electromagnetic fields when it is active.

By the same token, the AMI machine measures the electrical conductivity, capacitance and polarization of skin tissue and fluids. Although the subtle energy itself is not being measured, like the pathways created from the passage of subatomic particles sent through the semiconductors, ki energy passage can be monitored and quantified by noting what it has affected. Electrodes are placed atop acupoints at the tips of the fingers and toes where meridians begin and end. The biochemical constituents of sodium, potassium, calcium chloride, etc. present in the liquid of the meridians can be measured electrically as they exist as ions. Thus, their passage through the meridians creates an electrical current. The AMI measures this current and therefore can detect the flow of ki energy. The AMI machine is now being used in a variety of universities, among them UCLA, the University of Virginia, the University of New Mexico as well as in research projects in Canada and Japan. These research centers are utilizing the AMI machine to identify the functioning of the corresponding internal organs to detect pre-disease states or vulnerability to disease as well as identifying the level of stress and therefore, the health and level of functioning of the immune system of the tested individual.

In the 40s, research confirmed that acupuncture points possess electrical conductivity. Voll, MD, utilizing a measuring instrument called the Dermatron, discovered that the electrical resistance of the skin decreases at acupuncture points. This phenomenon was standardized and is reliable with healthy individuals. The instrument and its assessment later were identified as the Electroacupuncture According to Voll (EAV) and is utilized to indicate the health or dysfunction of organs and tissues. Many related instruments have developed to not only identify and diagnose but also to treat dysfunction (Goldberg Group, 1994).

The study conducted through the auspices of the National Center for Alternative and Complementary Medicine at Harvard-Beth Israel on distance intention also documented the transfer of energy from a "sensitive" or "healer" to an unaware subject in a metal isolation room.

In summary, much of what has been measured in attempts to "capture" the human energy field, document it and translate its empirical reality in Western laboratories has produced a list of components. These are: extremely low electromagnetic frequency, sonic waves, thermal, electrostatic ions, and visual elements which substantiate the presence of this bioplasmic phenomena. The research to date suggests this elusive subtle life force consists of minute elements that demonstrate the same characteristic as subatomic particles and are fluid-like in nature. However, many at the forefront of this documenting research believe that this phenomenon is composed of as yet undiscovered energy. It is clear that this phenomenon has a higher frequency or vibration than normal matter.

Harvard's research substantiated the power of distance intention sent to unknowing subjects who were in eletrostaticly shielded rooms. The scientific validation that positive energy or prayer could be sent and affect another from great distance had this medical center schedule a conference with the spiritual leaders in various religions to address the question from their perspectives. Clearly the rift among science, Western religion and Eastern paradigms of spirituality, mysticism and health may begin to be finally closing and the new physics may just be the glue.

QUANTUM PHYSICS AND ENERGY MEDICINE

Neurophysiologist Karl Pribram from Stanford, quantum physicist and former protégé of Albert Einstein, David Bohm and others are beginning to collaborate on integrative models which can attempt to explain what the dualistic Cartesian Western mind has been unable to get a handle on. Bohm and others posit that there are subtle energies at a subquantum level (subatomic level) that have still eluded scientific detection. Even now, scientists are still only being able to describe how various fields like electric or gravitational "behave." They have been unable, given the limitations of current scientific linguistics and syntax, to actually relate what these fields are! It is not surprising that the human energy field is being met with the same limitations of cognition. Whether the answer can be found in holo-

graphic universe theory which parallels much of Eastern philosophy of an infinite interconnectedness or in newer models, it behooves holistic health practitioners to integrate the paradigm of energy medicine into their theory and practice.

Elaborating holographic theory, Talbot (1991) writes, "In principle the whole past and implications for the whole future are enfolded in each small region of space and time (p. 50). As long as the formlessness and breathtaking freedom of the beyond remain frightening to us, we will continue to dream a hologram for ourselves that is comfortably solid and well defined. The conceptual pigeonholes we use to parse out the universe are of our own making. They do not exist "out there" for "out there" is only the invisible totality. We are, as the aborigines say, just learning how to survive in infinity" (p. 302).

Ukrainian quantum physicists have been studying the "giga energy" of DNA. They have discovered that human DNA vibrates at 52-78 Gigahertz, animals at 47 and plants at 42. These scientists assert that this vibration is the electromagnetic support for system for "chi."

Three models of the human energy field are discussed: Meridians, chakras, and auric fields:

MERIDIANS

The human body is viewed as both matter and as a system of bioenergy which "performs autonomously an exchange of energy in each cell throughout the numerous connective systems without becoming subject to the control of the nervous system" (Motoyama, 2000, p. 2). This bioenergy is called C'hi in Chinese medicine and combines with breath to circulate throughout the body. It is organized in Chinese medicine into twelve regular and eight irregular pathways called meridians (see Figure 7-1). Each meridian is an energy transportation system. It supplies energy and is connected to the functioning of the organ with which it shares the same name. This multilevel network connects these organ systems to the body surface either on the chest, back or arms and legs. Of the 12 major trunk meridians, there is thought to be a corresponding pairing yin yang (receptive/active) relationship. They act to balance each other. If the corresponding meridian cannot balance the other than disease ensues:

Yin Meridians	Yang Meridians
Lung	Large intestine
Spleen	Stomach
Heart	Small intestine
Kidney	Urinary bladder
Heart constrictor	Triple heater
Liver	Gall bladder

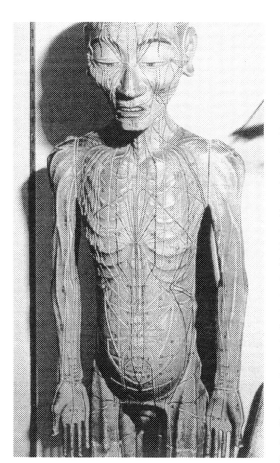

Figure 7-1. Accupunture meridians.

Additionally, there are divergent meridians that arise from each of the major 12. Muscle network meridians also distribute chi from the major twelve superficially to muscles, tendons, and joints. Even more superficial, are the skin layer meridians believed to relate to the sensory nervous system. Eight more meridians or vessels are the interconnecting links among the major twelve. A system of 15 collateral meridians arise from each of the 12 organ meridians, the governor and conception meridians and one from the spleen branch out horizontally and vertically. This complete meridian system is an elaborate network reflecting and influencing the balance and well-being of the individual.

Meridian theory entails not only the presence of these energy pathways but approaches to the diagnosis and treatment of illness and imbalance. Dysfunction is indicated along the specific points on the meridian. A human organ releases c'hi. This energy delivers information about the functioning of the organ through the quality and strength of the energy. For example, if the stomach is in distress, there will be an indication of this imbalance along the stomach meridian. Energy may gather in the meridian in the anterior or posterior point of the body at the Bo point and Yu respectively. This phenomenon is utilized by acupuncturists to diagnose and evaluate healthy clearing and flow. Acupuncture is the art and science of inserting fine needles into specific points along the meridians for the prevention and treatment of disease as well as for the reduction and elimination of pain. These meridians have end points at the tips of fingers and toes called Sei. The energy emitted from these well Sei points has been utilized by healers and focused upon in foot and hand reflexology.

Chinese call life energy Qi or C'hi and associate it with force, power and breath. C'hi carries "bioinformation" and has been employed by acupuncture, acupressure and regulated by martial arts such as Qigong to improve health, calm the mind, condition the body for fighting through moving the Qi, expelling old energy and absorbing new and generally nourishing life. T'ai chi cha'uan or taiji quan is a choreography of 108 flowing meditational movements which cultivates Qi. All of these Chinese-based alternative and complimentary systems have grown in acceptance and involvement in the West since the 70s.

NADIS

Yoga teachings relate that prana energy is absorbed through the solar plexus chakra and distributed throughout the body through nadis, which correspond to acupuncture meridians. There are 14 main nadis with thousands of tributaries. The three main channels are: the shushumna which draws energy from the chakras and runs along the spinal column (which corresponds to the governor vessel meridian) and the ida and pingala which are on either side of the shushumna, crisscross each other like the snakes in the caduceus and end in the nostrils (the presence of these two main nadis is the rationale behind pranayama breath practices primarily utilizing breathing through the nostrils). The gross nadi system as described in *Ayar Veda* and the meridian system as put down in *Yellow Emperor*–considered the first text in meridian theory–although separately conceptualized, appear to be virtually identical in definition.

CHAKRAS

Based upon Indian Aruvedic and specifically yogic literature, chakras are several energy centers located in the body. Chakra in Sanskrit means wheel of light. Each center is located close to the midline of the body and are spinning vortices of energy, which like the meridians, connect to organs, glands, and physiologic systems and extend out of the body into energy fields (see Figure 7-2).

The chakras receive energy from the human energy fields and spin clockwise sending it into the physical body. Each chakra radiates wavelengths associated with colors; each oscillates, has a certain magnitude, and frequency which is detected in the extremely low frequency electromagnetic field.

Their purpose is to maintain and regulate the physical, emotional, mental and spiritual aspects within an individual. Each chakra has its own specific communication function. They send measurable energy through the physical body that can often be felt through the senses. "The chakras are dimensional portals within the subtle bodies which take in and process energy of higher vibrational nature so that it may be properly assimilated and used to transform the physical body" (Gerber, 1988, p. 370). Many who use this paradigm in their work believe that the psyche and spirit are also utilizing the chakras in the receiving, processing, analyzing and transmitting of information for mental and soulspiritual understanding. For this purpose, chakras connect to mental and causal energetic fields.

Kundalini energy is experienced as an explosive life force that assists in the alignment and clearing of the chakras as well as in the raising of consciousness. In addition to kundalini, quanta (energy that moves at slower than light speed) or tachyons (energy that moves faster than the speed of light) are considered to be the spiraling energy within the chakra itself.

The lower 7 chakras are centrally located from caudal to cephlad. Many systems consider them to have both anterior and posterior loci (Brennon, 1987; Dale, 1996). In the physical realm they are thought to be affected by and influence certain organs and systems. In the astral realm (discussed in the section on auric fields), they are associated with certain emotions, psychological tendencies and intuitive abilities (see Figure 7-3 for the delineation of each chakra in relation to physical location and related organ systems; associated color frequency, elements, sym-

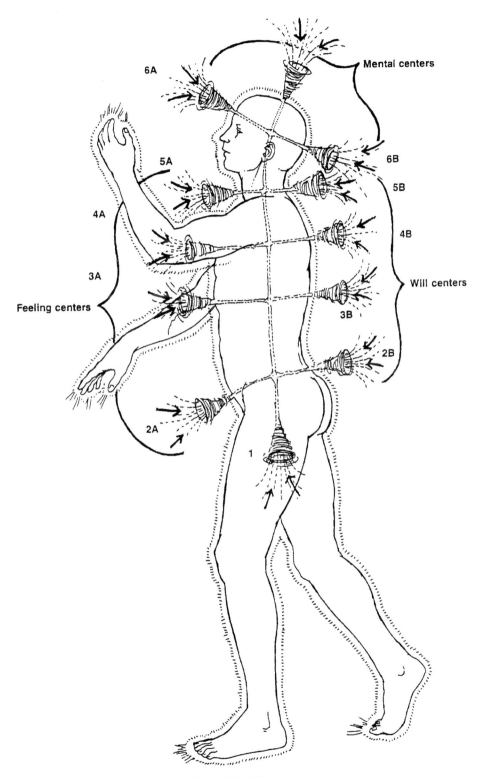

Figure 7-2. Chakras.

bols and foods: psychological aspects and imbalances; functions and lessons; related instinct; glands and secretions; and related illness associated with unhealthy chakra activity) (Brennon, 1987; Karagulla & Kunz, 1989; Villodo, 2000; Juduth, 1996; Myss, 2000; Motoyama, 1995; Dale, 1996).

1st Chakra-Root-Muladhara

Considered the 1st chakra, the root chakra is located at the base of the spine. Here is where the kundalini is awakened which lies metaphorically like a coiled snake at the base of the spine. Activation or the awakening of the kundalini is a spiritual practice in and of itself. Many descriptions have been written about this process which can be highly painful if done incorrectly (Krishna, Motoyama, 1995). This coccygeal center is related to the physical world. Its energy extends through the legs and feet and connects individuals to the earth. When the root chakra spins in health, an experience of being grounded, assertive and powerful in the physical realm is present. The will to survive and the vitality to sustain life are generated here. Its programming comes from the family and the individual's mechanisms of surviving within the family system. Primal memories are stored here. It is a physical/tactile sensation-based chakra. Without an active root chakra, an individual will be less present and active in the world. These individuals are cut off from the experience of the abundance in the world and life and often have a scarcity mentality. A first chakra fixated person is self-absorbed and caught in the material realm. Food, shelter, money and material possessions are focused upon. They often express their emotional imbalance through physicalization or somatization in various stress-based illnesses. These individuals find it difficult to delay gratification of any kind and can be easily violent and may need to control the environment and individuals around them.

2nd Chakra-Sacral-Svadhisthana

The sacral chakra is located in the lower abdomen and is considered to be the source of feelings and sexual creative drive. The posterior sacral chakra is associated with strong sexual desire while the anterior lower abdomen chakra addresses the emotional aspect and the capacity to give and receive. The 2nd chakra is in charge of the secretion of adrenaline from the sympathetic "fight" response. Here the first and second chakra act together to produce rage addicts and hypervigilance bullies. This chakra also is the source of the "flight, freeze and faint" sympathetic responses as well. Instead of Eros driven by the desire to connect, a dysfunctional 2nd chakra emanates fear that precludes the capacity to love and intimately relate. The need to control through money and sex and the confusion of sex with love are, with healthy 2nd chakra functioning, replaced with harmonious relationships and feelings of tolerance, the passion to connect and create, and to give and receive.

Women's strength resides in her hips and thighs; it is also felt that women are better able to express feelings, particularly the ones that reside in the second chakra which are in service to relationship rather than the male driven first chakra assertion and aggression. Whenever there exists dysfunction in the 2nd chakra area, these relationally-based feelings for self and others can become blocked or stored from early family patterning resulting in such dynamics as codependency or martyrdom. Blocks in creativity are also detected here.

3rd Chakra-Solar Plexus-Manipura

The third chakra located at the belly or solar plexus is the seat of the sense of self. With the discovery of the actual neuopysiological biochemical presence of "gut feelings," object relations developmental therapists have confirmed that the sense of self is "enteroceptive" (in the stomach). Infants develop this body-felt confirmation of an experience of a sense of self by feeling filled with nurturence through the ingestion of milk from a loving object (primary caregiver). This sense of fullness aids in activating and maintaining the health and well-being of the manipura chakra. In this chakra, individuals are connected to their own uniqueness and posteriorly to personal will. Anteriorly, the vulnerable sense of self stores judgements and beliefs about the core self. Self-esteem or unworthiness resides here. It is therefore the source of personal power and will. When core self seeks connection on a deep level, individuals feel as if there is a connecting thread or cord which joins them at this 3rd chakra often producing a psychic connection that exists beyond time and space. This phenomenon may be associated to the early mother-child umbilical connection. These energetic connections may serve as negative relational contracts and extend across time (Dale, 1996).

This diaphragmatic center is also associated with psychological health and well being. A deeper connection into the core of this chakra allows for a connection to the Self—the organizing principle of wholeness from which individuals' life purpose can be accessed. When inner child work can heal injury to self-esteem, access to the Self and Selfless individuation can occur. "When you want to improve the world, bring balance to your 3rd chakra" (Villoldo, 2000, p. 89).

4th Chakra-Heart-Anahata

The heart chakra is located at the cardiac plexus and is the locus of the energy to connect to all beings through love and compassion. It is the processor of energy from upper and lower chakras. Native American Cherokee tradition states that real transformation must therefore occur at a heart chakra level. Here is where prana is received through the breath and sent through out the body. Fourth chakra energy affects what is circulated to every cell of the body. From this heart chakra each human is valued for their uniqueness and their universal connection to the Light. The fourth chakra gives energy to the thymus, one of the sources of the development of the lymphocytes called T-cells that attack cancer and other cells that do not belong in the body. A healthy open-heart chakra energizes the immune system and encourages individuals to "stop falling in love and become love itself" (Villoldo, 2000, p. 92).

One model sees the vibration of the heart chakra as initially green. As the individual evolves and alchemically integrates lower chakras (red) with the upper chakra (white), pink has been seen in this center. When this occurs the individual has shifted from "my family's and cultural collective's will be done" (1st chakra), through "my will be done" (3rd chakra) to "Thy will be done" (4th–10th chakras).

5th Chakra-Throat-Vishuddha

The 5th chakra relates to the capacity to express with truth, not to blame, but rather to take responsibility for one's own life and actions. Additionally the 5th chakra is associated with receiving guidance as well. The capacity to take in what is given without contaminating it with past experiences or future obsessions is a sign of a healthy chakra. This center is also related to work and the capacity to experience fulfillment and to take responsibility for one's success or failure. Spiritually, it is the center from which the capacity to express and receive without visual confirmation or words is stored. An ever-expanding relationship to the world and existence also means that individuals are able to detach from what they expressed when it relates to the greater good. Holding on to ideas, rigidifying them in dogmas, and being unable to expand understanding through receiving knowledge from another is suggestive of a blocked throat chakra. Open chakras can channel information through clairaudience (clear thinking) which can aid in soul guidance regarding what an individual is meant to do as well as assistance in the support of healing another.

6th Chakra-Third Wye-Ajna

The third eye is associated with the capacity for wisdom and intuition. One of it's target responsibilities is the pituitary gland which is considered the command center for most hormonal and endocrine functions that affect cellular genetics as well as brain functioning. If the chakra spins counter clockwise, mental confusion ensues. Individuals' images or cognitions regarding reality are clogged with the past or contaminated with created fantasies of reality frequently based upon dysfunctional 1st–3rd chakras. Unable to see the present, they cannot adequately understand themselves and their relationship to the world. Posteriorly, the chakra gives energy to creative ideas and their implementation on the world. It facilitates the access to visioning the future based upon life path information.

Spiritually, a healthy supported 6th chakra allows individuals to clairvoyantly see the divine universality in all things and to comfortably experience the knowing that individuals "have a body rather than are some 'body.'" Transpersonal states, satori, peak experiences and ecstatic states are accessed and inform an ever-expanding understanding of the many layers of coexisting reality. With a developed imbalance in, disconnection, or denial of the lower chakras, individuals could be pulled from grace producing upper chakras into the shadow of material wealth, sexual acting out, or fame and status cravings of dysfunctional first chakras. This is due to the fact that those who focus too much on the higher chakras without continued connection to the lower centers lose consciousness of them and are eventually pulled into their shadow side. Many gurus, roshi and spiritual leaders in the West have succumbed to the lower

chakra-driven Western culture.

7th Chakra-Crown-Sahasrana

The crown chakra is related to individuals' access to spirituality that is a personal experience of numinous transcendent grace. The 7th chakra receives energy through the top of the head. This energy is connected to higher consciousness reminding each individual that they are part of a universal Divine Source. A functional crown chakra draws in the vision of the future and what is the soul's purpose in this lifetime. Conversely, a closed crown chakra produces dogmatic concretized rigid religious beliefs or a blocked experience of spirituality all together. These people frequently think that those experiencing transcendental experiences are "making it up," "emotionally disturbed," or are needing some cosmic caretaker and can't accept the limitations of mortality. "Individuals who master the gifts of this chakra understand that the river flows beyond form and formlessness, beyond existence and nonexistence" (Villildo, 2000, p. 102).

8th Chakra-Above the Head-Atman

The 8th chakra is located about an inch and a half above the head. It is believed to be the door in and out of this time/space reality. It is the portal into the archetypal–or universal knowing–that Jung spoke about (Jung, CW *Mysterium conunctionis*). As such, it is the source of all past knowledge including karmic memory. It is said to contain the Akashic records (the records of all that an individual has experienced or been through during their lifetimes).

9th Chakra

Residing above the head it is considered the source of creation, soul and spirit. Experiencing this chakra is an experience of being one with the Light.

10th Chakra

Some systems have a 10th chakra that resides one to four feet under the feet. It is elemental in nature and is the energy that serves individual grounding and every day reality-based information. It supports individuals' ability to deal with day-to-day situations. It aids in the centering of the 7 body chakras through drawing up and securing the related subtle energy.

AURAS: THE HUMAN ENERGY FIELD

Auras are part of the human energy field that surrounds the entire body. Some theories suggest that each chakra corresponded to an auric field (see Figure 7-4). Others state that there are 3 important layers. Starting closest to the body, they are: the etheric or vital; the energy blueprint which guides and shapes the growth of the body, the astral or emotional body which holds trauma and other emotionally charged phenomenon that can be triggered and transferred onto another who enters the field, and the mental body associated with thought forms and the causal or soul bodies (Brennon, 1988; Talbot, Karagiulla and Kunz, 1989). These concepts have emerged from theosophical literature and are seen as the energetic "personality" of the individual. These fields interact among themselves as well as the universal energy field of which they are a part.

Etheric Body

The primary task of the etheric field is to transfer universal energy to the individual field (the human physical body). The individual field is vitalized by life force–vital energy from the etheric field that enters the body through the energy portals of the chakras. It is the closest to the human body and disintegrates when the body dies. This field has been described as a pale blue-gray or violet gray gently luminous heat wave-like flowing phenomena which typically extends between two to three inches beyond the periphery of the body.

Astral Body

The astral field is considered the energetic vehicle of feeling and functions at a high frequency. This aura is a moving picture of all one feels whether expressed or not. It is generally considered to be the field that encompasses a person's personal space. It is approximately 15 to 18 inches beyond the physical body and is multicolored. The periphery of the emotional human energy field is clear. This is what, in the psychotherapy and recovery field, is known as the external boundary. If an individual enters a person's emotional field, she/he can get contaminated by unintegrated or unhealed emotionally-charged relationally-based trauma. When that happens, the person entering into the other's field will have their emotional field affected by the others. In these instances, these individuals feel "slimed" as if they are being experienced not as who they are but as the emotionally-charged imprint of a significant relationship that existed earlier in the person's life now held in the person's astral body. These transferences occur when individuals respond to such frequencies due to their own histories as subjects or objects of these emotionally-charged roles and behaviors. Like attracts like or its reciprocal in this energetic plane. So it behooves individuals to ensure that they reduce the possibility of projecting or transferring onto another or of receiving others' projections by sealing their astral auric field.

Sensitives can see more instinctual feelings related to aggression, survival and sexuality at the lower portion of the astral field and emotions such as love and compassion higher up closer to the heart. Those who utilize the somatic countertransference technique discussed in the former chapter are picking up information from this energetic field.

Chakras	Location, Organs & Systems	Color & Elements Foods Symbols	Psychological aspects	Psychological imbalance	Functions & Lessons	Instinct	Glands & secretions	Related illnesses & diseases
1st Root Base **Muladhara** **Instinctual body**	Spinal base (coccyx) Adrenals Kidneys Spinal column Rectum Legs, bones Feet Urinary system Immune system	Red Earth Masculine Source of Kundalini Proteins Meats Bull, Ox Snake Scorpio Dragon Saturn Earth	Safety, Feeding, Shelter, Survival, Self Preservation Grounding Stability Security Stillness Courage Patience Healthy Boundaries	Depression Hoarding Greed Predatory Behavior, Violence, Abandonment Issues, Narcissism Self-centered Battering Boundaryless Victim	Gives vitality to the physical body Matters pertaining to the physical world and the physical body Anger management Gives support Attraction of opposites	Survival Security from the material realm Life force "I have" "I feel physically"	Adrenals	Chronic fatigue Tension in spine Constipation Chronic low back pain Varicose veins Rectal cancer Immune-related disorders Sciatica Obesity
2nd Chakra Sacral **Svadhisthana** **Emotional body**	Lower abdomen Pelvis Sexual organs Intestines Bladder Digestion Urination Sexual potency	Orange Water Feminine Liquids, fruits and vegetables Fish Neptune Moon	Feelings Fear Passion Power Aggression Creativity Sexual love Tolerance Change Surrender Family connection Sweetness	Bulling Blame Guilt Hatred Jealousy Food, sex, Alcohol addictions Desire to possess Disconnection to feelings	Procreation Issues of money and sex Issues of power and control Capacity to create Ethics and honor Giving and receiving Working harmoniously with others	Reproduction Oral drives Sexual Instinctual drives of the unconscious Procreation Desire "I feel emotionally"	Ovaries Testicles Sex hormones	Chronic low back pain Sciatica Ob/gyn problems Urinary and prostate dysfunction Sexual dysfunction Impotence
3rd Chakra Solar Plexus **Manipura** **Mental Body**	Solar plexus Abdomen Stomach Upper intestines Liver Gallbladder Pancreas	Yellow Fire or Air Masculine Starches Bird Ram	Locus of core self/inner child Self-connection, esteem, & confidence Trust Personal	Fear Intimidation Sensitive to criticism Powerful inner judge Personality disorders	Self-connection and care Care of others Capacity to make decisions Personal honor Capacity to	Power instinct Will "I can" "I want" "I think"	Pancreas Adrenals Digestive secretions	Arthritis Gastric or duodenal Ulcers Intestinal illnesses Diabetes Indigestion

	Body	Color / Element / Planet	Qualities	Dysfunction	Higher qualities	Affirmation	Glands	Physical dysfunction
3rd cont.	Spleen Middle spine Nervous system Muscular system Autonomic nervous system Digestive system	Mars Sun	power Will Self awareness and control Personal unconscious Dreams Imagination Thoughts Judgements Humor	Abandonment Sense of emptiness Anorexia Bulimia	digest or process material Personal transform-tion Individuation			Liver dysfunction Hepatitis Digestive problems
4th Chakra **Heart Chakra** **Anahata** **Astral body**	Heart Lungs Diaphragm Thymus Shoulders Arms Hands Ribs/breasts Circulatory system	Green Rose Air or earth Feminine Green fruits & vegetables Mammals Birds Venus	Love Hatred Grief Anger Commitment Artistic & scientific genius Clairvoyance Equilibrium	Resentment Bitterness Loneliness Inability to love Too giving Betrayal Unexpressed grief	Compassion Forgiveness Trust Hope Universal love Realization of the interconnect-edness of all things	Instinct to love "I love"	Thymus glandular secretions	Heart disease Heart attack Asthma Allergies Lung cancer Emphysema Pneumonia Breast cancer
5th Chakra **Throat Chakra** **Visuddha** **Spiritual body**	Throat Thyroid Mouth Neck vertebra Esophagus Larynx Medulla Oblongata hypothalamus Respiratory system	Indigo Sky blue Ether Masculine Blue & Purple fruits & vegetables Humans Lion Mercury	Integration Peace Expressed truth Loyalty Honesty Reliability Kindness	Depression Blocked expression Communication problems Lack of discrimination Judgement Criticism	Expression in speech & arts Communica-tion Capacity to make decisions Capacity to mindfully detach	Psychic Expression "I speak"	Thyroid Parathyroid secretions	TMJ Swollen glands Laryngitis Thyroid problems Throat cancer Speech pathology Hearing impairment
6th Chakra **Third eye** **Forehead** **Ajna** **Celestial body**	Midbrain Eyes, ears, nose Pituitary Gland Hormonal systems Autonomic	Violet Dark blue Light or radium Feminine Blue/purple fruits &	Self evaluation Intellect Emotional intelligence Intuition Wisdom Insight	Dissociative ADD ADHD Disembodied soul Detached from the world	Openness to ideas Learn from experience Soul realization Seeing and doing one's	Truth "I see" "I love"	Pituitary secretions in charge of hormonal secretions	Headaches Eye problems Brain tumors Neurological disturbances Learning disabilities

6th cont.	nervous system	vegetables Mind altering substances Owl Spirits Jupiter	Channeling ability Enlighten-ment	Delusion	calling Self-actualization Soul realization Seeing nonduality	universally" "I intuit"		Seizures Weak or blocked celestial Light
7th Chakra Crown Sahasrara Ketheric body	Cerebral cortex Skin Skeletal system Organs & tissues of entire body	White Purple Pure energy Androgynous Fasting All life forms Uranus	Faith Inspiration Spirituality Devotion Divine knowing Bliss Mindfulness Conscious-ness Idealism	Mystical depression Confusion Alienation Senility Alzheimer's Paranoia Psychosis	Ability to trust life Humanitarianism Selfless service Ability to see the bigger picture Oneness with the Infinite	Universal ethics "I know" "I am"	Pineal gland secretions	Energetic disorders Extreme Sensitivity to light, sound or other environment factors
8th Chakra Atman	Resides a few inches above the head Soul Architect of the body	Gold	Timelessness Invisibility	Cosmic horror (caught between the world of spirit & matter) Caught in the *bardo* planes	Experience of deep union with the Creator Out of body experiences Astral travel	Transcend-ence "I transcend"	None	Templates of disease
9th Chakra	None	Translucent white light Spirit	None	None	None	Liberation "I am infinite"	None	None

Figure 7-3. Chakra charts.

The Mental Body

The mental energetic field interpenetrates the etheric and astral fields and extends about three feet beyond the physical body. The higher frequency and luminosity of this field can be experienced when ideas are charged with this mental energy. Whether right or wrong, others' thoughts can transform another's view. By the same token, habitual automatic negative thinking can keep individuals caught in old thought forms. These thought forms are often constructed of visual imagery as well as abstract cognitions. The power of thought forms are based upon their dynamism rather than static immutable images or stories.

The Causal Body

The causal body is considered to be the energy of the soul or spirit. It is likened to Jung's concept of the Self–the organizing principle of wholeness. It is causal because the soul/Self is the fundamental cause or essence of an individual's being. The causal body is that which exists throughout eternity. It provides the continuity of existence. This self-actualizing spiritual energy exists across lifetimes. It is part of universal consciousness from which comes agape, compassion, serenity, sartori, and intuitive and psychic abilities. It holds the karma and also the universality of the collective or archetypal. Sensitives see this spiritual human energy field as a pale translucent energy bubble.

GENERAL CONCEPTS

An individual is seen as a system of interdependent force fields that are responsive to changes in consciousness.(Karagiulla, Kunz, 1989). A field is defined as a "continuous condition of space" (p. 27). Consciousness, energy and matter are interconnected. Individuals are all connected to the universe through the continuous exchange of energy and consciousness through the various human energy fields and physical mindbody. These fields regulate the human energy system maintaining the tao or balance in mindbody and soulspirit.

Health

Health is clearly a multidimensional interrelated process. Health from an energetic point of view is seen as the natural flow of this subtle energy through the nadis and meridians. The chakras are aligned and all spinning clockwise (with some exceptions such as a period of time around female menstruation). When the chakras are spinning appropriately, they send energy to the corresponding nadi or meridian. The lower chakras 1-3 spin at lower frequencies. The higher ones spin at progressively higher rates. The more activity in the higher chakras the higher the state of consciousness of the individual. The color of the chakras indicate health as well, such as red in the 1st chakra indicating the capacity to stand up and assert oneself; clear yellow in the third identifying the capacity to know what one truly wants and thinks; or blue/indigo in the 6th reflecting the capacity to intuit (Bruyere, 1994).

Healthy etheric fields are described as "a luminous web of fine bright lines of force which, in a healthy person, stand out at right angles to the surface of the skin" (Kunz, p. 30).

Dysfunction, Illness, and Trauma

Pathology can develop at a number of levels. Studies utilizing the AMI and other measurement devices have shown evidence of abnormalities in the meridian activity even before the manifestation of physical symptoms of illness. Such signs demonstrate instability, excitation or weakness of meridian function. In terms of the human energy fields, holes in the auric fields can be present with energy leaking out. Leakage in the

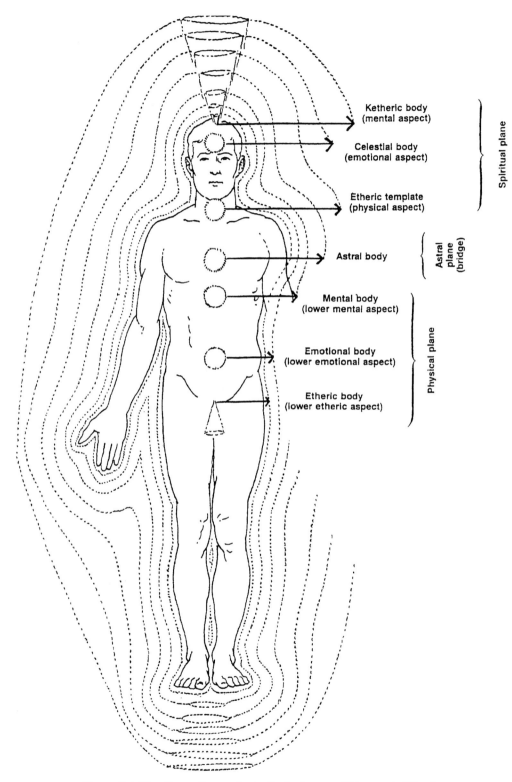

Figure 7-4. The Seven Layer Auric Body System (Diagnostic View).

etheric field decreases the amount of life force available physically and can produce a chronic fatigue. Sensitives report tears in the etheric web or separations from the human body. Misalignments can occur between the etheric, astral and mental fields as is found in autism. Dysrhythmia in the energy fields produces a lack of harmony among the physical, emotional and mental aspects. This is seen in severe emotional dysfunction such as psychosis. Chronic emotional distur-bances such as rage, cause disordered distur-bances on the astral or emotional human energy fields, while depression and fear cut down the normal flow of energy. Anxiety typically localizes around the solar plexus and in several cases, the emotional energy field can be seen flowing inward toward the physical body inhibiting the normal free flow of energy surrounding the body.

Chakras may be displaced, blocked, trun-cated, leaking, too cold or overheated. They may be spinning counterclockwise sending needed energy from the body that energeti-cally supports the psychological dysfunction of projection. Their color and hence their frequency may be dull or gray; the rhyth-micity may be dysrhythmic, the rate of spin too fast or slow; its form and size may be too small or wilted. Depending upon which chakra is not within normal range, the prac-titioner can be alerted as to related organs, systems, mental and emotional issues which may be potentially or currently dysfunction-al (see Chakra chart for specifics).

Healing

Healing occurs when energy is unblocked, cleared, and charged, realigned or balanced thus creating an environment for health and recovery. As a person's level of consciousness is altered-expanded, recog-nizable changes also occur in the nervous system (Motoyama, 1978, p. 64). When a person is calm, energy flows evenly and smoothly and the etheric energy field is straightened. From the perspective of yoga, health and healing occurs when the chakras are awakened and are spinning clockwise allowing energy to flow into the body.

There are several methods for these processes as each Indian school of yoga has its own focus. Chakra meditation and con-centration, the development of prana, asanas or postures, the chanting of tones are a few vehicles. These methods can aid in:

- grounding–the experience of being fully in the body rooted on the earth capable of receiving energy from the earth
- opening blocked and or appropriately sealing the energy center for protection
- aligning–centering and adjusting the placement of energy fields and chakras.

Healing is seen as working with the "quanta, the energy units capable of going back and forth between the visible and invis-ible, that are able to become or connect with an organic cell, feeling, thought or piece of our soul" (Dale, 1996, p. 14).

HEALERS

Well-known healers have been tested to have an excess of energy in the heart merid-ian and in the manipura (3rd) chakra (Motoyama, 1990). Those therapists who employ the somatic countertransference receive the emotional energy into the manipura chakra. Energy Medicine profes-sionals such as polarity practitioners and Reiki Masters have been able to break through the limitations of their senses to a high sense perception. Energy practitioners who use their hands in healing are found throughout the world. These healers are transmitters of etheric energy. Their heart chakras are open and the universal love energetically travels down their arms into and through their hands. Clairvoyants or medical intuitives typically refers to those capable of being sensitive to "seeing" or per-ceiving the etheric and/or emotional energy fields.

SUMMARY

The awareness, movement and healthy processing of bioenergy has existed in the East for 5000 years and has become gradually accepted in the West largely because of the success of acupuncture. Now yoga, tai c'hi, and qi qong are gaining in interest as are forms of energy healing such as polarity, craniosacral, Reiki and therapeutic touch. With the understanding of the influence of this subtle body energy on prevention and recovery of physically and emotionally driven trauma and illness as well as its involvement in psychospiritual enlightenment comes the comprehension of the fundamental source of life itself. Bioenergy medicine is seen to join mindbody and soulspirit, medicine and spirituality and may just be the portal to a greater understanding of how the universe works.

Practitioners and consultants in the field of integrative holistic health whether energy healers or not bring their own energetic field into the work with clients. It is vital that this paradigm be understood and included in the consciousness that surrounds the work and the client-practitioner bi-personal healing vessel.

REFERENCES

Becker, R. and Seldon, G. (1987). *The Body Electric: Electromagnitism and the foundation of life.* New York: William Morrow and Co., Inc.

Brennan, B. (1988). *Hands of light: A guide to healing through the human energy field.* New York: Bantam Books.

Bruyere, R. (1994). *Wheels of Light-Chakras auras and the healing energy of the body.* New York: Fireside Books.

Dale, C. (1996). *New Chakra Healing.* St Paul, MN: Llewellyn Publications.

Gerber, R.(1988). *Vibrational medicine.* Santa Fe, NM: Bear & Co.

Judith, A. (1996). *Wheels of light.* St Paul, MN: Llewellyn Publications.

Karagulla, S. & Kunz, D. (1989). *The Chakras and human energy fields.* Wheaton, IL: The Theosophical Publishing House.

Motoyama, H. with Brown, R. (1978). *Science and evolution of consciousness: Chakras, Ki and Psi.* Brookline, MA: Autumn Press.

_____. (1990). *Toward a supraconscious. Meditation theory and practice.* Berkeley: Asian Humanities Press.

_____. (1995). *Theories of the Chakras.* Wheaton, IL: Quest Books.

Legion of Light. (1988). *Chakra Awareness Guide.* Mt. Shasta: CA: Legion of Light Products.

Myss, C. (1996). *Anatomy of the Spirit.* New York: Harmony Books

Talbot, M. (1991). *The Holographic Universe.* New York: HarperCollins Pub.

Tsuei, J. (1996). Scientific Evidence In Support of Acupuncture and Meridian Theory: Introduction. In *Engineering in Medicine and Biology Magazine,* Vol. 15, No. 3.

Villolodo, A. (2000). *Shaman. Healer, Sage: How to Heal yourself with the Energy Medicine of the Americas.* New York: Harmony Books.

CIHS Newsletter. (2000 & 2001). Encinitas, CA: California Institute for Human Sciences. Vol. VIII. NO. 2, Vol. VII, No. 4.

Chapter 8

SPIRITUALITY, THE TRANSPERSONAL AND ERA III MEDICINE

"In the beginning of civilization healers, priests and scientists were one in the same with coherent unifying beliefs. Cartesian duality and Newtonian materialism theoretically fragmented a unified universe." (Motoyama, 1990, p. 29)

EVEN MORE ELUSIVE than bioenergy is the experience of grace and numen, and yet this palpable being-in-relation with the transpersonal holds practitioners and clients alike in a compassionate loving interconnectedness which some believe is the *sine qua non* of healing. When this ineffable spiritual experience is awakened, both practitioner and client are blessed, bathed and transformed. The word "holistic" derives from the same root as "health," "healing" and "holy." This should come as no surprise since from the dawn of civilization the medicine wo/man, priest/ess, and shaman were simultaneously the medical doctor, herbalist, energy practitioner, counselor, and spiritual leader of their community. What is surprising is that the Western analytic, scientific left brain, in an effort to deepen understanding through specialization, severed and fragmented these identities. This has resulted in incomplete and often contradictory recommendations. It is only now in this current millenium that the new identity of holistic health practitioner and consultant has emerged to reunite these roles again, coordinate, and integrate the healing of a client.

SPIRITUALITY

Being religious has typically been associated with the identification with a particular institutionalized religion, practice, or discipline. Spirituality, on the other hand, defines characteristics irrespective of whether or not the individual is affiliated with a specific group. These are, for example: a sense of love, compassion and empathy for self and others, a sense of something greater than the self or collective human species, and a meaning of existence that transcends empirical reality. Spirit as defined in dictionaries comes from life force.

SPIRITUAL HEATH IS SEEN AS:
- An ongoing experience of well-being and inner peace
- An experience of self locus of control over a person's life
- A sense of personal empowerment
- The capacity for intimacy with oneself, others, and a higher divine grace
- The presence of meaning, calling and or purpose in a person's life
- An experience of hopefulness and a view

of the glass as half full

- Belief in a philosophy which provides an integrative wholeness to a person's life, behavior and activities
- A connectedness to nature and in the underlying unity of all things providing an ethical responsibility to the well-being of the planet
- Belief that there is a power greater or more fundamental than the individual
- A capacity for agape or compassionate love, acceptance, and peace regarding self and other
- The capacity to allow and experience the power of mystery to transform
- The capacity to forgive
- The capacity for faith
- The capacity to know what is in personal power to change and let go of what is not, and the wisdom to know the difference
- The capacity to shift from personal needs and issues to the bigger picture

Studies have shown that those with strong spiritual-religious beliefs recover sooner, stay alive longer and are less depressed and anxious. Research has documented that those who attend church or synagogues stay healthy longer (Hafen et al., Sagan, 1987). The numerous support 12-step recovery groups that have developed from the AA model stressing surrendering to a Higher Power attest to aiding many in the recovery from addictions (Pelletier, 2000).

Faith and its capacity to heal have been researched along with the placebo effect of drugs and physicians relating positive prognoses to patients. Startling replicable evidence has been documented proving the power of a person's faith to recover and stay healthy (Hafen, et al 1996, Hall, 2001, Dossey, 1998).

Spiritual healing is an ongoing journey that affects the mindbody occurring one step at a time. Most all beliefs recognize that individuals are inherently spiritual, religions; and spiritual disciplines can help individuals remember who they truly are. The path may take a person to a temenos such as a temple or church or to a spiritual teacher or a holistic health practitioner or transpersonal counselor, or the journey may be entirely inward.

However, not all who identify themselves as religious and/or spiritual may be positively influenced by their belief system. For example, those who adhere to a judgmental God who views humans as sinners tend to be more depressed and anxious. Dogma that relate to people that they deserve to suffer and that all life is suffering can view disease as a punishment or part of a living hell that they should expect to experience. Some religions encourage ritual suicide and wars. Others, who identify as being spiritual, are using it as a rationalization for their lack of responsibility and inability to have grounded engagement in reality and interpersonal relationships. Many reinvent the concept of nonattachment to help support their survival mechanisms of *de*tachment, isolation, avoidance, lack of a capacity to commit and passive aggression. These individuals may fear intimacy with themselves and others. They are unable to connect to or express feelings nor empathetically relate to others. This fear has the reverse effect on healing and wellness. Additionally, those who involve themselves in a religion or spiritual practice in search of being a pedistaled model of, for example: the all-giving Blessed Virgin, the martyred Christ, the perfect yoga "pretzel body" or the one who can meditate longer have clearly fallen off the razor's edge of grace. A different god motivates them. Vanity, pride, status and power are all false gods and frequently call to those who began a spiritual path particularly if others idealize them (Cope, 2000, Lewis, 1993).

EASTERN TRADITIONS

Much of Eastern practices that have strongly influenced Alternative and Complimentary medicine are based in the capacity to co-exist in the Einsteinian frame of simultaneous multiple dimensions of reality. The quest in Buddhism and the Hindu yogic philosophy is to become a nonjudgmental nonattached to outcome witness. This mindfulness appropriately holds and returns to consciousness and the experience of the underlying, undifferentiated unity of all existence. All believe that we have a body rather than we are a body, and that even in the yoga model, "the more deeply we penetrate the phenomenal world (the body, the earth) with our attention, the more we discover that the world and its forms are full of God—indeed, are God . . ." (Cope, 2000, p. 268).

Yoga

Yoga is not just a series of asanas or stretches; it is a spiritual discipline. It has been defined as "a means of achieving union with the inner true self, the God within" (Motoyama, 1995, p. 30). Yoga is sanskrit for yoke signifying the union between individual and the divine. Yoga's purpose is to reunify individuals with divine consciousness that is experienced in the state of Samadhi. This is supported though eight disciplines:

- Yama (abstaining from violence, lying, stealing, and greed)
- Niyama (undertaking virtuous behavior through purification, contentment, asceticism, chanting and worship)
- Asana (Yogic postures. Hatha yoga seeks to join the shakti energy lying coiled like a snake at the base of the spine with shiva the stillpoint of pure consciousness.)
- Pranayama (Abdominal, chest and yogic breathing exercises); Bandhas (postures which hold and tighten); and Mudras (exercises which awaken the chakras and kundalini to bring about control of the prana)
- Pratyahara (Shifting away from desire associated with the 5 senses)
- Dharana (Concentration)
- Dhyana (Meditation)

- Samadhi (Spiritual union)

The paradigm upholds the process of reincarnation through lifetimes chained to desire and attachment. Through detachment, individuals can let go of self-alienation and remember who they are—God. The yoga philosophy states that each human has an eternal core soul or Atman that dwells in the Brahman or infinite divine cosmos. Through repeated experiences with samadhi, individuals are reminded of their pure nature: the union of consciousness and energy. Spirit derives from the Latin meaning "Breath" and Yoga, which focuses on Prana as the source of life, and may just provide the closest psyiologic link.

Psychologically speaking Cope (2000) contends that most Western religions do not "confront the unconscious" (p. 138). The personal unconscious can trap an individual in webs of history and fears or attachments to future outcomes. The capacity to be fully present in the moment without bringing the past or the future along with its associated thoughts, feelings, and roles is part of an Eastern spiritual point of view.

Consciousness allows the disciplined pilgrim an experience of divine presence. Instead of worshiping at an altar, the yoga mat becomes the altar with the worshiper being that which is worshiped in the moment within the stillpoint of Samadhi.

Buddhism

Buddhism roughly 2500 years old, held that life is full of suffering as long as individuals are attached to needed outcomes. Individuals continue to reincarnate until they find the way to end this suffering. This end is Enlightenment. To this end various forms of meditation have been created to quiet desires and the busy mind. Westerners, who spent substantial amounts of time in Asian monasteries or with Roshi's of zen meditation, and Tibetan and Vietnamese monks have brought these spiritual disciplines to the West. They have provided one of the most powerful influences upon spirituality in integrative holistic health. Meditation has been considered the heart of Buddhism. Siddhartha was initially trained in the sramanic tradition of Yoga that focused on the direct personal experience of the infinite cosmic consciousness through asceticism and yogic meditations. Sitting meditation has developed from yogic practice.

Through meditation and other spiritual disciplines individuals come to experience the myth of duality. Everything in all times is considered to be part of the undifferentiated consciousness. Abbot Loori states it clearly:

> Every particle, every event is interpenetrated, codependent, mutually arising, with mutual causality. What happens to one thing happens to all things. That is the nature of the universe, the nature of the self. That is Buddha-nature: that is who we are. Whether we realize it or not, that is the way the world functions. When we live our lives out of the deluded notion of separateness, inevitably we clash with the natural law of the universe. We run into difficulty, pain, misfortune and suffering. And that too is one big pearl. (1996, p. 2)

THE TRANSPERSONAL PARADIGM IN WESTERN PSYCHOLOGY

Unlike theoretical models that stem from psychodynamic, cognitive-behavioral, or even existential-humanistic approaches, the transpersonal frame upholds that there is more to an individual's identity than his/her intrapsychic or interpersonal realms. Their view of the individual transcends empirical phenomena to include concepts such as soul, karma, spiritual connection and consciousness.

With a transpersonal perspective, the therapy process encompasses definitions from psychodynamic, cognitive, and humanistic approaches that address recovery from maladaptive and abusive childhood histories

that lock individuals into dysfunctional thinking, outmoded survival patterns, and a disconnection to what the individual truly believes. These approaches see health as the ability of an individual to be fully present, capable of discovering one's own values and meaning in life, able to connect to and be intimate with the self and others, and to manifest an ego-based objective engagement with the empirical. Additionally, a transpersonal perspective includes a gradual shifting of the primacy of the ego to one in which the individual disidentifies from the personal to focus upon the greater good and the bigger picture. This is a picture which moves beyond physical reality to espouse other realities such as those found in energetic field theory, connection with those in spirit and with what has been identified as the pure Consciousness, the Light, the Source, and/or God.

Transpersonally speaking, dysfunction occurs when individuals believe that all that exists is what is empirically present. "If I can't see it; it doesn't exist." Science has attempted to amend this assumption by asserting that phenomena does exist by virtue of the effect they have upon the observable; such as found in subatomic particle research. However, most Westerners believe that a transpersonal view is a matter of faith rather than anything that has any scientific or experiential substantiation. Many transpersonal holistic health therapists and practitioners believe that this inability to experience the transpersonal in the West or for that matter in any culture, would inhibit an individual's capacity to unfold personal spiritual essence, karmic or soul path or to move beyond a self focus. Thus, techniques of active imagination through visualization, ritual, the use of the arts, spiritual quests and awareness trainings, as well as Eastern meditational practices are encouraged in order to avail individuals numinous experiences of the transpersonal. Such states as mystical or transcendental experiences, satori, or St. Francis-like ecstatic states are supported by many approaches as they serve to awaken the person to greater consciousness or enlightenment. These states all have similar characteristics; (Barber, 1976) among them are: "an experience of unity, . . . a feeling of identifying with all things, . . . the experience of timelessness and spacelessness, . . . a sense of having been in touch with ultimate reality". . . an experience of grace, joy and peace, . . . a feeling of the divine, and an inability to put the experience into words (pp. 415–417).

Many of the other traditional approaches in psychotherapy find the above altered states examples of dissociative or psychotic episodes or at best, reductively interpret them.

C.G. Jung and Individuation

Carl Jung is considered the first of the European/Euro American psychotherapists to bring the transpersonal into the field of psychotherapy. Jung expanded the psychoanalytic concept of the unconscious as receptacle of repressed drives, split-off parts of the self, and trauma to include an archetypal layer of the unconscious. It is through the inner journey that the analysand accesses the collective unconscious and taps into the universal pool of wisdom. This connection is seen outwardly through synchronistic phenomena such as astrology and the I Ching and events which cannot be explained by rational cause and effect logic as well as through archetypal images, themes, sounds and movement for which art, drama, music, and dance provide the sacred containers. This spiritual connection also presents itself internally through dreams, visions, active imagination, and meditation practices (Jung, CW 9.1).

Jung, unlike the Eastern influenced transpersonal therapists, saw the process of therapy as individuation i.e., "the process by which a person becomes a psychological 'individual'; that is, a separate, indivisible unity or 'whole'" (Jung, CW 9.1, p. 275). Instead of

disidentifying with duality, Jung felt it was vital to be in relation to the archetypal lest the individual gets too close, identifies with it and becomes inflated. Myths such as found in the motifs of Icarus, Medusa, and Prometheus point the way to the devastating results of attempting to liken oneself to the gods. The danger of inflation has also demonstrated itself with Hitler, Jim Jones, and the numerous priests, gurus and spiritual teachers who like Icarus, crashed because they felt they were "above" human limitations and ethics. Thus, the concept of an ego–Self axis (Edinger, 1982) is viewed as the ideal relationship to the transpersonal. This highly Western view maintains that one should stay at a humble respectful distance or axis as Edinger identified it. And yet Jung saw the self-actualizing power of the archetype of the Self, the transpersonal organizing principle of wholeness, as having a profound effect on the ego.

The Self–sometimes seen as Jung's concept for the threshold into Consciousness–often takes the unknowing pilgrim into personal spiritual journeys described as "dark nights of the soul." An individual may be struck with a life-threatening illness or lose everything that was thought to be dear as in the story of Job. This so-called "defeat of the ego" can shake loose all of that which individuals have identified prior and move them into a liminal phase where they are no longer who they are and not yet who they will become (Lewis, 1993). This disidentification process reoccurs throughout adult life stages. Each time individuals let go of more of their egocentric needs, they are seen to gradually receive universal wisdom. This is the process of healing that may or may not be associated to a cure.

Assagioli and Psychosynthesis

Although Roberto Assagioli was a contemporary of Jung's, his work did not receive larger attention until the 1970s. Psychosynthesis "is a name for the conscious attempt to cooperate with the natural process of personal development . . . to perfect itself" (Carter-Haar, Synthesis, Vol 1, 1975, p. 116). This approach asserts that each individual has a "transpersonal essence" and that it is each individual's purpose to manifest this. Assagioli adopted Jung's concepts of the Transpersonal Self and the collective unconscious and added the concept of the superconscious from which emerge impulses for "altruistic love and will, humanitarian action, artistic and scientific inspiration, philosophic and spiritual insight, and the drive for purpose and meaning in life" (Ibid., p. 116).

Dysfunction occurs, in addition to those identified in the psychodynamic, existential-humanistic, and cognitive-behavioral Western frames, when an individual is unconscious of or unable to manifest his or her sublime highest nature. Similar to the Jungian view, transpersonal stage work of psychosynthesis can result in a person caring more about the community, the environment, and the transpersonal and living in a state of grace. This approach utilizes visualization and imaginal dialogues with intrapsychic subpersonalities, one of which is identified as the supraconsciousness. It is considered the spiritual access to the infinite wisdom of the cosmic consciousness.

Maslow, Vaughan, Walsh, Groff, Tart and Transpersonal Psychotherapy

It's unclear just who coined the term transpersonal. It appeared in the fifties but really acquired a larger usage in the late sixties with the formation of the *Journal of Transpersonal Psychology* and with Tart's *Transpersonal Psychologies* in the mid-seventies. Out of the humanistic ideal of Maslow's self-actualizing person capable of so-called peak experiences evolved a foundational philosophy for an Association of Transpersonal Psychology. Influenced as well by Eastern traditions such as Taoism, Buddhism,

Sufiism, Hinduism as well as Native American shamanic frames, a more culturally universal approach continued to develop. From this synthesis, transcendental dimensions of existence and experience, soul connected unfolding of what one is meant to do, the involvement in a spiritual path, and the disidentification with thoughts and limited world views are seen as major concepts identifying health.

Regarding the need for disidentification, Walsh and Vaughn conceptualized dysfunction as occurring when individuals believe that they are what they think. Walsh and Vaughn (Boorstein, 1991) write, "When the individual identifies with mental content, this content is transformed into the context within which he or she interprets other content, determines reality, adopts a logic, and is motivated" (p. 17). No cognitive therapist would disagree with this assumption, but transpersonal psychotherapists do something very different with this premise. Rather than utilizing charts, rational discussions and behavioral techniques with the goal of having the individual "think something different," the transpersonal therapist supports the individual's transcendence from all identification thereby lifting them from their own world view to one in which "the individual would presumably identify with both everything and nothing" (Walsh & Vaughn in Boorstein, 1991).

Neo-transpersonal Approaches to Psychotherapy

The first wave of the human potential movement of the sixties and seventies gave way to the second wave of new age in the eighties and nineties. The belief in Buddhist and Hindu systems in the first wave supported such approaches as mindfulness and past life regression and therapy. Additionally shamanic practices from a variety of native cultures around the world have rekindled spiritual channeling, soul retrieval and active imagination techniques, which, like those of psychosynthesis, draw the individual into contact with sentient beings.

Those who adhere to the existence of past lives, believe that individuals may at times need to heal from abuse either they or others committed in former lifetimes thus expanding the individuals' consciousness and clearing their karma. Utilizing much of the same techniques that are employed in today's recovery models (Lewis 1993, 2000), therapists support individuals' deeper discovery of the etiology of survival patterns and the repeated reexperiencing the same karmic lessons. This healing is often at a soul level and must always be respectful of the fact that karmic clearing has its own time frame.

Shamanism views individuals as capable of existing both in ordinary and in nonordinary states of reality. Vital for well-being is the maintenance of one's personal power (Harner, 1982). Individuals with diminished power are seen as "dis-spirited" and often experience harmful intrusions that can energetically reduce the individual's life force. Individuals are encouraged to employ active imagination to enter into "shamanic states of consciousness" and channel power animals or more human-like spiritual beings. Holistic health practitioners who support era three medicine, such as those trained in medical intuition (see the following chapter) or the somatic countertransference (Lewis, 1986, 1988, 1992, 1993, 1996), can draw connections to shamans who would receive the disease of their patients diagnosis and/or release them from their suffering or possession.

Channeling, or the capacity to intuitively receive on behalf of the client through nonordinary means, is receiving greater acceptance and tolerance. Here therapists empty themselves similar to the preparation needed for meditation. Information can be received through synchronistic events or simply as thoughts that seem to intuitively emerge out of nowhere to be utilized as the therapist sees fit in service to the healing and expanded consciousness of the client (see the following chapter).

SACRED ALCHEMY: THE WESTERN JUDEO-CHRISTIAN PROCESS OF SPIRITUAL HEALING

To the outsider, alchemy was considered a science that chemically sought to change baser materials or *prima materia* into gold. In fact, most of the alchemists in the West were utilizing this chemical paradigm as a guise in order to cloak their spiritual journey from the baser experience of duality and unconsciousness to that of spiritual union and consciousness. Alchemists believed that the heavens and earth, inner and outer were all interconnected and the *opus* or work was about finding and experiencing universal spiritual truth. C.G. Jung became fascinated with these mystics and sought out as many ancient texts as could be found. This was difficult at best due to the fact that most alchemists obfuscated their notes, for they realized that it was only through the experience of the process itself that the spiritual pilgrim could ever transform.

Thus, alchemists would hide their experience in esoteric language or statements of simple chemical procedures. Frequently, alchemical texts or lexicons would be destroyed lest irreverent seekers debase the material. Thus, the seeker must first be the holistic health practitioner his or herself because unless the practitioner/healer has a spiritual relationship to the divine, the grace needed for expanded consciousness for the creation of a sacred space or *temenos* will not be assured within the healing container. But committing to being a seeker whether practitioner or client is no easy venture. Edinger (1978) in his discussion of the opus or alchemical work quotes from an old text entitled *The ordinal of Alchemy*:

Anyone who gives himself up to the search must therefore expect to meet with much vexation of spirit. He will frequently have to change his course in consequence of new discoveries which he makes. . . . The devil will do his utmost to frustrate your search by one or another of these stumbling blocks, namely haste, despair, or deception. He who is in a hurry will complete his work neither in a month, nor yet in a year: and in his art it will always be true that the man who is in a hurry will never be without matter of complaint.

If the enemy does not prevail against you by hurry, he will assault you with despondency, and will be constantly putting into your minds discouraging thoughts, how those who seek this art are many, while they are few that find it, and how those who fail are often wiser men than yourself. He will then ask you what hope there can be of your attaining the grand *arcanum*: moreover, he will vex you with doubts whether your master is himself possessed of the secret which he professes to impart to you: or whether he is not concealing from you the best part of that which he knows.

The third enemy against whom you must guard is deceit, and this is perhaps the more dangerous of the two. The servants whom you must employ to feed your furnaces are frequently most untrustworthy. Some are careless and go to sleep when they should be attending to the fire: others are depraved, and do all harm they can. This *arcanum* should be regarded not only as a truly great, but a most holy art. Therefore, if any man desire to reach this great and unspeakable mystery, he must remember that it is obtained not only by the might of man, but by the grace of God, and that not our will or desire, but only the mercy of the Most High, can bestow it upon us. (p. 5)

Thus, the therapist/practitioner/alchemist/ spiritual seeker must first center themselves through meditation or prayer to hold the mindbody soulspirit connection from moment-to-moment in the therapeutic or consulting process. When patients begin their own alchemical journey in their quest toward the gold of Self-hood, they may find themselves in a darkened hell with a diagnosis of a potential debilitating or life-threatening disease, they may complain of migraines or other stress-related disorders, they may be experiencing depression or anxiety or may be undergoing midlife transition in which age or life events have put a halt to who they envisioned themselves to be. The holistic health practitioner needs to maintain the bridge between the physical and psychic manifestations of their distress and the deeper spiritual meaning which can facilitate their transforming the baser material of physical and emotional disease into the healing gold of meaning and sacred union.

This dual nature of suffering is reflected in the first illustration of the *Rosarium Philosophorum* series published in 1550. It is of the mercurial fountain, symbolic of the opus or spiritual work. The liquid has been called "the water of life" but it is also poisonous as well. Illness, be it psychological or physical, and trauma, be it inflicted on the body or psyche, can destroy a person or transform them through healing and deeper meaning and connection to the sacred (see Figure 8-1, *The Alchemy of Mindbody and Soulspirit*).

The experience of the quest toward the gold of Consciousness, is symbolically depicted as the *uroboris*–the oldest symbol` in alchemy representing the opus itself. The snake or dragon devours itself, dies and rises again. This symbol of the self-impregnating and self-destroying manifests the paradox of the therapeutic work. Clients with stress-related autoimmune diseases and others who maintain high levels of tension in their musculature making them susceptible to back strains and pains may just be "uroborically" communicating with themselves. Through self-destroying the individual may be alerted to a process that must be allowed to die in order for healing and well-being to be resurrected from the ashes of their old patterns (see Figure 8-2, The *uroboris*).

	PRIMA MATERIA	SOLUTIO	CALCINATIO	COAGULATIO	SEPARATIO	CONUNCTIO	MORTIFICATIO PUTRIFICATIO	SUBLIMATIO
SYMBOLIC	PRIME MATTER CRASHING	FLOOD DROWNING	BURNING FIRE	SOLIDIFY EARTH MATTER	DIVIDING SEEING FROM A DISTANCE	UNION JOINING OF OPPOSITES	DEATH DESCENT UNDER GROUND	HEIGHT ASCENT
	BLACK	WASHING	HEAT	IMPRISONMENT	DUALITY	MARRIAGE	BLACKNESS	AIR
	MUD	DISSOLVING	JUDGEMENT	DENSITY	JUDGEMENT	COITUS	CORPSE	PURIFICATION
		WATER	RED	LIMITATION			DEFEAT	
MIND	DEPRESSION	INTOXICATING ADDICTIONS	RAGE	FIXATION	DISSOCIATION	ECSTATIC STATE	SUICIDAL	JOY BLISS
	CHAOTIC THOUGHTS	FLOODING OF UNCONSCIOUS MATERIAL	FRUSTRATION	CLOSED SYSTEM EMESHED FAMILY	ISOLATION INSULTATION	GROUP ATTACHMENTS	BORDERLINE DEPRESSION	LOVE COMPASSION
	ANXIETY	PSYCHOSIS	ASSERTION	RIGIDITY	DISTANCING	LOVE/EROS	FEAR	INSPIRED
	INNOCENCE	NARCISSISM		DENIAL	DIFERENTIATION	LOYALTY FAITH	HOPELESS HELPLESS	WISE
			AGGRESSION	OBSESSIVE-COMPULSIVE	AWARENESS	CONTROL OVER OTHERS	LIMBO LIMINALITY	
BODY	DISEASE	CIRCULATORY AILMENTS	FEVER	BODY	SURGERY	SEXUAL DYSFUNCTION	ROTTING GANGREEN	HEALING
	PAIN	URINARY TRACT	RASHES	CONSTIPTATION	EXTRACTION	SEXUAL UNION	SELF MUTILIATION	THE BODY RISES FROM THE BED IN HEALTH
	LOWR GI AILMENTS	LYMPAHATIC SYSTEMS	INFLAMATION	HYPER COAGUATION	DISMEMBER-MENT	ORGAN REPLACEMENT	POISONING	
		DIARRHEA	LOW BACK PAIN	OBESITY	BRAIN/BODY SPLIT		WOUND	
		SWELLING	HEART BURN					
BIOENERGY SOUL/SPIRIT	HELL	BAPTISM	PURGATORY	EUCHARISTIC BODY	MINDFULNESS AWARENESS	PREGNANCY	SUFFERING	SHAMANISM
	CAUGHT IN MAYA	COMMUNION WINE	HELL	BLOCKED CHAKRAS & MERIDIANS	SOUL OUT OF BODY	ONE WITH NATURE	SACRIFICE	ASENSION OF SOUL SPIRIT
		MICKVAH	SACRIFICE		NON ATTACHMENT	SPIRITUAL UNION	SOUL/SPIRIT HAS LEFT THE BODY	ASTRO TRAVELING
						MYSTICAL UNION	BARDO	REVELATION
		BIO ENERGY FIELDS LEAKS	PURIFICATION			SARTORI	SHAMANIC DESCENT	SAMSADHI
		BIO ENERGY FIELD CLEANSING	REDEMPTION			CHRISTIAN COMMUNION		BODHISATTVA

Figure 8-1. The alchemy of mindbody and soulspirit.

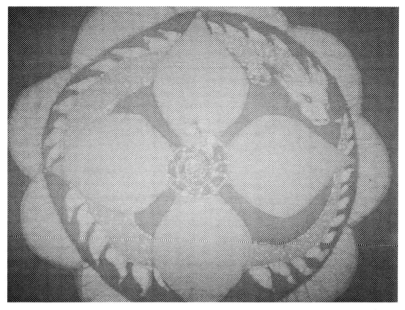

Figure 8-2. The Uroboris.

This is batik created by a client without any understanding of the symbol. This expression of her initial journey points to its completion as well. In the center spiral there emerges a butterfly–the symbol of the soul's transformative power.

Stages of Alchemy

PRIMA MATERIA. In alchemy, the *prima materia* or prime matter is the original substance: the current state of the mindbody and soul spirit of the client. Typically this "base state" is despised, rejected and devaluated. An individual in chronic pain frequently comes to a practitioner hating their pain wanting to do anything but notice it. Likewise others want to get rid of their disease, addiction, depression or anxiety. Some want to dull their minds with drugs or disown their bodies by feeding their yearnings for connections with sugared, caffeinated, nutrition poor diets or beating it with a physical exercise regime that creates hardened armored "fighting machines." Edinger (1985) writes regarding this substance, "those aspects of ourselves most painful and most humiliating are the very ones to be brought forward and worked on" (p. 11).

These clients come in because they have crashed. Their doctors have given them ultimatums. They are "dis-abled" and cannot work. Their psychological state and/or addictions have isolated them from interpersonal relationships. They find themselves with a life-threatening disease. So they come to the holistic health care practitioner/consultant or center seeking to have someone else cure them as in era one medicine. What they find are era II and III practitioners who require them to be mindful and conscious. Hopefully, putting the locus of control in others has been unsuccessful enough so that they are willing to begin the healing process. When this happens, they symbolically experience their own *prima materia*. They may find themselves dreaming about falling into mud, the ocean, or having an uncontrollable bowel movement. Synchronistically, they might experience car trouble, computer crashing, septic problems or other home-related difficulty. In Einsteinian medicine, an appreciation of the interconnectedness of all things is recognized. Even though there is no cause and effect relationship between an individual's distress and the surrounding nonhuman items, a relationship can, nontheless, exist. Many believe the tenant, "there are no coincidences."

SOLUTIO. *Solutio* is the chemical process within the alchemical opus in which the solid is flooded and dissolves. The *aqua permans* or divine water dissolves boundaries. Psychologically this corresponds to an experience of the symbol of the oceanic liquid unconscious washing over the existing personality. Like the annual flooding of the Nile, it refertilizes the psyche and helps expand the consciousness. But sometimes this solutio is more like a title wave as in trauma flashbacks and requires the practitioner to help create a dam that allows for some flow without drowning the limbic system. Some are caught in this state through intoxication as in addictions. Physiologically, others are flooded with viruses and bacteria; still others have chronic swelling.

With too little access to *solutio*, others are caught in a desert-like state. Some find themselves so rational that they are cut off from the expression or flow of their feelings. They are too dammed up. They lack the capacity to cry or gently communicate. Still others find themselves with a malfunctioning circulatory, lymphatic or urinary system. Kidney stones or hardening of the arteries may block the flow. Migraines are produced by a vasodilatation in reaction to initial vasoconstriction. The body needs to be bathed inside and out.

Spiritually, meditation and rituals have been employed to cleanse the soul and energetic fields through holy water and envisioned White Light. Other practices seek to dissolve into the undifferentiated cosmic unity such as found in mystical and Eastern traditions.

CALCINATIO. *Calcinatio* represents the chemical process of burning or heating up. Symbolically, it can be experienced as a dry-

ing up of portions of the oceanic unconscious thus augmenting more landmass to consciousness. Psychologically, calcinatio can appear when the client has "had enough" of a given behavior or life choice, and with assertion 'stop' who they were in order to become who they truly are. Others have an overabundance of calcinatio and in type "A" style, tend to have a "fight" response to everything. Without a sufficient amount of fiery calcinatio, individuals could be victims, responding in flight, faint or freeze.

Somatically speaking, *calcinatio* can be seen in rashes and blushing which occurs when individuals are seen. Individuals with inflammations, heartburn and fevers are experiencing this alchemical process often synchronistically the same time they are psychologically saying "no" to some behavior or person.

Without the needed passion, their ideas, needs and feelings may be lost in the shuffle. The calcinatio may be purifying such as the fire that doesn't consume or spiritually the fires of purgatory that burn off the superfluities of unconsciousness, attachment to desire and/or sin. Spiritual disciplines which include meditation and yogic asanas require the student to notice without judgement and breath into any pain or bodily burning sensations.

COAGULATIO. *Coagulatio* is that alchemical process that is the solidifying or cooling down producing cohesiveness. Psychologically this occurs after the old conscious pattern is dissolved or thrown into the flames of transformation. What remain starts to take shape and have weighted relevance to the individual. It is a process that, by its very nature, encourages embodiment and physical self-calming. Too much coagulatio, however, and individuals can be intractable, stubborn, controlling and rigid. This holding on to history or yesterdays survival behaviors can produce a rigidity that literally has to crack in order for change to occur. Too little and individuals are not grounded. They seem to lack a well-boundaried mediating ego or seem to fly off with inspiration without realistically addressing the feasibility or embodied hard work it would take.

In terms of somatic complaints, they often lack flexibility and are easily injured with strains and back pain. Their arteries are susceptible to clogging, as are their bowels. They eat a great deal of bulk and have a tendency to be overweight. Heaviness fills them psychologically and physically.

Spiritually, they may be caught in a limited understanding. They may concretize or literalize spiritual texts intended for metaphoric understanding. Their chakras or chi may be blocked. Mystical, surrender may be difficult, but, with just enough, they may be able to ground others with calm and presence.

SEPARATIO. *Separatio* is the chemical process that divides and separates the elements. Psychologically this is a crucial dynamic that allows individuals the ability to distinguish between what is truly them and what belongs to another. This boundary helps separate one individual's projections of disowned parts of themselves form another. It also keeps one from accepting or sending transferred former relationships. Intrapsychically, separatio provides the needed awareness so as not to be possessed by complexes that would contaminate the ego's capacity to mediate rationally. Knowing that an inner critic may not have an accurate hold on a person's behavior is vital if the people are to express themselves freely.

Somatically, era I medicine addresses *separatio with* reference to surgical procedures of extractions of tumors and infected organs. Bio-energetically, practitioners clear, balance and align chakras separating what does not belong.

Spiritually, separatio, produces the needed mindfulness that without judgement notices the busy mind and returns to the breath or yogic asana. Separation in Yoga is seen "as an effort to separate the atman (the reality) from the non-atman (The apparent)

and to unite the individual soul with the reality that underlies the universe. This process is called *viveka* which literally means separating out" (Cope, 2000, p. 103) .

CONIUNCTIO. *Coniunctio* represents to the union of opposites. This occurs first in the process of claiming all of who one is. Thus, personal projections are reclaimed and joined. Often this occurs in dreams of interpersonal reunion, marriage or sexual union. If the person has denied this intrapsychic part that needs to be integrated, however, it might initially appear as an angry figure chasing the person or attempting to "get into" their consciousness symbolized by trying to break into their homes or cars. Dreamwork can easily transform them into lovers (Lewis, 1993, 2000). Psychologically that which joins disparate intrapsychic parts of the self or interpersonally joins individuals to one another in partnerships, marriages or among a group can be an experience of communion. Coniunctio allows for the experience of a gestalted totality that is that the whole is more than the sum of its parts. Figure 8-3 from the seventeenth century text depicts the coital union of opposites within an alchemical vessel. The soulspirit baby hovers above waiting for its rebirth. *Eros* or the energy of connection and relatedness comes from the heart and is manifested in such qualities as loyalty, patriotism, a sense of family or community, and what some have called "group mind."

From the perspective of the body, the organs of procreation are targeted with issues of sexuality and sexual dysfunction. The willingness of the body to receive–to join with the breath, food or another. The capacity to become pregnant and to experience the "dual unity" between the mother and infant during the first few months of life requires bodily as well as emotional attunement.

Spiritually, the *mysterium coniunctionis, hieros gamos* or mystical union is the quest of many religious beliefs. From the ecstatic state of St. Francis, to the satori experience

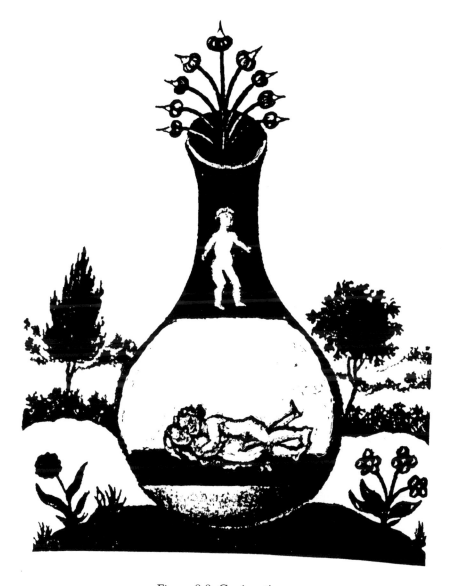

Figure 8-3. Coniunctio.

of at-one-ment, the experience of being one in the Light, to spiritually return to or mystically remember that one is Divine Consciousness is the goal of spiritual alchemy. Mystical union only can be sustained if individuals have first experienced personal union with themselves producing a metaphoric androgyny.

MORTIFICATIO AND PUTRIFICATIO. Once polarized and unconscious parts of the self have been mindfully brought into awareness through separatio, they are then dissolved in *solutio* or brought into union with opposing parts in *coniunctio*. Once in union the gestational process within the psyche brings about a death or *mortificatio* of the former two which can result in a state of limbo in which the person is neither who they were nor who they will be. Individuals in this liminal state describe experiences that prior persona identities feel like they are being stripped away. They report that old ways of thinking, feeling and behaving are going through a decaying process akin to putrefaction or *putrificatio*. Depression is common as individuals are mourning the loss of who they were, but the suffering is not without meaning, for it is part of the transformational process.

This death-like limbo state is midway into the powerful great round of the death-rebirth archetypal theme that occurs every time an individual developmentally moves into an evolved state of being. Individuals die to being a child in order to be born into adulthood. For several years they go through a liminal adolescent phase filled with mood swings as they remove and try on new identities and ways of being like a change in wardrobe.

Mid-life brings with it one of the most profound rites of passage in which everything previously held as fixed is questioned. Once again ways of thinking and feeling, relationships and work identities that individuals have cleaved to like a beloved can be renounced. In this death phase, old survival behaviors can feel rotten as their new more powerful connection to their core brings a deeper integrity toward the new birth of a more whole sense of self.

Middlescence, as well, entails a letting go of the virility and competitive edge for men and the fertile sexual beauty and maternity of the childbearing years for women. This death often brings what has been identified as a "free fall" which can entail a panic. Until men and women realize the freedom this gives them, they can feel as if they have been thrown in to the scrap heap of a youth culture that is fearful of the aging process.

In the final rebirth phase, a woman is able to let go of the childbearer and love goddess images, and claim her croneship. The post-menopausal woman has acquired deep serenity, power, wisdom, and depth of love and spirituality.

In men, being able to let go of the burden

of pretending to fit the male stereotype is a "putrificatio" that eventually feels freeing. Gone is the strength, gone the lithe body and tight stomach, gone the competitive edge. Contemplative, observant and knowing he has come through the retirement panic, i.e. that he was what he did. Now he is truly free. In rebirth, men have no need for excuses anymore and women have no more apologies that have to be said (Lewis, 2000).

On a somatic level, *mortificatio* relates to organ and system malfunction and putrification of the lack of the body to regenerate or recuperate. Heart attacks, amputations, surgical removals of organs, paralysis as well as potential debilitating diseases and cancer can all feel like deaths in terms of individuals' fantasies that they are impenetrable and immortal. Here resurrection and rebirth is more a question of healing rather than curing.

Spiritually, mortificatio is described "as the dark night of the soul." Some endure suffering like Job with trauma and stress coming at them from many directions. It can be a time when individuals can feel that "God is not with them" or is "punishing them by making them sick." It is akin to the journey in Exodus through the wilderness. Often individuals receive just enough to make it through the day. Like manna from heaven, they survive "one day at a time." From a Christian perspective, it can be a time of Lent when Christ was in the wilderness strengthening his faith. For others, the journey is one of deeper suffering as Christ's was on the cross. Here too, individuals can feel that their God has forsaken them.

Others feel an experience of grace, that, like the Catholic parable of "Footprints in the Sand," God is metaphorically carrying them through the dark time. Still others consciously choose this mortificatio rite of passage and enter into monasteries, ashrams, meditation retreats or spiritual quests in nature. They experience the *putrificatio* of the disciplined asceticism of letting go in order to surrender to mystical union and become one with the

Light.

Shamanic traditions often have a phase of initiation which entails the individual leaving the world as is known by them, journeying into the wild or descending into the under-world. Shamanism frequently entails a descent into the underworld to meet power animals, ancestors, or spiritual beings. Here individuals may gestate in deep meditation or receive guidance or instruction The symbolism of dismemberment appears in shamanic drawings. This symbolic experience of being ripped apart only to be reunified anew is a powerful metaphor for spiritual seekers.

SUBLIMATIO. Like Christ's resurrection and Siddhartha's experience of Bodhisattva, the alchemical goal is the gold of the Divine essence. It is literally a rising up which occurs when individuals feel reanimated emotionally, have positive thoughts, and physically feel healthy (Lewis, 1993).

Psychologically, *sublimatio*, is experienced as a revelation, a coming to great clarity or what Jung called the "transcendent function." Individuals can feel like they are being pulled apart, by not knowing which way to choose. Often when individuals surrender to a wiser will, a third dynamic rises up and transcends the other two options. In sublimatio clients and practitioners alike feel light-hearted, elated and joyous. Fourth-heart chakra and fifth-throat chakra support expression of love and compassion. Sublimatio is also reflective in the capacity to see from a distance. This larger perspective allows the seeker to see the bigger picture.

On a body level, sublimatio can literally be seen when persons' spirits rise as they feel well enough to fully live their life. They will "rise" out of the bed. Recovery as well as healing is a sublimatio experience. Individuals who feel that the interventions they and others have been making on their behalf are working will regain a sense of control of their health and return to a sense of well-being.

On a spiritual level, this may be seen as enlightenment, being in the presence of the Light or God, or mystically becoming or reexperiencing the truth that one is one with the Light. Christians refer to an experience of Christ as being "with Him, through Him, and in Him" encompassing the Judaic "I-Thou" relationship that Martin Buber spoke of (with Him and through Him) as well as the mystical ecstatic states of St. Francis of Assisi, Buddha, Roshis and Yogi masters (in Him). For those that are dying, the gold of the alchemical process is rising into eternal grace upon death from the Christian point of view. From the Eastern perspective of rein-carnation, the grand *circulatio* occurs and the *opus* begins again when the soul is returned to earth.

ROLE OF THE HOLISTIC HEALTH PRACTITIONER

Cross-culturally, numerous spiritual practices support the belief that experiences with the transpersonal assist in individuals' healing as well as their spiritual awareness and unfolding. Various sects of Judaism, Christianity, Hinduism, Islam, Buddhism, Taoism, Sikhism, as well as shamanic traditions all adhere to this premise (Smart & Hecht, 1982). Since for the Western world, those in alternative and complimentary medicine have for many become the modern priests and shamans integrating mind body and spirit, it is understandable that many practitioners incorporate a transpersonal paradigm.

Indeed, not only do practitioners have to be sensitive about working with spiritually and culturally diverse individuals, but we must also recognize that, when working within the imagination and consciousness, the expression of an individual's archetypal unconscious can transcend the individual's particular religion and spiritual world views. The holistic health practitioner must then be aware of and facile in a variety of religious traditions, transpersonal beliefs, and spiritual practices. Additionally, the CAM health care provider must not only be conceptually aware but also knowledgeable in the images, themes, and somatizations, that can emerge from the collective unconscious and supra consciousness and out through the portals of the client's mindbody. These so-called psychic and somatic symbols and metaphors of transformation (Jung, CW, vol.) as well as rituals, mythelogems, and rites of passage must, with humility, be understood and properly utilized for the profound vehicles of healing they are.

> When therapists sit in relation to the archetypal, transpersonal wisdom of wholeness can flow into and through their body and into the therapy vessel and help constellate the patient's own connection to the wisdom of spiritual consciousness. Embodied expression from both the personal and archetypal unconscious is needed in order for transformation to occur. The dance between the personal and archetypal is, thus, a crucial pas de deux in anyone's life who seeks the human quest toward consciousness. (Lewis, 1993, p.175)

It is strongly advised that all practitioners utilizing a spiritual perspective be involved in some form of spiritual discipline or religious practice themselves. For example, if holistic health facilitators employ yoga or any form of meditation in their work with clients, they need to have an integral practice in their own life.

CONCLUSION

The influence of spirituality in holistic health occurs when both practitioner/consultant and client have a connection to themselves. This first requires knowing the core self or child within. From this connection, individuals may then be able to open themselves to that which is eternal within them: to their soul, divinity or Light. This access is the threshold to transpersonal grace. Individuals may pray, receive inner guidance and healing. They may be able to experience presence and sustain expanded mindful consciousness. Living in moment-to-moment presence, nonattached from having to repeat their history or needing the future to be a certain way, individuals are then able to feel and express loving acceptance. Understanding that everything changes, individuals can then surrender to the alchemical cycles of evolution. Their sphere of influence expands from loving compassion toward self, to an intimate other, to family, community, nature, and the planet and finally to that which is fundamental to all that exists.

What matters more than curing in holistic health is healing. Healing can only occur through grace. People come to holistic health practitioners because they don't want to suffer any more, because they want their pain, fear, physical or mental distress to go away. What they discover is something far more powerful and significant. It is that they are neither their pain nor their suffering, nor is the holistic health care provider going to bring them happiness. That is an inside job that emerges with a deep inner path, life purpose, and spiritual connection.

REFERENCES

Arts in Psychotherapy Journal. (1992). Vol. 15, No. 4.

Barber, T. (1976). *Advances in altered states of consciousness & human potential.* New York: Psychological Dimensions, Inc.

Boorstein, S. (1991). *Transpersonal Psychotherapy.* Stanford, CA: JTP Books.

Carter-Haar, B. (1975). What is psychosynthesis? *Synthesis,* Vol. 1, No. 2, pp. 115–118.

Edinger, E. (1985). *Anatomy of the psyche.* LaSalle, IL: Open Court.

Edinger, E. (1982). *Ego and archetype.* New York: Penguin Books.

Harner, M. (1982). *The way of the shaman.* New York: Bantam Books.

Jerusalem Bible.

Jung, C.G. (1969). *The archetypes and the collective unconscious. CW, Vol. 9* Part 1. Princeton, NJ: Princeton University Press.

Jung, C.G. (1963). *Mysterium coniunctionis. CW, Vol. 14.* Princeton, NJ: Princeton University Press.

Jung, C.G. (1969). *Symbols of transformation. CW Vol. 5.* Princeton, NJ: Princeton University Press.

Lewis, P. (1993). *Creative transformation: The healing power of the arts.* Wilmette, IL: Chiron Publishing.

Lewis, P. (1996). Depth psychotherapy in dance/movement therapy. *American Journal of Dance Therapy*, Vol. 18, No. 2, Fall/Winter, 95–114.

Lewis, P. (1986). *Theoretical approaches in dance-movement therapy.* Vol. II. Dubuque, IA: Kendall/Hunt Pub.

Lewis, P. (1988). The transformative process in the imaginal realm. *Arts in Psychotherapy Journal.* Vol. 15. pp. 309–316.

Lewis. P. (1992). The transference and counter-transference in arts psychotherapy. *Arts in Psychotherapy Journal.* Vol. 15, No. 4.

Lewis, P. & Johnson, D. (2000). *Current approaches in drama therapy.* Springfield, IL: Charles C Thomas Pub.

Loori, A. & Daido, J. (1996). Husuan-sha's one bright pearl: Dharma discourse. *Mountain Record.* Fall.

Pelletier, K. (2000). *The best alternative medicine.* New York: Simon & Schuster.

Sagan, L. (1987). *The health of nations.* New York: Basic Books.

Smart, N. & Hecht, R. (1982). *Sacred texts of the world: A universal anthology.* New York: Crossroad Publishing Company.

Walsh, R. & Vaughan, F. (1993). *Paths beyond ego the transpersonal vision.* Los Angeles: Jeremy P. Tarcher/Perigee Books.

Chapter 9

SPIRITUAL HEALING IN ERA III MEDICINE

CHARLOTTE GREENE

CULTURES AND RELIGIONS in all times and places have grappled with the reality of spiritual healing. On all continents spiritual healing has emerged in one form or another and this has led to a wide variety of ever-evolving healing practices. Despite what current thought dominated the times, it has maintained its presence as a valuable and viable force of healing.

There has never been one single form of spiritual healing that is endemic to all people. Everyone has his or her own interpretation. There continues to be contention as to who really understands the "truth" of this form of healing. The questions that are asked today about its origin and methods are not new. As long as spiritual healing has existed, the same questions reemerge over and over again with great passion from the true seekers or critics. What is spiritual healing? How does it relate to current thought today? What was it in the past? What are healing energies? Where do they come from? What is a spiritual healer? Can anyone heal? What is the documenting evidence?

The search for this knowledge has taken many into the history of religions, sciences, and spiritual cultures from around the world. In the last three centuries, there has been much debate between scientific and spiritually-based organizations as to what really

constitutes healing. Since the sixties, people have become increasingly dedicated to incorporating more holistic, spiritual themes into their practices. The personal experiences of these seekers have led them away from the mechanistic traditional medical model to a more spiritual perspective. Some compliment medicine while others consider themselves alternative. There have always been extreme positions in the defining process of "healing" with the majority somewhere in the middle seeking their own understanding without the need to depend on others to define it for them. Today, spiritual healing is a vital component of many alternative and complementary practices.

SPIRITUAL HEALING: A DEFINITION

At the National Institute of Health's Alternative Medicine web site has a link to *Expanded Dictionary of Metaphysical Healers: Alternative-Medicine, Paranormal Healing, and Related Methods.* Jack Raso, the director at the American Council on Science defines spiritual healing as a "Form of channeling and energy medicine (vibrational medicine) that allegedly involves the 'transference' (commonly through the hands) of 'healing energy' from its spiritual source to one who needs help. Its theory posits a 'spiritual body.'"

The American Heritage Dictionary definition of healing is, "Heal: To restore to health or soundness; cure. To restore (a person) to spiritual wholeness" "of having the nature of spirit; not tangible or material. Of, concerned with, or affecting the soul." And 'spiritual' is defined as "Of, relating to, consisting of, or having the nature of spirit: not tangible or material. Of, concerned with, of affecting the soul. Of, from, or pertaining to God; deific. Of or belonging to a church or religion; sacred." 'Spirit' is defined as "The vital principle or animating force traditionally believed to be within living beings. The soul as considered to be departing from the body at death." Spiritual healing, according to this definition, is healing that restores a person to good health and the source of the healing is the 'spirit' found throughout all life.

> Never the spirit was born;
> the spirit shall cease to be never;
> Never the time it was not;
> End and beginning are dreams;
> Earthless and deathless and changeless
> abideth the spirit forever;
> Death hath not touched it at all,
> dead though the house of seems!
> *Song Celestial*, Bhagavad-Gita

SPIRIT

The word "spirit" or "soul" seem at times to be interchangeable yet these words are a common denominator to which people can relate. Even though spirit and soul translate into many other words depending on the culture or religious belief system their meaning remains the same. The spirit of spiritual refers to the source of the healing power and has been translated by various belief systems as Life Force, God, Buddha, Infinite Spirit, Eternal Light, Collective Consciousness, etc.

No matter how it is defined, it is generally agreed that spirit is the energy behind the healing.

The belief in Western culture that healing is not just about the body, or the mind, or the soul, but about these three components working in harmony with one another to create maximum health, has grown since the sixties. Carl Jung suggested that there is a natural drive in all people towards wellness. This "urge to oneness" or individuation is quintessentially spiritual and underlies the visions of all great religious traditions. It is the need to return or somehow reconnect with the Absolute, the Divine, with God. This urge towards greater wholeness is the most elemental quality of prayer and prayerfulness–the feeling that one is being drawn toward something higher, greater, and deeper (Jones, 1999).

This urge seems to be reflected in those who are doing so much to help those in the traditional medical field to awaken themselves to a more integral connection to the divine. This is the struggle of transition: to be freed from limited thinking, to carry the old ways into the new, and to be strong enough to stand up to those who would suffocate their research and efforts to bring humanity into a greater state of consciousness.

At Harvard Medical School's Department of Continuing Education, the Mind/Body Medical Institute of Beth Israel Deaconess Medical Center and Harvard Medical School, Dr. Herbert Benson began offering clinical training programs in mind/body medicine. His focus is on the integration of modern medicine, cognitive therapy, nutrition, exercise, relaxation techniques, spirituality and self-empowerment. When speaking about spirituality in *The Powers and Biology of Belief,* he states "We seem to be hard-wired to believe in something 'beyond' as a species because it has survival value." Benson feels that individuals have a biological need to believe in God.

Dr. Benson discovered that after a traditional medical foundation he still had some questions about healing that led him to study and to write about the mind's function in the healing process. For him, healing was beginning to take on a new form. In his mind something else was calling him to move beyond the traditional science of healing and to begin to question other aspects of the "self" as to their importance in getting well. Encouraged by Harvard University to pursue this area of thought, he wrote *The Relaxation Response* in 1975 based on his findings in his study of meditation. In essence, through his extensive studies at Harvard's Thorndike Laboratory and at Beth Israel Hospital in Boston, he was able to explain how the mind plays a crucial part in the healing process. His understanding of the history of cultural and religious practices is that meditation can control the stress response of the body and thus measurable decreases in heart rate, oxygen consumption, rate of breathing and blood flow could be observed. In his book he states, "The relaxation response is not a technique. It's a physiological state brought about by many techniques."

ERA III MEDICINE

This mind/body/spirit healing, which is known worldwide under the general heading of spiritual healing is becoming more of an integral part of many individuals' lives. The scientific medical paradigm continues to transition to a fuller appreciation in how all aspects, the body, mind, and soul work together. Larry Dossey, M.D.'s *Reinventing Medicine* gives historical insight into the evolution of healing from the eighteen hundreds to today (1999).

Dossey studied traditional medicine and helped to establish the Dallas Diagnostic Association. He served as Chief of Staff of Medical City Dallas Hospital. During this time he witnessed what many call "miracle cures" for medical conditions that defied traditional medicine. His interest turned to the search for a meaning of the interaction of the mind, body and spirit. He began to study religion, philosophy, meditation, oriental literature, parapsychology and quantum physics. He now explains how modern medicine since the eighteen hundreds is divided into three separate parts called eras (see Chapter 1, Figure 1-1).

Era III medicine expands mind/body medicine into many other levels of consciousness. It includes contact with the collective unconscious. Era III paradigms defy the traditional thinking of time and space. This expanded paradigm is identified as temporal nonlocality. The terms "local" and "nonlocal" come from physics, and were chosen so that they would relate more to those in the medical field. Dossey felt terms such as "one mind," "universal mind," or "collective consciousness" have too much "metaphysical baggage."

Spiritual healing thrives in this "nonlocal" category. He sees that the mind can work outside of the body. This nonlocal mind has the ability to travel through space and time without physical boundaries. Healing prayer can be directed to someone at any distance, as distance is not an issue. Era III opens the door to the creativity and intuition of the eternal spirit.

INTUITION AND MEDICAL INTUITIVES

Intuition has been describe as originating from the: "higher self," "higher consciousness," "creative mind," "essence," or "Godlike energy." Wisdom from this intuitive power can help an individual heal the self– the whole self: mind, body, and spirit. This is the faculty that all spiritual healers develop to some degree. Overcoming fear of ridicule, being wrong, and/or judgment from the self or others have been stumbling blocks in the development of healers for a long time. Many feel that intuition originates from an inner source, a higher self, expanded consciousness, soul or spirit.

The term "medical intuitives" is currently used to describe those who in the past have been called psychic diagnosticians, mediums, spiritual healers, and telepathic-clairvoyants. Medical intuitives are able to attune themselves to a person's physical, mental, and spiritual conditions and intuitively sense what the problem is. Some are considered highly intuitive medical doctors, nurses, psychiatrists, psychologists, and energy healers; others are specifically identified as medical intuitives and are consultants in the traditional and alternative health field.

As has been stated, intuition is a natural component of an individual's psyche. If it is developed as a medical tool, it can be of great service to all beings, the same as any other healing ability that one has. Some do not limit their diagnostic skills just to humans, as once this ability is developed it can be used with any form of life. Because the human sensory abilities develop in different ways from person to person, there exists a wide variety of approaches to this field. Sessions are held in person or from a distance, over the phone or by letter. Most intuitives only require a name, age, and/or address for the person they are treating; some need to hear the person's voice or be in the physical presence of the person. The attunement is typically to the energy in the levels of consciousness surrounding and permeating the physical body.

The following are some well-known medical intuitives:

Caroline Myss

Caroline Myss, Ph.D., a medical intuitive, states, "Intuition is the ability to interpret the energetic information that is always a part of every aspect of life and to use that energetic information for making wise choices—not safe, but wise. Intuition does not promise an end to all pain; in fact pain and pleasure should not even factor into our understanding of intuition. Intuitive ability has much

more to do with learning to rely upon our natural wisdom than it does with developing a means of protection." Myss believes that illness is a fact of life and that there is great wisdom in learning to respond to the innate intuitive sense that individuals are in a situation that is causing them to lose power. She stresses that individuals must be courageous and that the "biggest block to intuitive development is the fear that comes with being clear-sighted, because clear-sightedness means that you must make clear choices. Choice means change, and change frightens people even more than dying" (Emery, 1999, p. 34).

Myss uses her highly developed intuition to diagnose illness and disease. She calls herself a "medical intuitive" and describes her recognition of her abilities as gradually developing over time. Her words easily mirror what many others have said about their intuitive abilities. After 14 years of practice with the support of her colleagues, she began to teach others how to develop their own abilities. Her resources are from several spiritual traditions including the Hindu chakras, the Christian sacraments, and the Kabala's Tree of Life. Through the help and collaboration with Norman Shealy, M.D., Ph.D., founder of the American Holistic Medical Association, she began to heighten her awareness of the exact vibrations of a specific disease and its location in a person's physiology. Each illness and body organ, she learned, has its own "frequency" or "vibrational pattern" (p. 21). From this awareness, she was able to accurately diagnose medical conditions that Shealy brought to her; and subsequently, developed her practice as a medical intuitive. Her style is not unlike many spiritual healers, who use an intuitive diagnostic process during their work.

Myss has learned to discern among mind, body and spiritual energies. "Experiences that carry emotional energy in our energy systems include: past and present relationships, both personal and professional; profound or traumatic experiences and memories; and belief patterns and attitudes, including all spiritual and superstitious beliefs. The emotions from these experiences become encoded in our biological systems and contribute to the formation of our cell tissue, which then generates a quality of energy that reflects those emotions. These energy impressions form an energy language, which carries literal and symbolic information that a medical intuitive can read" (p. 34).

Positive as well as negative energy registers as a memory in cell tissue as well as in the energy field. Sometimes the energy images are quite literal and sometimes they arc symbolic. They all emit a vibration that can be translated into words. An area of the body that is not well will emit a frequency that is not in tune with the rest of the body (p. 37).

In Era III medicine, Myss is a pioneer in the field of energy medicine and human consciousness. Medical intuition can help physicians and other heath practitioners treat the underlying cause as well as the symptoms.

Edgar Casey

One of the leading medical intuitives of all times was Edgar Cayce (1877–1945). At the time he was called a telepathic-clairvoyant. A telepathic person is one who is psychic or intuitive and a clairvoyant is one who sees clearly into other levels of consciousness. For 43 years he helped many to find what the cause of their illness was and to recommend a cure. This he often did in a trance state. Trance states are similar to hypnotic states, where the mind is not in contact with the physical world. In this condition appearing to be asleep, he would bring information from "universal sources" (those in the spirit world who had some knowledge of a particular condition).

He was called the "sleeping prophet," as he often appeared to be asleep except for the sound of his voice. "He described events of the future with almost as great a clarity as he discussed the physiological functioning of an ailing human body that might be 2000 miles away. In this state he apparently had communication with the unconscious minds of people everywhere but specifically with the mind of that person for whom he was giving a reading (Carter & McGarey, 1972).

McGarey MD, comments, "His work with illnesses of the human body has provided me with the most fascinating and potentially important information that I have found in the 14,500 readings he gave over a period of some 40 years. Some 9000 of these readings dealt with human illness and its correction. The manner in which he was able to describe conditions with such accuracy—illnesses and points of strength of which he had no conscious awareness—has within it implications that are not easily avoided to all those involved in the field of healing. I realize that most physicians do not relish the idea of commenting publicly on the validity of psychic data—especially when this is dealt with in depth. But then most medical doctors have never either studied or experienced psychic happenings. However, one studying the Cayce material must at some point deal with these concepts of the unusual qualities of the mind and the destiny of the soul as a timeless voyager in putting to rest the unique phenomenon that Mr. Cayce presents to us in his life and experiences" (1972, p. 13).

Cayce's psychic ability appears to have emerged quite spontaneously. At twenty-one, Cayce developed a gradual paralysis of the throat that threatened the loss of his voice. When doctors were unable to find a cause for this condition, he entered a deep hypnotic sleep. Once in a self-induced trance, he was able to contact spiritual sources that recommended a cure, which successfully repaired his throat muscles. It was after this experience that he was able to enter this trance at will to give medical readings. These psychic readings constitute one of the largest and most impressive accounts of psychic perception to emanate from a single individual. Together with their records, correspondence, and reports, they have been cross-indexed under thousands of subject headings and housed at the Virginia Beach headquarters of the Association for Research and Enlightenment (A.R.E.), which Cayce founded in 1931. The readings are available to anyone who wishes to explore this vast storehouse. They are used by thousands of people each year, including students, writers, investigators, practitioners of holistic medicine, and psychologists (see Edgar Cayce Books World Database: *http://www.edgarcayce.com*).

Harry Edwards

Harry Edwards, a popular healer from England, had another approach. His belief was that the healing guides alone are the administrators of the diagnosis and healing energies. "It is the guide who is able to make the diagnosis in order to know the character of the healing energies the patient needs. Thus, the diagnosis is the responsibility of the guide and not the healer. This leads to the view, that it is not essential for the healer to make a diagnosis. At the same time the healer wishes to play an intelligent part in the healing, and the suggestions that follow may provide the means of attaining this" (Edwards, 1963, p. 90).

The means by which healers receive knowledge of the cause and nature of the sickness will vary according to the manner in which the guides can use the healer. A common form of diagnosing the area of trouble is when the healer places his hand over the affected part. Both the healer and the patient become aware of a strong heat emanating from the healer's hands that appears to penetrate into the patient's body. This heat is healing energy and cannot be measured with a thermometer even though both feel it. Through this connection of energy the hands relay information to the mind of the healer. The guides have the means of knowing the cause and nature of the disease or trouble and to transmit healing energies.

There is another aspect that can be associated with "diagnosis." This is when some healers appear to "take on" the conditions (symptoms) of the patients. Edwards and others are concerned about this method, as these can be difficult impressions to handle. In many healing practices students are taught about "spiritual boundary issues." They learn to receive information in a manner that will not harm them. Once there has been sufficient training and practice, spiritual healers seldom "hold" symptoms within their body. They know that once they feel them they can use the power of their mind to release them.

INDIGENOUS AND SHAMANIC HEALING PRACTICES

In *The Power to Heal*, Smolan, Moffit, and Naythons M.D (1990) explain some of the indigenous history of spiritual healing "Health is a state of balance, of harmony, and for most societies it is something holy. As a result, traditional medicine acts on two quite different levels. Ailments may be treated by herbal baths and massage, the administration of medicinal plants, physical isolation of the patient in a sacred place and, in certain traditions, an animal sacrifice so that the patient may return to the earth a gift of life's vital energy. But almost invariably it is intervention on the spiritual plane that ultimately determines a patient's fate, and for this the healers must often sail away on the wings of a trance to distant realms where they may work their deeds of magical rescue."

They continue, "For the Native American shaman the vehicle to the gods is the sweat lodge, the rhythm of drums, the pain of ordeal, and the arrows of the magic plants. The Huichol ingest peyote, the tracks of the little deer. Tibetan healers meditate the fate of their patients by ritually transforming themselves into Tantric deities capable of influencing the passage of time. African priests also become gods, often demonstrating their omnipotence by handling burning embers. In the high Andes of Peru, traditional healers divine the future and diagnose aliments by eating the coca leaves, a sacred practice reserved only for those who have survived a lightning strike. In such traditions, there is no rigid separation between the sacred and the secular, and thus every act of the healer becomes a prayer for the entire community, every ritual a form of collective preventive medicine" (1990, p. 12).

MEDIUMS, CHANNELERS AND THE HISTORY AND PRACTICE OF WESTERN SPIRITUALISM

March 31, 1848 marks the beginning of Modern Spiritualism. All major religions in history began with some form of psychic, mystical or intuitive event. Spiritualism was no exception although it was rather unique. In upper state New York, the Fox sisters experienced such unusual physical phenomena that the public flocked to their home to experience and reexperience the same remarkable event.

Over a period of time the two sisters devised a simple communicational code with the source of rappings created by a non-physical source. By this means they were able to hold a "conversation" with a man in spirit who told them that his name was Charles B. Rosna. He had been a traveling salesman staying with some people called Bell, in that same cottage, some years before the Fox family had moved in. He told the Fox sisters that he had been murdered, that his stock and personal belongings had been stolen and that his body was buried in the cellar. He also mentioned a tin box that was with his body. This event stimulated the curiosity of many people who were interested in similar phenomena and soon they too were able to communicate with spirits that

were traditionally felt to be "dead." Even though there was much skepticism and the Fox sisters were considered to be frauds by many investigators, in 1904, the cellar of the Fox home was dug up and the peddler's remains were found along with the tin box.

Thus, many had their consciousness awakened to the fact that there was life beyond the death of the body and that one could communicate with those who had passed. These "communicators" are called "mediums" and the skill of this form of communication is called "mediumship." People gathered together in "circles" and used a medium to receive messages from their loved ones. The communication skills began to include other methods to translate messages. Some mediums can see spirits in the spirit world, others can hear them, and others just receive sensory impressions that they translate into words. Many employ a combination of these skills in their work. Spiritualist mediums were enormously popular for many years in the 1800s, but lost favor in the heyday of the mechanistic Newtonian era. This example of Era III consciousness now called mediumship or channeling is experiencing an international revival.

Even though mediumship has sometimes been equated with "parlor games" by critics, Spiritualist mediums take their gift quite seriously. Through spiritual meditation, they are guided into other levels of consciousness where they receive information on behalf of another. These guides are spirits who are gifted in communication and wish to be of service on earth.

In India, it is common to speak with the divas (good spirit), and pitris (or departed human spirits). In China, the worship of ancestors is still practiced. Western beliefs date back to Plato who postulated that each person has a particular spirit with him to be his tutor and guide during mortal life. Judeo-Christian faith upholds the interventions of the Lord or angels of the Lord in human affairs.

Spiritualism as a Religious Belief

Spiritualism began as a movement and then became an organized religion. It seeks to encourage individuality of the expression of one's spirituality. It does not ask anyone to believe based on faith alone. In this religion is a belief in "Infinite Intelligence." This denotes a nonpersonal, nonphysical word that means the same as "God." God is not a "he" or a "she" but is simply the "intelligent consciousness" or "spirit" that is the motivating force throughout all of life. Spiritualists recognize the infinite intelligence and the creator of natural law as God yet honor the beliefs of all religions. This God is a loving God, not an angry God of the past that judges and punishes if they don't behave as the religion dictated. Spiritualism allows for the study and discussion of all religions and uses the resulting wisdom in their lectures and books. They state that they have no dogma or creed, but focus on 10 principles that they live by and that these principles are not cast in stone, but can be changed at any time by the majority. One such truth is the belief that religion's spiritual purpose is to bring one closer to the "source," the infinite intelligence that many call God. How they get there is up to each one. It isn't necessary to be involved in mediumship or healing to belong to Spiritualism.

Spiritualism teaches tolerance and compassion for all people and for all of life. These are important attributes to develop as a spiritual healer. Healing in Spiritualism began in the mid 1900s when groups of people wanted to include healing into the Sunday services. Not all services are conducted in churches. Many rent other places such as halls or meet in someone's home. Training then began for healers. Healing sanctuaries opened and flourished. When the Era I medical model became a more commanding force spiritual healing stepped into the background but did not disappear. Orthodox science and traditional religions were increasingly antagonistic to some forms of mediumship and healing and convinced many to abandon this way of life. Thus Era I medicine took hold for a while. But this did not last and as the shift into Era II occurred, Spiritualism began to be popular again.

In a general sense, Spiritualists believe that all people can heal and have "spirit" within them. They mirror the teachings of Harry Edwards, the English spiritual healer/medium, and others that stress that all one needs to do is recognize the "desire to help" and to develop their spiritual selves to become an effective spiritual healer; prayer and meditation being important aspects of this sacred process.

Spiritual Healing and Mediumship in Spiritualism

Harry Edwards, the famous English Spiritual Healer, believed that anyone could do healing work. For as Jesus is said to have proclaimed in the New Testament, "Go forth and heal as I do," meant to him that the healing power was available to all. His books contain not only spiritual guidelines for healing but also references to anatomy, legal regulations, ethical considerations, hygienic procedures, healing tools, and other techniques that have been used in the past during the healing treatments.

He states that a spiritual healer is one that has the innate desire for the sick to be made well and so "they give their love and sympathy, thus helping to create the right 'conditions' to assist the healing." That is, he speaks about creating a comfortable atmosphere for the patient ensuring contact from the spiritual energies to the spirit-self of the patient. Edwards looks at the whole picture of healing not just the act of giving and receiving (1974, p. 103).

HANDS-ON SPIRITUAL HEALING

Hands are used to treat the area of sickness as Edward suggests "they will be the terminal for the transmission of the healing force." Here the maintenance of attunement to the spiritual source and to the spirit of the patient is key. Many forms of hands-on healing use passes and specific hand positions to heal; however, it is the "intent" of the healing process that does the healing. The rest is for the benefit of the healer and not necessarily for the benefit of the healing process. In the laying-on-of hands, the hands become an extension of the healer's mind that focuses on and channels from the spiritual realm.

DISTANT SPIRITUAL HEALING

"Absent Healing," or "Distant Healing" part of Dossey's Era lll medicine occurs when the healer is a distance from the patient. Some call it "Divine Healing" or "Prayer Healing." It is considered to be intangible or impersonal by some. Individuals have written to healers such as Edwards who administered his Absent Healing Method. Since 1948, over 15 million healing letters have been received and answered. Edwards (1974) was not interested in being studied by scientists but considered his success substantiated and recorded the thousands of letters he received to validate the results of his work.

Era III medicine is common to all religions through various forms of prayer. It has been used for centuries to ask for healing in the form of divine intervention. Many spiritual healers also emphasize the importance of "self-healing" either through prayer or hands-on healing.

SPIRITUAL ATTUNEMENT

"The act of healing, which produces a change within the physical body, demands not only knowledge of the manipulation of spirit forces but also their coordination with the physical forces that govern the human anatomy. We are, therefore, forced to the conclusion that the operating mind must be a non-physical one; a spirit mind that has acquired greater wisdom than man possesses. These spirit operators we call the 'healing guides'. What we can do (as healers), and this is of primary importance, is to train ourselves to attune to Spirit and so become more useful instruments of the spirit healing operators." (Edwards, 1974, pp. 78–79)

He emphasizes the need for attunement to establish a state of affinity with the spirit guides. Meditation and prayerful thoughts addressed to God is the way to attune to the healing guides. He stresses that an altered state of grace be engaged when communicating to the spirit world for healing or for mediumship. This quality of the healing experience was fundamental to his philosophy.

"Attunement is a subtle state between consciousness and spirit awareness, very difficult to describe in words. Attunement is so natural that there are rarely any physical symptoms by which to recognize it. One does not get hot or cold, or feel any physical sensation. There should, however, be consciousness of a feeling different from normality, which is often more readily appreciated when returning to normal full consciousness after emerging from the state of attunement" (Edwards, 1974, p. 85). During the process of attunement one's intuition becomes heightened. Awareness is developed of "finer energies." The word "intuition" and "psychic" are interchangeable.

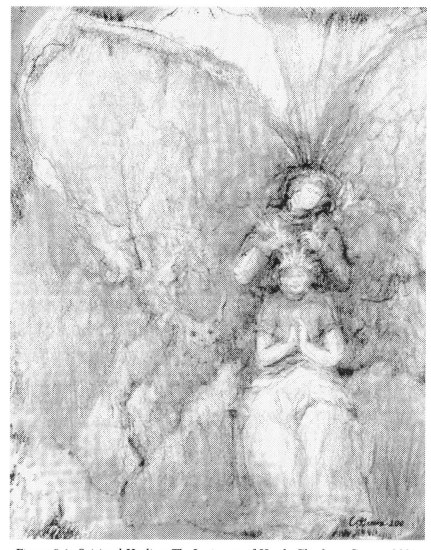

Figure 9-1. *Spiritual Healing: The Laying-on-of-Hands,* Charlotte Greene 2001.

MEDITATION

Meditation, often experienced as spiritual attunement, is an important component of spiritual healing. It was first recorded in 1500 B.C. from the Vedas, scriptures that reflect the ancient meditation practices in India. In the Eastern tradition, meditation is a process by which one attains "enlightenment." It is a growth-producing experience along intellectual, philosophical, and, most importantly, existential (soul healing) dimensions.

Through meditation the brain's order of processing appears to give way to the intuitive mode producing extraordinary awareness. It is during this time of awareness that one is able to fully connect to one's spirit and access the healing energies. This is an important aspect of all spiritual healing practices both for the healer and the receiver. Some call it contacting the "higher self." For some, meditation has been experienced as prayer.

Benson sees meditation as a form of healing and states:

- A meditation that does not bring in the life of spirit is no meditation.

- A meditation that does not lead to growth of character or creativity is no meditation.

- A meditation that does not lead to soul healing is not mediation.

- The goal of meditation is not just to get more ideas–it is to obtain the power to think!

- The goal of mediation is not just to get more good feelings–it is to tap the power to love!

- The goal of mediation is not just to slow down our heartbeat or breathe more deeply–it is to contact the power to act!

NATURAL LAW

"Natural Law" is a term that is used quite often in reference to "God" and also to science. It was the nature of the period prior to Era I to often refer to "life" following God's law and that science interpreted God's law as scientific reality. Due to the drastic transformation of how scientists viewed "science" during Era I compared to what was "known" to be true before that, there was much confusion about the definition of science and its role in religion. Even though Era I brought a change in the definition of "natural law" many did not change their own beliefs and continue today to view Natural Law as it was prior to and during the 1800s.

In *Having Their Way with Science*, Erika Dyson (1997) discusses the relationship of science to religion. She states, "By approaching the natural world as the creation of a benevolent God, and by insisting that science was the best way of discovering God's will within that creation, nineteenth-century scientists offered rational support of Christianity while putting themselves in a position of social importance with Protestant America. The religious significance of scientists' work gave Protestant Christians ample reason to support science and to hold scientists accountable for conducting their

research properly, as shoddy work could have damaging theological consequences. This was the science to which American Spiritualists appealed, a science already deeply invested in supporting religious ideas and which presented itself as answerable to Protestant Christian theology" (p. 22).

Today, other belief systems as well as Spiritualism base their paradigms of health and healing upon a universal divine or conscious natural laws or principles. Deepak Chopra, (1994) speaks of Natural Law. He blends physics and philosophy, the practical and the spiritual, venerable Eastern wisdom and cutting-edge Western science.

The following represent some of the most common Natural Laws:

The Law of Giving and Receiving

The universe operates "through dynamic exchange. Nothing is static. Your body is in dynamic and constant exchange with the body of the universe; your mind is dynamically interacting with the mind of the cosmos; your energy is an expression of cosmic energy" (Chopra, 1994, 27). "In every seed is the promise of thousands of forests. But the seed must not be hoarded; it must give its intelligence to the fertile ground. Through its giving, its unseen energy flows into material

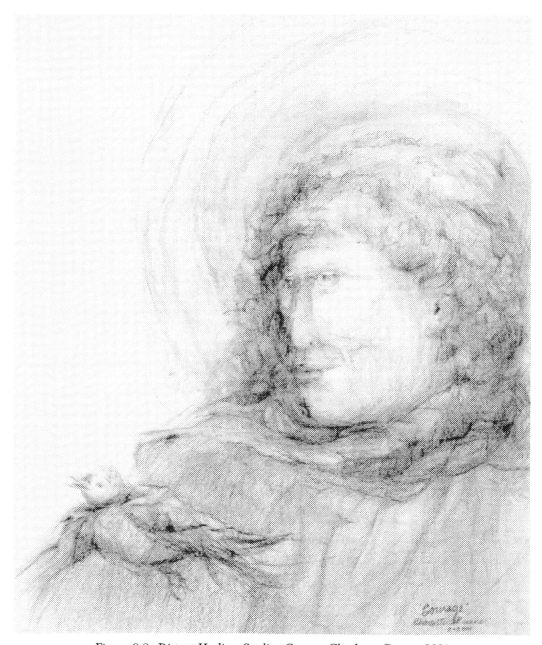

Figure 9-2. *Distant Healing: Sending Courage,* Charlotte Greene 2001.

manifestation." The more you give, the more you will receive because you will keep the abundance of the universe circulating. He describes "abundance" as not just being about material wealth, but the "abundance of all things" including one's spiritual path.

The Law of Cause and Effect

Thoughts whether they be prayers or limited beliefs have the power to transform. Discussing the Laws of Cause and Effect, Chopra and others talk about the choice individuals make in their everyday life that affect themselves and others and emphasizes the responsibility they have to make the choices that will do no harm. This stresses that the thoughts and behaviors that an individual generates into the universal energy field of which everything is a part affects everything. Thus, personal responsibility and clarity of intention is vital.

The Law of Pure Potentiality

"The source of all creation is pure consciousness . . . pure potentiality seeking expression from the unmanifest to the manifest. And when we realize that our true Self is one of pure potentiality, we align with the power that manifests everything in the universe" (Chopra, p. 7). He also calls this law the Law of Unity, as underlying the potential of the diversity of life is the unity of the undifferentiated totality. This potential and knowledge of unity frees all who are conscious from suffering and fear.

The Law of Least Effort

"Nature's intelligence functions with effortless ease . . . with carefreeness, harmony, and love. And when we harness the forces of harmony, joy, and love, we create success and good fortune with effortless ease" (Chopra, p. 51). Staying in the present moment and focusing on the "here and now" allows individuals the experience of "life flowing with effortless ease." This law encourages individuals to accept what is and take responsibility for perceived problems in every moment. In this way there is the possibility for transformation.

The Law of Intention and Desire

"Inherent in every intention and desire is the mechanics for its fulfillment . . . intention and desire in the field of pure potentiality have infinite organizing power. And when

we introduce an intention in the fertile ground of pure potentiality, we put this infinite organizing power to work for us" (Chopra, p. 65).

It is this law that many spiritual healers experience as key. When their intent is to use spiritual forces to heal and to do no harm, and to send the healing energies to the cause of the problem, the result is that this infinite organizing power works for us.

The Law of Attraction

The Law of Attraction basically states that similar vibrations attract one another. These vibrations can be from material objects, thought and emotional expression, as well as spiritual energies from many levels of consciousness. "Like attracts like" what you think is reflected back to you. All thought is energy. All energy influences and attracts its own vibration. This can have positive or negative effects. "Be careful what you ask for you may just get it" is an old adage. Psychotherapists have long known that if a client cannot imagine a positive future, they will probably not avail themselves of it. Conversely, if a future can be imagined, it will most certainly aid in its unfolding.

The Law of Balance

Everything in life seeks equilibrium. This law applies to all living things. In healing, the spiritual energy goes to the cause of the problem so that balance is restored in the mind, body, and spirit.

The Law of Freedom

Individuals have the freedom to choose how they respond to any given situation. Physically they may not have choice, but emotionally and spiritually they do. This law is also reflected in the Law of Cause and Effect.

The Law of Motion or Vibration

Everything is in continuous motion. Everything is vibrating at a different rate. This applies to thought and physical matter. Healing energy can affect the vibrations of diseased parts of the body and help those parts to change their vibration to a more harmonious state. In the process of communicating with spirit, meditation helps to change the vibration of the mind, body and spirit. The focus then moves away from the slower vibration of the physical world to the faster vibration of the spirit world.

The Law of Love

Love is the energy of the healing force. Living this law involves living with the highest form of energy that can help humans and all life balance existence on any plane of consciousness. It is the opposite of fear and is the basis of spiritual healing and mediumship.

The Law of Conservation of Energy

Matter and energy are interchangeable and the total amount of energy and matter in the universe is constant. This is a principle in Physics.

SUMMARY

Though the methods of reasoning and wording of the Natural Laws have changed throughout our history, it seems that their individual concepts are basically the same. They consistently are found to be at the root of philosophical, medical, religious, and spiritual research for as long as we have written records. Medical science has not been able to prove that all illnesses can only be addressed with pharmaceuticals and surgical interventions, and spiritual healers also cannot prove to be the only avenue to wellness. Yet, the knowledge that has come through both scientific medical research and spiritual healing has been invaluable in helping "certain" conditions to heal. Once again, in time there is an opportunity to encourage the emergence of a more holistic approach to healing. Natural Laws help to understand that as a community of beings on this earth, humans have more to learn about life than their immediate perceptions may tell them.

Spiritualism asks individuals to be receptive to unlimited potentials rather than to get stuck in personal beliefs, to take responsibility for personal choices, and to believe in the unlimited power of Spirit. Era III medicine invites all to be receptive to the unlimited possibilities of existence.

REFERENCES

American Heritage Dictionary. (1985). Boston: Houghton Mifflin.

Benson, H., M.D. (1975). *The Relaxation Response.* New York: William Morrow and Company.

Carroll, B. E. (1997). *Spiritualism in Antebellum America.* Bloomington & Indianapolis, IN: Indiana University Press.

Carter, M. & McCarey, W. (1972). *Edgar Cayce on Healing.* New York: Coronet Communications, Inc.

Chopra, D. (1994). *The Seven Spiritual Laws of Success.* San Rafael: Amber-Allen Press and New World Library.

De Swarte, L. (1999). *The Principles of Spiritualism.* Hammersmith: Thorsons/HarperCollins.

Dossey, L. (1999). *Reinventing Medicine.* New York: HarperCollins.

_____. (1993). *Healing Words.* New York: HarperCollins.

Dyson, E. (1997). *Having Their Way with Science, Nineteenth-Century Natural Theology, The Spiritualis Movement and the Mediumship of Cora L. V. Richmond.* Thesis. Holyoke: Mt. Holyoke College.

Edgar Cayce Books World Database *www.edgarcayce.com.*

Edwards, H. (1963). *The Power of Spiritual Healing.* London: The Healer Publishing Co. LTD.

_____. (1974). *A Guide to Understanding and the Practice of Spiritual Healing.* Tiptree: The Anchor Press Ltd.

Emery, M. (1999). *The Intuitive Healer, Accessing Your Inner Physician.* New York: St. Martin's Press.

Goldberg, B. (1997). *Soul Healing.* St. Paul: Llewellyn Publications.

The Great Books (1952). *Galen/Hippocrities.* Chicago/London/Toronto/Geneva: Encyclopedia Britannica, Inc.

Jones, P. (1999). *Conscious Life, Prayer and Meditation in the World Religions & Science.* Conscious Life e-magazine *www.conscious-life.com.*

_____. (1999). *Interfaith Spirituality.* Conscious Life e-magazine *www.consciouslife.com.*

Myss, C. (1996). *Anatomy of the spirit.* New York: Harmony Books.

National Institute for Health, Alternative Medicine, (2001). *Spirituality and mediation. www.hsl.mcmaster.ca/tomflem/altmed.html.*

Rasso, J. (2001). *Expanded dictionary of alternative-medicine methods. www..acsh.org/dictionary /s.html.*

Redwood, D. (1995). *An interview with people who make a difference: An interview with Larry Dossey.* Health World Online *www.healthy. net.*

Smolan, R., Moffitt, P., Naythons, M. (1990). *The power to heal, ancient arts & modern medicine.* New York: Prentice Hall Press.

Tompkins, P. and Bird C. (1973). *The secret life of plants.* New York: Harper & Row.

Chapter 10

TOWARD AN INTEGRATIVE HOLISTIC HEALTH THEORETICAL MODEL

A new spirit is required for a new science—one that does not seek to dominate or control, or impose its views on nature, but is tempered by respect, the desire for harmony and compassion for all things. Such an activity must retain the scientific passion for truth and understanding while, at the same time, seeking to celebrate nature and restore the harmony of the planet, society, and each individual.

(Pert, D., 1992, pp. 191–205)

THE INQUIRY AND PURPOSE OF THE STUDY

THE PURPOSE OF THIS RESEARCH is to uncover a unifying theory of holistic health. This theory is termed implicit in that it represents fundamental conceptual constructs among the most widely used frames of reference in alternative and complementary medicine. It is hoped that this integrated theory will provide an ever-expanding foundation or trunk upon which the various approaches or branches can be supported, feel a connection to the whole, and be able to draw from the strength that comes from a sense of commonality. The achievement of this goal is based on the understanding and integration of the meaning of the major ways of knowing integrative alternative and complementary approaches to traditional medicine in United States and Europe through the use of phenomenological qualitative research.

The fundamental paradigms in Era II, Era III and Einsteinian medicine that support hundreds of holistic approaches are conceptually discussed. The data was then analyzed through a phenomenological coding process based upon its relationship to predetermined theoretical questions as well as allowing the data to elucidate new categories of conceptual formulations (Lewis, 1978, 1986; McMillan, Schumacher, 1997; Straus, Corbin 1998).

REVIEW OF LITERATURE

This research design and methodology has been utilized in the elucidation of a body of knowledge in creative arts therapy fields. In 1978, a phenomenological research study was conducted in dance therapy and in 2000 in the field of drama therapy, utilizing the most widely employed theoretical approaches in each field. The subject/author/therapists responded to conceptual questions regarding their theoretical base entailing (1) the view of the individual, the health dysfunction continuum and the embodied creative arts therapy, (2) the method of identification and evaluation of the health dysfunction continuum, (3) the therapeutic process, and (4) the role of the therapist. Responses to these questions were extrapolated from the protocols in the form of natural meaning units. The situated concepts were cleared of any language that couched them in the specific idiom related to the approach. The unsituated themes were then organized and synthesized to produce a fundamental body of knowledge in the fields of dance therapy and drama therapy (Lewis, 1978, 1986, 2000).

SELECTION OF SUBJECTS AND DESIGN

The qualitative research analyzed the major paradigms in:
Era II: Mindbody medicine:
1. Stress and the autonomic nervous system
2. Psychoneuroimmunology
3. The biopsychology of solid emotion
4. The biophysiology of liquid emotion
5. Trauma and brain development and neurophysiology
6. The psychology of body movement
7. Imagination and the personal and collective unconscious
8. Nutrition and health

Einsteinian medicine:
1. Bioenergy medicine
   a. Meridians
   b. Chakras
   c. Human energy fields
2. Spiritual energy healing

Era III: Eternal medicine
1. Spirituality
2. Transpersonal psychotherapy
3. Western Spirituality
4. Alchemy

5. Eastern Mystical approaches
6. Indigenous shamanic practices
7. Spiritualism, mediumship and channeling
8. Distance intention and prayer
9. Medical intuition

Based on an understanding of theoretical constructs of theory building in the field of integrative alternative and complimentary medicine and discussions generated at the Institute for Healing and Wellness and the Institute for Body, Mind and Spirituality, the following questions were asked of chapters 1-9:

• What is the conceptual view of the individual?
• What is the conceptual experience of human development?
• What is the conceptual experience of health?
• What is the conceptual experience of diminished health, dis-ease, or dysfunction?
• What is the conceptual experience of the methods of identifying and evaluating health and its diminishment?
• What is the conceptual experience of healing?
• What is the conceptual experience of the role of the holistic health practitioner and consultant?
• What is the conceptual experience of the setting?
• What is the conceptual experience of the stages of the healing process?

Comparative Analysis

Phenomenological data analysis integrates the operations of organizing, analyzing, and interpreting the data. The following represents the steps in this qualitative research process.

STEP 1. Each protocol or chapter was read first to get a sense of the whole in a process of immersion that requires both objectivity and sensitivity. "Objectivity is necessary to arrive at an impartial and accurate interpretation of events. Sensitivity is required to perceive the subtle nuances and meanings in data and to organize the connections between concepts" (Strauss and Corbin, 1998, pp. 42–43).

STEP 2. Conceptual constructs situated in the language of the particular approach are then arranged according to the predetermined research questions in a frame of reference summary for each of the nine chapters. Because theoretical sampling is cumulative, each theoretical approach chapter builds from and adds to the previous protocol and analysis. In the initial stating of concepts from the first chapters, it was important to generate as many concepts as possible as it was unclear which constructs would be germane to a large proportion of the paradigms researched.

STEP 3 AND 4. The conceptual constructs from the frame of reference summaries are then unsituated. That is they are cleared of any language which couched them in the specific idiom related to the approach, organized according to Era II, III, or Einsteinian medicine primacy. They are then placed on a grid in which nine paradigms could be cataloged as either agreeing or not agreeing to the particular conceptual construct.

STEP 5. The theoretical concepts on the grid are then further reduced and densified. During the process, subcategories began to reveal themselves as the conceptual meaning units group themselves around topic areas.

STEP 6 AND 9. The grid was then consolidated. The concepts were retransposed back into pros to provide the summary description of the implicit theoretical body of knowledge in integrative complimentary and alternative holistic health (see Figure 10-1).

SUMMARY OF THE IMPLICIT PARADIGMS IN INTEGRATIVE COMPLIMENTARY AND ALTERNATIVE HOLISTIC HEALTH

View of an Individual

INTERCONNECTED UNITY. The human being is seen as a multidimensional organism with a physical mindbody, a consciousness/soulspirit, and an energetic realm. The mindbody, soulspirit and bioenergy are an interrelated whole affecting and influencing each other for the purpose of maintaining and regulating the physical, emotional, mental and spiritual aspects of an individual.

UNIQUE AND UNDIFFERENTIATED NATURE. Individuals are both unique and part of an infinite unified Consciousness. Individuals have an eternal soul or transpersonal essence and a sense of personal self that develops within a lifetime. The sense of self is composed of gut feeling neuropeptides, the somatic imagination, and bioenergy. It is activated and grown by an attuned and developmentally sensitive primary caregiver.

Development and the Principle of Self-Actualization

There is a dynamic identified as self-actualization within each individual that moves them toward health, development, and consciousness. This dynamic attempts to reveal information in the mindbody personal and collective/archetypal/universal unconscious. The personal unconscious stores trauma, unaccepted parts of the self as well as the

Key Concepts in the Fundamental Body of Knowledge in Era II, Era III and Einsteinian Integrative Holistic Health	Mindbody ANS & Stress	Psycho-neuor-immun-ology	Molecular & CNS Emotion & Trauma	Body Posture & Move-ment	Nutrition	Western Psychology & Judeo-Christian Spirituality	Bioenergy & Human Energy Fields	Eastern & Indigenous Traditions Of Spirituality	Spiritual Healing & Distance Intention
View of an Individual									
Era II Mindbody medicine									
The mind and body are an interrelated whole.	X	X	X	X	X	X	X	X	X
The individual is both conscious and unconscious.	X	X	X	X		X	X	X	X
The personal unconscious receives trauma and unaccepted parts of the self as well as holds all of who an individual is meant to be.		X	X	X		X	X	X	X
The mind affects the body and the body affects the mind.	X	X	X	X	X	X	X	X	X
The flow of the contraction of muscle tissue can identify temperament, hypothalamic affective reactions to safety and danger as well as rhythmically be associated with various stages of development.	X			X		X			
The flow of shape of body movement are responses to safety and danger, a person's internalized representations of early relation-ships and reactions to the present.				X		X			
The brain monitors and can alter the immune system.	X	X	X			X			
Individuals have a liquid nervous system made up of chemicals that enhance or inhibit neural transmission that, in turn, modulate arousal, mood and attention.		X	X						

Key Concepts in the Fundamental Body of Knowledge in Era II, Era III and Einsteinian Integrative Holistic Health	Mindbody ANS & Stress	Psycho-neuor-immun-ology	Molecular & CNS Emotion & Trauma	Body Posture & Move-ment	Nutrition	Western Psychology & Judeo-Christian Spirituality	Bioenergy & Human Energy Fields	Eastern & Indigenous Traditions Of Spirituality	Spiritual Healing & Distance Intention
The immune system is seen as a floating endocrine system that communicates with the nervous system through liquid peptides.		X	X						
The immune system helps define an individual's sense of self by accepting what is kin and repelling what is not.		X	X						
Body responses including ANS and molecular emotions occur whether the person is having thoughts and feelings based upon imaginings or external reality.	X	X	X	X		X	X		X
Emotions are the liquid information messengers that link mindbody systems.			X						
Gut feelings or somatic markers assign value or positive or negative reactions to an individual's emotional integrity and the safeness of others and the environment.	X	X	X	X		X	X		
Pheromones are transmitted by air from one person to another affecting reproductive behavior.			X						
Incoming stimuli from the senses is first filtered through the amygdala in the limbic system before entering the neocortex. If any element of the stimuli is associated with a prior emotionally charged memory, it will be sent to the cortex as a match. This can result in *emotional hyjacking.*		X	X	X					

Key Concepts in the Fundamental Body of Knowledge in Era II, Era III and Einsteinian Integrative Holistic Health	Mindbody ANS & Stress	Psycho-neuor-immun-ology	Molecular & CNS Emotion & Trauma	Body Posture & Move-ment	Nutrition	Western Psychology & Judeo-Christian Spirituality	Bioenergy & Human Energy Fields	Eastern & Indigenous Traditions Of Spirituality	Spiritual Healing & Distance Intention
Early pre and neo natal memory is stored in the limbic system as emotional arousals without images.			X						
Thought and feelings have and take up both psychic and bioenergy.			X	X		X	X	X	X
The imagination is the doorway into the unconscious and the spiritual and is the realm of healing and transformation.	X	X	X			X		X	
Each individual is biochemically individual and requires an individually tailored diet.					X				
Einsteinian Medicine The human is seen as a multidimensional organism with a physical realm and an energetic realm.							X	X	X
An individual is composed of bioenergetic systems of life-sustaining energy. These systems receive, store, exchange and circulate energy through pathways, centers, and fields surrounding the body for the purpose of maintaining and regulating the physical, emotional, mental and spiritual aspects within an individual.							X	X	X
The human energy fields are felt to consist of subatomic particles or subquantum energies that are at a higher frequency or vibration than normal matter. It affects sonic, thermal and electrostatic ions.							X	X	X

Key Concepts in the Fundamental Body of Knowledge in Era II, Era III and Einsteinian Integrative Holistic Health	Mindbody ANS & Stress	Psycho-neuor-immun-ology	Molecular & CNS Emotion & Trauma	Body Posture & Move-ment	Nutrition	Western Psychology & Judeo-Christian Spirituality	Bioenergy & Human Energy Fields	Eastern & Indigenous Traditions Of Spirituality	Spiritual Healing & Distance Intention
An individual is seen as a system of inter-dependent force fields that are responsive to changes in consciousness.							X	X	X
Consciousness, energy and matter interconnect in humans as well as all life forms.							X	X	X
Individuals are connected to the universe through a continuous exchange of energy.							X	X	X
Era III Medicine: View of Individual The collective, archetypal or universal unconscious is an individual's access to the infinite all knowing Source.					X				
There is a dynamic within each individual that moves them toward consciousness, Self-actualization and attempts to reveal material that is in the mindbody unconscious.						X	X	X	X
The individual is viewed as a transpersonal essence.						X	X	X	X
Consciousness is separate from the brain and is free from embodied space and time.						X	X	X	X
The individual is viewed as having an eternal soul.						X	X	X	X
The individual is part of the undifferentiated essence of divine Conscious, Light or pure consciousness.									X

Key Concepts in the Fundamental Body of Knowledge in Era II, Era III and Einsteinian Integrative Holistic Health	Mindbody ANS & Stress	Psycho-neuor-immun-ology	Molecular & CNS Emotion & Trauma	Body Posture & Move-ment	Nutrition	Western Psychology & Judeo-Christian Spirituality	Bioenergy & Human Energy Fields	Eastern & Indigenous Traditions Of Spirituality	Spiritual Healing & Distance Intention
Underlying the diversity of individuals is the unity of the all pervasive Spirit.								X	X
Individuals exist in both ordinary and non-ordinary states of reality.						X	X	X	X
There is a dynamic exchange between each individual and the universe that means that an individual being, including their thoughts, affects the entire universe.							X	X	X
View of Human Development									
Era II Mindbody Medicine Development is seen as a progression through various stages with earlier phases providing foundations for higher levels.	X	X	X	X		X		X	
Key interpersonal and environmental elements are needed for each phase to be integrated in healthy development.	X	X	X	X		X			
Stress and trauma can cause regression to earlier insufficiently integrated developmental phases resulting in childlike behavior.	X		X	X		X			
If healthy ego, body and external boundaries do not develop, they are replaced with childhood survival behaviors that often continue beyond their need into adulthood.	X		X	X		X			

Key Concepts in the Fundamental Body of Knowledge in Era II, Era III and Einsteinian Integrative Holistic Health	Mindbody ANS & Stress	Psycho-neuor-immun-ology	Molecular & CNS Emotion & Trauma	Body Posture & Move-ment	Nutrition	Western Psychology & Judeo-Christian Spirituality	Bioenergy & Human Energy Fields	Eastern & Indigenous Traditions Of Spirituality	Spiritual Healing & Distance Intention
A realistic sense of self develops in relationship to an attuned and developmentally sensitive primary caregiver.	X		X	X		X			
Era III Medicine: Spiritual Development Through adulthood individuals go through many death-rebirth cycles which gradually move them through adult stage development into middle age, middlessence, aging and dying.				X		X			
Development gradually shifts the individual into an ego-Self axis in which individuals shift their focus from theirs and their family's needs to the needs of humanity, the planet and Consciousness.						X		X	
The individual is moved toward higher states of evolution through an inner dynamic process of self-actualization.						X		X	X
The developmental shift to the primacy of the Self is experienced as a defeat or death of the ego.						X		X	
Soulspirits are seen to develop over many lifetimes toward full consciousness.								X	
View of Health									
Era II: Mindbody Health Health is seen in the spontaneous adaptively appropriate movement and verbal expression of an individual.	X	X	X	X		X			

Key Concepts in the Fundamental Body of Knowledge in Era II, Era III and Einsteinian Integrative Holistic Health	Mindbody ANS & Stress	Psycho-neuor-immun-ology	Molecular & CNS Emotion & Trauma	Body Posture & Move-ment	Nutrition	Western Psychology & Judeo-Christian Spirituality	Bioenergy & Human Energy Fields	Eastern & Indigenous Traditions Of Spirituality	Spiritual Healing & Distance Intention
Health is the adaptive use of the relaxation response and other increases the in strength of the immune system.	X	X	X			X			X
Health is the capacity to be in touch with and expressive of personal emotions that produce a stronger immune system and faster recovery.	X	X	X	X		X			
Health is the capacity for internal boundaries that discriminate fantasy from reality and discriminates what belongs to the individual from what does not.			X	X					
Healthy is the capacity to experience personal locus of control, hope, and meaning n life.	X	X	X	X		X			
Health is the capacity to perceive rather than judge, to accept, forgive and let go of attachment to outcome.						X		X	
Health is the capacity to be fully present in the moment.	X		X	X		X	X	X	X
Health is the capacity for intimacy with one's essential core, others and spiritually.				X		X		X	X
Health is seen in the capacity to appropriately accept, forgive, have a positive outlook which makes meaning and supports the ccmmon good.	X	X	X	X		X		X	X
Health is the capacity for ego, body and external space boundaries that serve discrimination, appropriate expression and protection.				X		X			

Key Concepts in the Fundamental Body of Knowledge in Era II, Era III and Einsteinian Integrative Holistic Health	Mindbody ANS & Stress	Psycho-neuro-immun-ology	Molecular & CNS Emotion & Trauma	Body Posture & Move-ment	Nutrition	Western Psychology & Judeo-Christian Spirituality	Bioenergy & Human Energy Fields	Eastern & Indigenous Traditions Of Spirituality	Spiritual Healing & Distance Intention
Supported involvement in interpersonal networks, pets and relation to nature promotes health and longevity.	X		X			X			
Conscious individually designed diet promotes and supports health.					X				
Health is the capacity for self-actualization and the natural transformational growing which comes from that ongoing experience.						X		X	
Health is the capacity to be fully spontaneously who one is.	X		X	X		X			
Health is eating a healthy diet of fresh seasonal chemical-free nutrient rich organic foods.					X				
Health is supported with an individually tailored diet direction which appropriately balances, builds, and/or cleanses and can change over time.					X				
Einsteinian Medicine Health is described as bioenergy systems which are balanced, aligned and have a natural flow or spin of energy.							X	X	X
Era III Medicine: Spiritual Health Health is the capacity to shift from self-focus to the bigger picture—from "my will be done to thy will be done"—from the primacy of personal needs to those of humanity and nature.						X		X	X

Key Concepts in the Fundamental Body of Knowledge in Era II, Era III and Einsteinian Integrative Holistic Health	Mindbody ANS & Stress	Psycho-neuor-immun-ology	Molecular & CNS Emotion & Trauma	Body Posture & Move-ment	Nutrition	Western Psychology & Judeo-Christian Spirituality	Bioenergy & Human Energy Fields	Eastern & Indigenous Traditions Of Spirituality	Spiritual Healing & Distance Intention
Spiritual health is seen in individuals who have faith and are connected to a greater eternal infinite Souce that gives deep meaning to their life.						X		X	X
Health is the capacity to flow without effort accepting what is and transforming what can evolve which is disharmonious to existence.	X					X		X	X
Health is the capacity for mindfulness, nonattachment and an expanding Consciousness that experiences the unity of all things.						X		X	X
Health is the capacity to transcend the view that one is a body or one's thoughts and identifies with everything and nothing.							X	X	X
Health is the capacity to evolve through various lifetimes toward full nonattached Consciousness.								X	X
Spiritual health is seen in the ongoing experience of well-being, peace, personal empowerment that surrenders to Divine Will or Consciousness.						X		X	X
Spiritual health is seen in the presence of meaning, calling, or purpose in one's life.						X		X	X
Health is seen in the experience and following of an integrative transcendental philosophy of life as a spiritual path.						X		X	X

Key Concepts in the Fundamental Body of Knowledge in Era II, Era III and Einsteinian Integrative Holistic Health	Mindbody ANS & Stress	Psycho-neuro-immun-ology	Molecular & CNS Emotion & Trauma	Body Posture & Move-ment	Nutrition	Western Psychology & Judeo-Christian Spirituality	Bioenergy & Human Energy Fields	Eastern & Indigenous Traditions Of Spirituality	Spiritual Healing & Distance Intention
Health is seen in a connection to nature and the underlying unity of all things which, in turn, provides an ethical responsibility to the well-being of the planet.						X		X	
Health is the experience that there is something greater than the self.		X				X		X	X
Health is seen in the capacity for compassionate love, acceptance, faith and forgiveness.	X		X			X		X	X
View of Diminished Health									
Era II Mindbody Medicine Diminished health is seen in physical and emotional complaints and symptoms.	X	X	X	X	X	X	X	X	X
Held tension areas in the body store emotional and physical trauma at a sensorimotor level leaving an individual vulnerable for physical trauma and illness.	X	X	X	X		X	X	X	X
Diminished health is seen in the somatization of distress.	X	X	X	X	X	X	X		X
Diminished health is seen in rigidly staying fixed in one state of the cyclic alchemical process of spiritual consciousness.						X		X	
Held planes in the body attitude may denote relational and self-formulation difficulties in the first 3 years of life.				X					

Key Concepts in the Fundamental Body of Knowledge in Era II, Era III and Einsteinian Integrative Holistic Health	Mindbody ANS & Stress	Psycho-neuor-immun-ology	Molecular & CNS Emotion & Trauma	Body Posture & Move-ment	Nutrition	Western Psychology & Judeo-Christian Spirituality	Bioenergy & Human Energy Fields	Eastern & Indigenous Traditions Of Spirituality	Spiritual Healing & Distance Intention
Chronic stress decreases the strength of the immune system.	X	X	X			X	X	X	X
Early childhood trauma affects the development of the brain. Trauma is seen as being stored in the sensorimotor: ANS, Limbic, and body's peripheral nervous system.			X						
The lack of interpersonal attunement results in isolation and the atrophy of emotions and emotional expression.			X	X		X			
Dysfunction is seen in the individuals who are judgmental, isolated and fearful.	X	X	X	X		X		X	X
Dysfunction occurs when cultural oppession and limited thinking impairs an individual's connection to and expression of themselves, appreciation of relatedness to others and the transpersonal.						X			
Some learning occurs via mirror neurons that replicate visually assimilated actions and behaviors of others without cognitive awareness.			X						
Thoughts are remembered better if actions are associated with them as movement produces neurtrophins resulting in increased neural connections.			X	X					
Negative imagining or re-remembering of trauma can reduce the potency of the immune system and place the mindbody in chronic stress as if the trauma were occurring in the moment.			X						

Key Concepts in the Fundamental Body of Knowledge in Era II, Era III and Einsteinian Integrative Holistic Health	Mindbody ANS & Stress	Psycho-neuor-immun-ology	Molecular & CNS Emotion & Trauma	Body Posture & Move-ment	Nutrition	Western Psychology & Judeo-Christian Spirituality	Bioenergy & Human Energy Fields	Eastern & Indigenous Traditions Of Spirituality	Spiritual Healing & Distance Intention
Afflicting thoughts and feelings such as hopelessness and fear can reduce the body's capacity to be healthy and heal.	X	X	X						
Diminished health occurs when the capacity to be fully present and have healthy boundaries are replaced with childhood survival behaviors and addictions.				X			X		
Childhood survival behaviors attack intimacy and connection to the core self, others and the transpersonal.	X	X	X	X		X		X	X
Diminished health is experienced with ongoing physical, emotional and/or spiritual abuse.			X	X		X	X	X	X
Dysfunctional connection to and sense of self occurs with nonnurturing, abandoning and/or enmeshed nonattuned primary caregivers in childhood.			X	X		X	X		
Diminished health occurs when individuals are isolated and lack others and/or pets to relate to.	X		X	X		X		X	X
In emotional hijacking of reoccurring imprinted trauma, the prefrontal cortex remains cool while the amygdala refires cutting off the capacity for cognitive reality testing and the capacity to learn to make adaptive decisions.			X					X	
Stress prevents molecular emotion from flowing freely where it is needed, producing physical responses to chronic stress.			X						

Key Concepts in the Fundamental Body of Knowledge in Era II, Era III and Einsteinian Integrative Holistic Health	Mindbody ANS & Stress	Psycho-neuor-immun-ology	Molecular & CNS Emotion & Trauma	Body Posture & Move-ment	Nutrition	Western Psychology & Judeo-Christian Spirituality	Bioenergy & Human Energy Fields	Eastern & Indigenous Traditions Of Spirituality	Spiritual Healing & Distance Intention
Dysfunction occurs when individuals focus solely on themselves.	X		X	X		X		X	
Diminished health occurs when individuals chronically ingest modified food products.					X				X
Diminished health results in being overdrawn nutritionally producing an unhealthy appearance, fatigue, pain and mood disorders.					X				
Einsteinian Medicine Dysfunction occurs when the body's bioenergy systems have holes and leaks in the fields, and/or weakness, imbalance, displacements, blocks, movements in the wrong direction and/or instability in the pathways and centers.							X	X	
Dysfunction occurs in the human energy fields with instability, excitation or weakness in meridian, chakra or auric fields.							X	X	X
Era III Medicine: Spiritual Distress Dysfunction is the inability to experience the transpersonal.						X		X	X
Dysfunction occurs when an individual holds a limited view of existence as being composed solely of empirical physical reality.						X	X	X	X
Dis-ease can occur when individuals adhere to a judgmental God who views them as sinners.	X			X		X		X	X

Key Concepts in the Fundamental Body of Knowledge in Era II, Era III and Einsteinian Integrative Holistic Health	Mindbody ANS & Stress	Psycho-neuor-immun-ology	Molecular & CNS Emotion & Trauma	Body Posture & Move-ment	Nutrition	Western Psychology & Judeo-Christian Spirituality	Bioenergy & Human Energy Fields	Eastern & Indigenous Traditions Of Spirituality	Spiritual Healing & Distance Intention
Dis-ease can occur when humans feel hopeless due to the belief that life is suffering.	X	X				X		X	X
Distress can occur when individuals feel they are being punished by God as the reason why they are sick.	X					X		X	
Distresses occur when individuals blame God for not being cured or for others being sick or dying.	X					X		X	X
Dis-ease occurs when individuals use spirituality as an excuse to isolate themselves or be judgmental of others.						X		X	X
Dis-ease occurs when individuals shift from humility to a grandiose identification with the Higher Power and function as if fundamental human values do not apply to them.				X		X		X	X
Disease is living in unconsciousness and the myth of duality.						X		X	X
Distress comes when individuals attach to their busy mind.						X	X	X	X
Unconsciousness is the experience that humans are their bodies or thoughts.							X	X	X
Dysfunction occurs when individuals believe that all that exists is solely on the empirical realm.						X	X	X	X

Key Concepts in the Fundamental Body of Knowledge in Era II, Era III and Einsteinian Integrative Holistic Health	Mindbody ANS & Stress	Psycho-neuor-immun-ology	Molecular & CNS Emotion & Trauma	Body Posture & Move-ment	Nutrition	Western Psychology & Judeo-Christian Spirituality	Bioenergy & Human Energy Fields	Eastern & Indigenous Traditions Of Spirituality	Spiritual Healing & Distance Intention
Dis-spirited individuals often experience harmful intrusions which can energetically reduce their life force.						X	X	X	X
Because of the interconnectedness of all things, an individual's distress can be synchronistically identified when phenomena in their environment break down, malfunction or go into distress.						X	X	X	X
Dysfunction occurs when emotionally charged energy becomes encoded in individual's biological systems and influences cell tissue and neurophysiologic responses.							X	X	X
View of the identification and evaluation of health and its diminishment									
Era II Mindbody and Medicine Observing the presence and degree of energetic, behavioral and/or neurophysiologic hyper and/or hypo-arousal produced in chronic stress is an identifying marker.	X	X	X	X	X	X	X	X	X
Observing the capacity of an individual to adapt to the moment as opposed to bringing the past into the present and responding on a mindbody neurophysiologic and/or energetic level in the present as if it were the past.	X	X	X	X	X	X	X	X	X
Observing body, posture and movement can indicate emotional maturity, healthy boundaries, personality and/or outmoded survival behaviors.	X		X	X	X	X			

Key Concepts in the Fundamental Body of Knowledge in Era II, Era III and Einsteinian Integrative Holistic Health	Mindbody ANS & Stress	Psycho-neuroimmun-ology	Molecular & CNS Emotion & Trauma	Body Posture & Move-ment	Nutrition	Western Psychology & Judeo-Christian Spirituality	Bioenergy & Human Energy Fields	Eastern & Indigenous Traditions Of Spirituality	Spiritual Healing & Distance Intention
Observing and tracking what gets the individual's attention.	X		X	X	X	X		X	
Through the use of the arts, dreams, visualization, hypnotic states and the translation of life into symbol and metaphor, an individual's unconscious can be accessed and the focus and direction of the individual's healing understood.			X	X		X		X	
Through the use of interviewing which identifies the history and current physical, emotional and spiritual condition of the individual.	X	X	X	X	X	X	X	X	X
Through an individual's response to a battery of mindbody and/or soulspirit questions.	X	X	X	X	X	X	X	X	X
Einsteinian Medicine Observing or feeling the energetic fields, pathways and centers in the body through touch, high sense intuition, applied kinesiology or special bioenergy diagnostic machines, physical, emotional, and spiritual distress can be identified.				X			X	X	X
Through noticing what gets energetically transferred or projected through the human energy field into the energetic field of the practitioner.						X	X	X	X
Era III Medicine Through receiving information regarding the presence of an individual's spiritual beliefs, their influence and application in personal philosophy, life path and daily life.	X					X		X	

Key Concepts in the Fundamental Body of Knowledge in Era II, Era III and Einsteinian Integrative Holistic Health	Mindbody ANS & Stress	Psycho-neuroimmunology	Molecular & CNS Emotion & Trauma	Body Posture & Move-ment	Nutrition	Western Psychology & Judeo-Christian Spirituality	Bioenergy & Human Energy Fields	Eastern & Indigenous Traditions Of Spirituality	Spiritual Healing & Distance Intention
Through receiving energy impressions that carries symbolic and literal information from the encoding of energy from cell tissue as well as energetic fields. Energy frequencies that are not in tune with the rest of the body are identified as problematic.							X	X	X
View of Healing									
Era II Mindbody Medicine Health practitioners of all fields address the minds: thoughts and feelings and body's somatic symptoms in both psychological and physical distress in their healing techniques.	X	X	X	X	X	X	X	X	X
Healing is a process of manipulating the body via cleaning, aligning, and adjusting as well as directing energy into and out of the body.	X						X	X	X
Healing occurs when unconscious material from a person's life is made conscious cleared, transformed and/or integrated into consciousness.	X		X	X		X	X	X	X
Healing can occur when consciousness of an individual or group can support another.	X					X	X	X	X
Healing can occur with sensorimotor processing.	X		X	X			X	X	X
Healing can occur without the involvement of the brain's cortex.	X	X	X	X		X	X	X	X

Key Concepts in the Fundamental Body of Knowledge in Era II, Era III and Einsteinian Integrative Holistic Health	Mindbody ANS & Stress	Psycho-neuro-immun-ology	Molecular & CNS Emotion & Trauma	Body Posture & Move-ment	Nutrition	Western Psychology & Judeo-Christian Spirituality	Bioenergy & Human Energy Fields	Eastern & Indigenous Traditions Of Spirituality	Spiritual Healing & Distance Intention
Healing can occur with imprinted trauma when the individual is encouraged to notice emotions, bodily sensations and any resultant thoughts separately, slowly and mindfully.	X		X	X				X	
Healing occurs in an ongoing individuation process in which individuals become more fully who they are.			X	X		X			
Healing occurs through the ingestion of food that contains nutrients, energetic properties, positively influences glands, organs and tissues, and provides nutrient diversity.					X				
Foods that are chemically free and nutrient rich enhance healing.					X				
Einsteinian Healing Healing occurs when human bioenergy is unblocked, cleared, charged, realigned and/or balanced.							X	X	X
Healing can occur through the practitioner transmitting or channeling energy into the bioenergy field of the client.							X	X	X
Spiritual Healing Spiritual healing in energy medicine is a form of channeling that involves the transference of healing energy from its spiritual source to one who needs help.							X	X	X

Key Concepts in the Fundamental Body of Knowledge in Era II, Era III and Einsteinian Integrative Holistic Health	Mindbody ANS & Stress	Psycho-neuro-immun-ology	Molecular & CNS Emotion & Trauma	Body Posture & Move-ment	Nutrition	Western Psychology & Judeo-Christian Spirituality	Bioenergy & Human Energy Fields	Eastern & Indigenous Traditions Of Spirituality	Spiritual Healing & Distance Intention
The spirit is the source of energy of spiritual healing.						X	X	X	X
Spiritual healing occurs when individuals experience peak, at-one-with-the-Source experiences in which the individual remembers or discovers their pure nature i.e., that they are part of divine Consciousness.	X					X	X	X	X
Spiritual healing occurs when an individual can experience mindfulness and presence.	X					X		X	
Spiritual healing occurs when an individual can let go of desiring and outcome.	X					X		X	X
Spiritual healing occurs when an individual experiences the myth of duality.	X					X		X	X
Spiritual healing occurs when an individual surrenders to a Higher Power and experiences divine love, forgiveness and acceptance.						X			X
Spiritual healing occurs when an individual shifts from the primacy of the ego to one in which the individual nonattaches from the personal to focus upon the greater good and the bigger picture.	X					X	X	X	X
Distance intentional healing occurs when the nonlocal mind is directed to someone for their health and well-being. This has been called prayer healing and distance healing.						X	X	X	X

Key Concepts in the Fundamental Body of Knowledge in Era II, Era III and Einsteinian Integrative Holistic Health	Mindbody ANS & Stress	Psycho-neuro-immun-ology	Molecular & CNS Emotion & Trauma	Body Posture & Move-ment	Nutrition	Western Psychology & Judeo-Christian Spirituality	Bioenergy & Human Energy Fields	Eastern & Indigenous Traditions Of Spirituality	Spiritual Healing & Distance Intention
The Role of the Holistic Health Practitioner									
Era II Mindbody Medicine									
The healer needs to attune to the clients' breath, movement, somatic unconscious to unconscious connection, and/or bioenergy.			X	X			X	X	X
The role of the therapist is to aid clients in the accessing of the unconscious—both personal and transpersonal, and through the use of the imagination, help individuals heal and expand their access to their Consciousness.			X	X		X			
Through sensitivity to the somatic unconscious to unconscious connection between client and holistic health practitioner, the clinician receives material in the form of energy, feelings, sensations and images of the client for the purpose of understanding, holding, healing and/or returning their split-off feelings, sensations or parts of the individuals personality.				X		X			
The role of the holistic health practitioner is to hold the client in compassionate unconditional positive regard and love.	X	X	X	X	X	X	X	X	X
Einsteinian Medicine Healing The holistic health practitioners who are trained in energy medicine have acute high sense perception and intuitive abilities which can sense, feel or see the state of an individual's bioenergy pathways, centers and/or fields.							X	X	X

Key Concepts in the Fundamental Body of Knowledge in Era II, Era III and Einsteinian Integrative Holistic Health	Mindbody ANS & Stress	Psycho-neuor-immun-ology	Molecular & CNS Emotion & Trauma	Body Posture & Move-ment	Nutrition	Western Psychology & Judeo-Christian Spirituality	Bioenergy & Human Energy Fields	Eastern & Indigenous Traditions Of Spirituality	Spiritual Healing & Distance Intention
The role of the healer is to transmit, clear, energize, and/or balance human bioenergy.							X	X	X
Era III Medicine: Eternal Medicine/ Spiritual Healer The role of the holistic health practitioner is to be the modern day priests, priestesses and shamans.						X	X	X	X
The therapsit holds the individual in compassionate unconditional love, grace and Light.						X	X	X	X
The holistic health practitioner employs intuition that accesses the transpersonal, archetypal, or infinite undifferentiated realm.						X	X	X	X
The role of the healer is to support the transendence from desire and attachment and identification so that the individual would identify with everything and nothing.	X							X	
The role of the clinician is to be sensitive to the uniqueness of the individual's world view, spiritual and cultural values both on a conscious and archetypal level.						X	X	X	X
It is the role of a holistic health Era III practitioner to be a spiritual seeker oneself.	X					X		X	X
The role of the holistic health practitioner/ consultant is to help the individual heal on a soul level sometimes requiring past life work.						X		X	X

Key Concepts in the Fundamental Body of Knowledge in Era II, Era III and Einsteinian Integrative Holistic Health	Mindbody ANS & Stress	Psycho-neuor-immun-ology	Molecular & CNS Emotion & Trauma	Body Posture & Move-ment	Nutrition	Western Psychology & Judeo-Christian Spirituality	Bioenergy & Human Energy Fields	Eastern & Indigenous Traditions Of Spirituality	Spiritual Healing & Distance Intention
Era III practitioners need to both open to personal and transpersonal information.						X	X	X	X
Spiritual healers utilize the capacity to receive information spiritually on behalf of their clients.						X	X	X	X
Spiritual healers utilize distance intention to receive information regarding a client and send love and positive healing to the client from a physical distance.						X	X	X	X
Medical intuitives, psychic diagnosticians, and mediums attune themselves to a person's physical, mental, and spiritual conditions to sense the problem.							X	X	X
Meditation experienced as spiritual attunement which produces nonlocal awareness is used in service to mindbody and soul healing.						X	X	X	X
Medical intuitives attune to the energy in the levels of consciousness surrounding and permeating the physical body.							X		X
The role of the spiritual healer is to utilize the innate spiritual faculty of intuition in order to connect to one's higher consciousness and wisdom in service to the health and healing of another.						X	X	X	X
The somatic countertransference telesomatically discerns among the mindbody and the spiritual.							X		X

Key Concepts in the Fundamental Body of Knowledge in Era II, Era III and Einsteinian Integrative Holistic Health	Mindbody ANS & Stress	Psycho-neuro-immun-ology	Molecular & CNS Emotion & Trauma	Body Posture & Move-ment	Nutrition	Western Psychology & Judeo-Christian Spirituality	Bioenergy & Human Energy Fields	Eastern & Indigenous Traditions Of Spirituality	Spiritual Healing & Distance Intention
The medical intuitive through channeling or mediumship enters into a trance-like state through contact with healing guides in spirit.	X						X		X
Setting Holistic health and healing occurs in a temenos or sacred space whether it be an office, in nature, or in a specific religious setting.						X	X	X	X
Since all realms exist in an interconnected undifferentiated unity; time, distance and physical space is less important than holding positive intention.						X	X	X	X
Stages of the Healing Process **Era II Mindbody Medicine** Through assessment of the mindbody, bioenergetic, and/or soul spirit status of the individual, the therapist and/or client come to the goals, techniques and alternative and or complimentary approaches to be employed.	X	X	X	X	X	X	X	X	X
The therapist notes any precautions based upon physical and psychological limitations and complications.	X	X	X	X	X	X	X	X	X
The holistic health practitioner and/or consultant recommends complimentary and/or alternative approaches and refers the individual to a practitioner or program.	X	X	X	X	X	X	X	X	X

Key Concepts in the Fundamental Body of Knowledge in Era II, Era III and Einsteinian Integrative Holistic Health	Mindbody ANS & Stress	Psychoneuroimmunology	Molecular & CNS Emotion & Trauma	Body Posture & Movement	Nutrition	Western Psychology & Judeo-Christian Spirituality	Bioenergy & Human Energy Fields	Eastern & Indigenous Traditions Of Spirituality	Spiritual Healing & Distance Intention
The holistic health practitioner engages in a holistic health healing process with a client or clients within which the practitioner has been fully trained.	X	X	X	X	X	X	X	X	X
Through mindbody techniques that employ the imagination, an individual comes to undergo healing process.	X	X	X	X		X		X	
The holistic health consultant continues to monitor the combination of holistic health modalities to insure a positive outcome in terms of healing and/or wellness.	X	X	X	X	X	X	X	X	X
The stages of the therapeutic process may include: (1) the processes of increasing awareness of the mindbody soulspirit and/or bioenergetic interrelated phenomena; (2) preparation via: accessing the unconscious, reducing the flooding, and/or increasing the energy for the healing process; (3) identifying the direction of the healing and/or the main-tenance of health and well-being; (4) the providing of engagement in the healing and health processes; and (5) followed by ongoing evaluation and possible alteration of the holistic health plan.	X	X	X	X	X	X	X	X	X
Einsteinian Therapeutic Process The bioenergy healer clears, energizes, and/or balances human bioenergy in the meridians, chakras and/or human energy fields.							X	X	X

Key Concepts in the Fundamental Body of Knowledge in Era II, Era III and Einsteinian Integrative Holistic Health	Mindbody ANS & Stress	Psycho-neuor-immun-ology	Molecular & CNS Emotion & Trauma	Body Posture & Move-ment	Nutrition	Western Psychology & Judeo-Christian Spirituality	Bioenergy & Human Energy Fields	Eastern & Indigenous Traditions Of Spirituality	Spiritual Healing & Distance Intention
Era III Therapeutic Process The Era III practitioner holds with grace the capacity for the person to evolve in their spiritual practice and awakening. Wherever possible, healing states of transpersonal unity are encouraged within the techniques of the healer.	X					X	X	X	X

Figure 10-1. Integrative body of knowledge in holistic health.

potential of who one is. The collective unconscious is the individual's access to the infinite all-knowing Source. The imagination is the doorway into the personal and archetypal/spiritual unconscious and serves self-actualization as well as healing and transformation.

Self-actualization moves an individual through a progression of various stages of development with earlier phases providing foundations for higher levels. Key interpersonal and environmental elements are needed for each phase to be integrated in healthy development. Stress and trauma can affect brain development and neurophysiologic functioning and can cause regression to earlier insufficiently integrated developmental phases resulting in childlike behavior. If healthy ego, body and external boundaries do not develop, they are replaced with childhood survival behaviors that often continue beyond their need into adulthood. These limited thoughts and behaviors are a result of core beliefs that are based in primal fear.

Throughout adulthood individuals go through many death-rebirth cycles which gradually move them through adult stage development into middle age, Middlescence, aging and dying. Development gradually shifts the individual into an ego-Self axis in which individuals alter their focus from theirs or their family's needs to the needs of humanity, the planet and Consciousness. The developmental shift to the primacy of nonattached undifferentiated oneness is experienced as a defeat or death of the ego.

Soulspirits are seen to develop over many lifetimes toward full Consciousness.

Neural, Liquid and Energetic Responses to Internal and External Stimuli

Early pre and neonatal memory is stored in the limbic system as emotional arousals without images or thoughts. Later, the mindbody receives information (stimuli from the senses from the outside world). This stimuli is first filtered through the amygdala in the limbic system (emotional center) of the midbrain before entering the neocortex. If any element of the stimuli is associated with prior emotionally charged memory, it will be sent to the cortex as a match. Additionally gut feelings and other somatic emotional markers produced by liquid molecular neuropeptides in the body assign value or positive or negative reactions to stimuli affecting the individual's emotional integrity and the assessment of the safeness of others and the environment. This liquid nervous system chemically enhances or inhibits neural transmission that, in turn, modulates arousal, mood and attention.

Internally, the mindbody receives information from the unconscious housing repressed trauma, thoughts and imaginings of the individual. The mindbody, not being able to decipher the difference between real and imagined external and internal stimuli regarding safety and danger, responds similarly to both. This may include activation of the limbic system, the autonomic nervous system, the molecular emotional system, and the bioenergetic system. The bioenergetic systems composed of subatomic or subquantum energies receive, store, exchange and circulate energy through pathways, centers and fields surrounding the body.

Responses to chronic real or imagined danger produce the sympathetic nervous systems response of chronic stress. Chronic stress reduces the functioning of the immune system and the energetic systems resulting in the body's susceptibility to illness, diminished ability to recover and maintain wellness. The immune system is seen as a floating endocrine system, which in turn, communicates with the nervous system through liquid peptides. Additionally, chronic stress and imprinted trauma affect the observable quality of flow and developmentally based rhythms of agonist and antagonist muscle systems and the shape that the body takes.

Health

Health is the capacity to be fully present in the moment capable of intimacy with one's essential core, others and spiritually. Health is the capacity for ego, body and external space boundaries that serve discrimination, appropriate expression and protection on mindbody and bioenergetic levels. These boundaries serve in the spontaneous adaptively appropriate movement and verbal expression of an individual both of which support and influence the adaptive use of the relaxation response that increases the strength of the immune system.

Health is the capacity to experience personal positive locus of control, hope, and meaning in life, to perceive rather than judge, to accept, forgive and let go of attachment to outcome. Health is maintained and supported by involvement in interpersonal networks, pets and relation to nature as well as a conscious individually designed diet of fresh seasonal chemical-free nutrient-rich organic foods which appropriately balances, builds, and/or cleanses the body over time.

Health is seen in bioenergy systems which are balanced, aligned and have a natural flow or spin of energy.

Health is the capacity to shift from a self-focus to the bigger picture—from "my will be done" to "thy will be done"—from the primacy of personal needs to those of humanity and nature. Surrendering to Divine Will or Consciousness gives deeper meaning to life and provides a sense of well-being, peace, personal empowerment and life purpose that flows effortlessly accepting what is and transforming what can evolve.

Additionally, health is the capacity for mindfulness, nonattachment and an expanding Consciousness that experiences the unity of all things and transcends the view that one is a body or one's thoughts and identifies with everything and nothing.

View of Diminished Health

Diminished health is seen in chronic stress, limited beliefs, physical and emotional complaints and symptoms. Diminished health is seen in being overdrawn nutritionally, producing an unhealthy appearance, fatigue, pain and mood disorders due to chronic ingestion of modified food products.

TRAUMA. Early childhood trauma of ongoing physical, emotional and/or spiritual abuses with nonnurturing, abandoning and/or enmeshed nonattuned primary caregivers in childhood affects the development and functioning of the brain. In emotional hijacking, reoccurring imprinted trauma results in the amygdala refiring cutting off the capacity for cognitive reality testing in the prefrontal cortex and the capacity to learn to make adaptive decisions. Negative imagining or rereremembering of trauma can reduce the potency of the immune system and place the mindbody in chronic stress as if the trauma were occurring in the moment. Trauma is seen as being stored in the sensorimotor: ANS, Limbic, and body's peripheral nervous system as well as held in body shape and tension areas in the body leaving an individual vulnerable for physical trauma and illness.

Childhood survival behaviors attack intimacy and connection to the core self, others and the transpersonal. Dysfunction continues to be caused when cultural oppression and limited thinking impairs individuals' connection to and expression of themselves, appreciation of relatedness to others and the transpersonal. This is seen in individuals who are judgmental, isolated and fearful, rigidly staying fixed in one state of the cyclic alchemical process of human development and spiritual Consciousness.

Additionally, Dysfunction occurs when the body's bioenergy systems have holes and leaks in the fields, show weakness, imbalance, displacements, blocks, movements in the wrong direction and/or instability in the pathways and centers. Dysfunction occurs when emotionally charged energy becomes encoded in individual's biological systems and influences cell tissue and neurophysiologic responses.

Dysfunction is the inability to experience the transpersonal as seen when an individual holds a limited view of existence as being composed solely of empirical physical reality. Distress comes when individuals attach to their busy mind and exist in unconsciousness and the myth of duality. Unconsciousness is the experience that humans are just their bodies or thoughts. Humans are everything and nothing; and because of the interconnectedness of all things, an individual's distress can be synchronistically identified when phenomena in their environment break down, malfunction or go into distress.

Certain religious beliefs can have a limiting, negative effect. For example, an adherence to a judgmental god who views them as sinners or to feeling hopeless due to the belief that life is suffering can produce distress. When individuals use spirituality as an excuse to isolate themselves or be judgmental of others, feel that they are being punished by god as the reason why they are sick or blame god or themselves for not having a complete cure are creating mindbody soulspirit distress and dis-ease.

View of the Identification and Evaluation of Health and its Diminishment

OBSERVATION. Integrative holistic health practitioners and consultants observe the presence and degree of energetic, behavioral and/or neurophysiologic imbalance, blocks, and hyper and/or hypoarousal produced in chronic stress as an identifying marker. The capacity of an individual to adapt to the moment as opposed to bringing the past or future into the present and responding on a mindbody neurophysiologic and/or ener-

getic level in the present as if it were the past or future, identifies the level of mindful presence. Observing and tracking what gets the individual's attention, tracing their core beliefs through their patterns of limited thinking as well as noting their body, posture and movement can indicate emotional maturity, healthy boundaries, personality and/or outmoded survival behaviors.

THE USE OF PSYCHOPHYSICAL ASSESSMENT. Most all professionals interview the potential client identifying the history and current physical, emotional and spiritual condition of the individual as well as any former or current medical, psychological, alternative and complimentary approaches they have experienced. Responses to a battery of mindbody and/or soulspirit questions are also employed for assessment (see Section II).

Through the use of body and movement assessment, the arts, dreams, visualization, hypnotic states and the translation of life into symbol and metaphor, an individual's unconscious can be accessed and the focus and direction of the individual's healing understood.

Bioenergy practitioners observe or feel the energetic fields, pathways and centers in the body through touch, high sense intuition, applied kinesiology or special bioenergy diagnostic machines. From this data physical, emotional, and spiritual distress can be identified. Some receive information on behalf of an individual through high sense intuition, the somatic countertransference or channeling.

View of Healing

Health practitioners of all CAM fields address the minds: thoughts and feelings and body's somatic symptoms of both psychological and physical distress in their healing techniques. Healing occurs when unconscious material from a person's life is made conscious, cleared, transformed and/or integrated into consciousness. With severe trauma this sometimes requires slow sensorimotor processing where the individual is encouraged to notice emotions, bodily sensations and any resultant thoughts separately, slowly and mindfully. Healing is seen as an ongoing individuation process in which individuals become more fully who they are.

Healing occurs through the ingestion of chemically-free and nutrient rich food that contains nutrients, energetic properties, positively influencing glands, organs and tissues, and providing nutrient diversity. Healing occurs through physical exercise that individually coordinates the aerobic, range of motion, and strength building and maintaining activity that is appropriate for each person.

Spiritual healing occurs when an individual surrenders to a Higher Power and experiences divine love, forgiveness and acceptance and/or shifts from the primacy of the ego to one in which the individual nonattaches from the personal to focus upon the greater good and the bigger picture. Here individuals experience peak, at-one-with-the-Source experiences in which the individual remembers or discovers the myth of duality and their pure nature i.e., that they are part of the Divine Consciousness. Individuals experience mindfulness and presence letting go of desiring and outcome.

Healing occurs when human bioenergy is unblocked, cleared, charged, realigned and/or balanced as well as directing energy into and out of the body. Healing can occur without the involvement of the brain's cortex. A form of channeling that involves the transference of healing energy from spiritual source to one who needs help can occur. Distance intentional healing occurs when the nonlocal mind is directed to someone for his or her health and well-being. This has been called prayer healing and distance healing.

The Role of the Holistic Health Practitioner

The role of the holistic health practitioner is to hold the client in compassionate unconditional positive regard and love and to receive information from a variety of levels for the purpose of creating an integrative holistic health program for the individual. Often alternative and complimentary practitioners are the modern day priests, priestesses and shamans. Thus, Era III practitioners need to be a spiritual seeker themselves.

Additionally, the clinician is to be sensitive to the uniqueness of the complexity of the client's symptoms, medical and nonmedical treatment, world view, and spiritual and cultural values both on a conscious and archetypal level.

ROLE AS RECEIVER OF INFORMATION. The practitioner must be in contact with physicians and any other health care providers to insure a safe and integrative approach. The practitioner may receive information and engages in supporting the healing of the client through a number of other avenues. The practitioner may attune to the client's breath, body, movement, somatic unconscious to unconscious connection, and/or bioenergy. Through telesomatic sensitivity to the somatic unconscious to unconscious connection between client and holistic health practitioner, the clinician may receive material in the form of energy, feelings, sensations and images of the client for the purpose of understanding, holding, healing and/or returning their split-off feelings, sensations or parts of the individual's personality. Bioenergy practitioners may have acute high sense perception and intuitive abilities that can sense, feel or see the state of individuals' bioenergy pathways, centers and/or fields.

Through channeling or mediumship, medical intuitives, psychic diagnosticians, and healers can enter into trance-like states through contact with healing guides in spirit. Meditation experienced as spiritual attunement which produces nonlocal awareness is used in service to mindbody and soul healing. The meditation aids in attuning to the vibration or energy in the levels of consciousness surrounding and permeating the physical body. Physical, mental, and spiritual conditions may be sensed.

ROLE AS INTERVENER. The holistic health therapist aid clients in the accessing of the unconscious–both personal and transpersonal. Through the use of the imagination, practitioners help individuals heal and expand their access to their Consciousness. Body-oriented practitioners transmit, clear, energize, and/or balance the human body and bioenergy. Trainers create personal exercise plans for individuals and specific population groups that maintain health and well-being, prolong active life and prevent trauma. Mindfulness-based practitioners support the transcendence from desire, attachment and identification so that the individual would identify with everything and nothing. Nutritionists, homeopaths, and herbalists suggest foods and substances for ingestion and monitor the process.

Setting

Holistic health and healing occurs in a temenos or sacred space whether it be an office, studio, gym, in nature, or in a specific religious setting. Since all realms exist in an interconnected undifferentiated unity, time, distance and physical space is fundamentally less important than holding positive intention. Thus, the fundamental setting is the sacred bipersonal field between the practitioner and client.

Stages of the Healing Process

Through assessment of the mindbody, bioenergetic, and/or soul spirit status of the individual, the therapist and/or client come to the goals, techniques and alternative and or complimentary approaches to be employed. The therapist notes any precautions based upon physical and psychological limitations and complications. The holistic health practitioner and/or consultant then recommends complimentary and/or alternative approaches and refers the individual to a practitioner or program and/or engages in a holistic health healing process with a client or clients within which the practitioner has been fully trained. The consultant continues to monitor the combination of holistic health modalities to insure a positive outcome in terms of healing and/or wellness.

The stages of the therapeutic process may include:

1. **Awareness:** the processes of increasing awareness of the mindbody soul-spirit and/or bioenergetic interrelated phenomena,
2. **Identification of goals:** the direction of the healing and/or the maintenance of health and well-being,
3. **Preparation via:** accessing the unconscious, reducing the flooding, entering into an altered state, creating a positive attitude or imagining about outcome; stretching or positioning the mindbody and/or increasing energy for the healing process;
4. **Involvement in approach(s):** the providing of engagement in the healing and health processes;
5. **Evaluation:** followed by ongoing evaluation and possible alteration of the holistic health plan.

Era III practitioners holds with grace the capacity for the person to evolve in their spiritual practice and awakening. Wherever possible healing states of transpersonal unity are encouraged within the techniques of the healer.

REFERENCES

Lewis, P. & Johnson, D. (2000). *Current approaches in drama therapy.* Springfield, IL: Charles C Thomas Pub.

Lewis-Bernstein, P. (1978). *Toward an implicit theory of dance movement therapy.* Dissertation. San Francisco: Saybrook Institute.

Lewis Bernstein, P. (1979). *8 Theoretical approaches in dance-movement therapy.* Dubuque: Kendall/Hunt.

Lewis, P. (1986). *Theoretical approaches in dance-movement therapy Vol. I.* Dubuque: Kendall/Hunt.

Lewis, P. (1984). *Theoretical approaches in dance-movement therapy Vol II.* Dubuque: Kendall/Hunt.

McMillan, J. & Schumacher, S. (1997). *Research in education.* New York: Addison Wesley Longman, Inc.

Strauss, A. & Corbin, J. (1998). *Basics of qualitative research.* Thousand Oaks, CA: Sage Publications, Inc.

Motoyama, H. & Brown, R. (1978). *Science and evolution of consciousness: Chakras, Ki and Psi.* Brookline, MA: Autumn Press.

Moustakas, C. (1990). *Heuristic research.* Thousand Oaks, CA: Sage Publications, Inc.

Pert, D. (1992). A science of harmony and gentle action. In Rubik, B. Ed. *The interrelationship between mind and matter.* Philadelphia: Center for Frontier Science at Temple University.

Rubik, B. Ed. (1992). *The interrelationship between mind and matter.* Philadelphia: Center for Frontier Science at Temple University.

Section II

INTEGRATIVE PROGRAMS
IN HOLISTIC HEALTH

Chapter 11

INTRODUCTION:
CREATING, IMPLEMENTING, ADMINISTRATING, PARTICIPATING, AND CONSULTING TO INTEGRATIVE HOLISTIC HEALTH PROGRAMS

THE FOLLOWING SECTION ADDRESSES the roles of the holistic health specialist in relation to integrative holistic health programs. Programs in this forum can be an integrated combination of alternative and or complementary modalities for a variety of populations and settings. Particular populations may include cancer patients and survivors, heart patients, those with chronic stress or illness such as chronic pain, those with emotional difficulties, or those who want to maintain wellness throughout their life span. They may be affiliated with a particular venue such as a hospital, educational setting, spiritual setting, corporate business, hotel, physical fitness gym or salon. Other health and wellness programs are freestanding, take referrals as well as walk-ins. They may be for profit or nonprofit, be hierarchical or cooperative. They may exist within one facility, have a central screening and referral system with modalities located elsewhere, or be a mutually referring loose consortium of holistic health practitioners. Programs may stay at a particular sight or travel depending on where the interest is such as targeting certain spiritual or vacation settings or geographic areas of need. New models are being created all the time as this field continues to expand.

Integrative programs minimally address mindbody health through stress reduction, relaxation, aerobic and yogic exercise and diet. Additionally they include forms of meditation, breath work and bioenergy clearing, balancing and healing. Spirituality, social support, psychological growth, creative expression and somatic-psychotherapy are encouraged if not provided. Health and wellness programs have extended beyond humans to include animals and eco-centers that value all life forms.

CREATING AND IMPLEMENTING

"Invisioning" a holistic center or program comes from a place of centered focus. Often founders and originators speak of being called or receiving an inner knowing or gnosis about what it is they are meant to do. Practitioners or co-innovators often find each other and feel as if they have known each other forever. Frequently these experiences come after individuals have done their personal work and/or have devoted themselves to a spiritual discipline for an extended period of time. If this is not the case, behaviors, limited beliefs and childhood-scripted patterns can interfere with the greater consciousness that is needed to hold a mindbody soulspirit program.

Conscious intention and spiritual access help commitment to the process. Universal law suggests that whatever individuals give energetic thought to will manifest. When this author asked spiritually how I might serve the greater good, I received that I should start a nonprofit for healing and wellness education, consultation and research. When I felt I needed a think tank of physicists, even though I knew none, within a week I had several around my dinner table discussing quantum physics, bioenergy and its documentation. When I was looking for a machine that would monitor chi and chakras, within 24 hours I got a call from a former graduate student who was getting his doctorate at an institute that had and trained people in such a research tool. Synchronicity, or the manifestation of phenomena that do not have a cause and effect relationship to each other but nonetheless have a powerful connection, occurs often when individuals are on the right path. There are no coincidences. The divine as well as human essence unfolds. Each individual knows what is true for them. The truth resonates in the third chakra or gut. Why are you reading this book now? What is it that is awakening in you or needs a jump-start into fruition or a reminder about why you are here?

Holistic health programs or centers do not flourish if the intention is misguided. They are not about making money, becoming successful or getting on the bandwagon of what is "in." These are false gods: money, status, and power will only eventually corrupt the vision. Any center that considers itself spiritually oriented must have a humble, centered, loving core of individuals fostering and midwifing the process. If the organization is hierarchical and the senior administrator is hooked in any way to the above false gods, the whole center, including every practitioner and client, will be adversely affected by this energy as it always trickles down in one form or another.

When founding a program and/or center it goes without saying that the originator must not only philosophically believe in the tenants and modalities, but also have a practice that has integrated these approaches. A disciplined form of meditation, exercise, and diet are fundamental. Ideally, all the major ways of knowing in Era II and III and in Einsteinian energy medicine are part of a program or center and are honored.

ESTABLISHING OR PARTICIPATING IN AN ORGANIZATIONAL SYSTEM

Affiliation

If a creator administrator wishes to affiliate with a particular organization such as a medical center, school, or exercise/health facility, a win/win integrated program proposal needs to be written up beforehand. It is best if the originator has research and experience to back up the proposal. Although making money is not the prime intention of the visionary, it is unfortunately often the major motivator of the organization. Thus, it is important when marketing the proposal that the holistic health presenter be knowledgeable about how the center could save or make money for them. For example, when presenting to a business, a probationary pilot study could be presented with a hypothesis that there would be a reduction in sick days for the participants. If the company were self-insured, they would be interested to know that holistic health programs have reduced psychiatric and medical hospitalizations and the prolonged use of medication.

Exercise facilities are always looking for new membership; hotels and spas are looking for customers. Not only would a holistic health center bring in revenue; it is highly marketable when individuals are looking to stay in a hotel or join a gym.

Nowadays, if a hospital does not have a wellness center, they are not keeping current. Patients will go elsewhere (here it would be useful to research documented evidence that hospitals' incomes have increased with such programs).

Freestanding

Some centers and programs are freestanding both for profit and nonprofit. Wellspace and Solutions described in this section are such successful day facilities. Centers such as these often offer courses and ongoing groups as well as individual sessions. Others such as Canyon Ranch in Arizona and the Berkshires in Massachusetts require residency.

Canyon Ranch is an example of a financially successful award-winning freestanding spa. As a model, it attempts to inspire those that come to transform their life-style through a variety of modalities including daily classes and/or individual appointments in:

- Exercise: Indoors: aerobics, fitness machines, pilates, aqua fitness, massage; outdoors: canoeing, cross-country skiing, ropes challenge, with private sports lessons and personal fitness training and exercise physiology counseling
- Health and healing services: medical and nursing consults, acupuncture, energy medicine: polarity, craniosacral, therapeutic touch; behavioral health, movement therapy, art and music therapy, and herbs and nutrition counseling
- Mindbody meditation: yoga, tai chi, chi Qung, sitting meditation and meditation counseling
- As well as relaxing facials, wraps and salon services.

After a medical intake, individuals speak to a nurse who helps them develop a program for their stay. Some come with a specific focus such as weight, stress, fatigue or pain management. No alcohol, smoking or cell phones. Individuals dine on chef-created healthy cuisine with a menu identifying calories, fat and fiber content of all items.

Of course with such exquisite vistas, richness and variety, this spa is only for the monetarily endowed, typically middle-aged who have a grasp on their mortality and the possibility that it may not be too late to make significant life-style changes.

When starting freestanding centers, pooling existing clients of participating practitioners can help provide the needed income for establishing a physical space if backers and funds are not readily available. Suffice it to say, there are many "holistic health centers" which purport to be integrative, but only rent space to alternative and complimentary practitioners. In these situations, the owner can be primarily interested in paying the rent. Practitioners can feel used. Some in these situations have complained that there develops competition among the therapist/facilitators. One practitioner felt uncomfortable that another renter was trying to get her client who was in the waiting room to set up an appointment for her modality. Self-referral is unethical no matter what holistic health practice an individual is trained, but the sense of desperation that that practitioner must have felt clearly influences the entire space and most probably trickled down from the so-called administrator.

What *makes* a center is not the name or even that the practitioners are in one physical space, it is the maintenance of communication among the practitioners with the focus upon the client or clients. Initial client presentations toward therapeutic and wellness goals, program development and referral, an ongoing case conference which evaluates and monitors individuals' groups' or systems' progress is key to developing or asking about when applying to a site. Collaboration meetings among practitioners regarding clients as well as supervision from a knowledgeable senior clinician or professional indicate that a program or center is, in fact, integrative.

Central Referral Consortium

Central referring systems typically focus on a particular population such as cancer support. Clients may hear by word of mouth or be referred by their physician. Marketing to medical specialists and specific hospital departments is vital and can be reciprocal thereby adding further inducement to referring sources. Practitioners and related programs are then suggested to screened individuals.

Mutual Collective Model

Even more decentralized, is the mutual collective model in which a group of holistic health practitioners located in their own space develop a referral collective. Familiar with each others work, they refer and collaborate on cases. Useful in this model are bi-monthly meetings in which cases are presented and ideas for joint collaboration on marketing, education, support groups, and time limited population-focused programs are discussed and initiated. Peer supervision or the use of a senior supervisor who may also screen and refer has proven successful in this model. This model can be used as a beginning step toward the eventual formation of a center that houses the collective. This model is nonhierarchical and mutually supportive of all involved.

ADMINISTRATION

Administration often requires juggling a variety of roles initially. As the center or program succeeds, these roles are taken over by others. Although some duties may be delegated to others, all of the following must be covered: business manager, accountant, creator of written advertising material, marketer, screener, advisor, supervisor, evaluator, and liaison to any larger system that the center is affiliated.

CFO and Marketer

Often the bane of health care professionals is the business side of a business. If someone is called to be a health care provider, having a business frame of reference is often the furthest skill from his or her repertoire. Although this work is not about making money, money needs to be made to support the practitioners and the program. No one should feel ripped off. Acquiring advice on the development of a business plan, financial backing, budget as well as a marketing strategy is vital. Personal referral sources are key. In all probability, all centers have a web site and target advertising sources.

Screener

Screening is vital to the admissions process. Screening encompasses an assessment of the client's basic level of mindbody soulspiritual health. Clients minimally need a strong enough ego and a basic intellectual level. Ego strength allows for grounded reality. A face-to-face interview is advised. Foundationally, the following should be explored:

ADVISING, TREATMENT PLANNING AND REFERRING

Once a decision to accept a client is made, the advisor will meet with the client to develop a treatment plan and program. The client must feel that they are collaborating in this process. If they are not invested in the plan, it is likely that it may not be successful. Sharing the vision of the program's success toward healing and wellness is half the process in meeting the co-created goals. A client may be ready to reduce chronic stress, but be unwilling at that time to tackle their diet. Thus, a wellness plan may have several stages and be renegotiated at any time.

Discussion regarding the limitations of the

Initial Screening—Consultation Questions

(General for all forms of alternative and complimentary medicine)

Current statistics:
Name
Address
Age
Employment
Ethnicity
Date of birth
Health insurance and range of coverage
Blood type
Place of birth
Citizenship
Sun sign

Why did you decide to see consultant/ practitioner/ program/ center?
What is/are the physical, emotional, energetic, interpersonal and/or spiritual complaint(s)?
When did problem(s) start and what was occurring at that time in your life?
What do you hope to receive from the program, treatment or consult?
What are your beliefs about this type of treatment?

The symptoms you are currently experiencing:
Physical symptoms you are experiencing
Emotional symptoms you are experiencing
Behavioral symptoms you are experiencing
Cognitive symptoms you are experiencing
Energetic symptoms you are experiencing
Interpersonal symptoms you are experiencing both at work/school and outside work

Any pain you have or are suffering?

Who referred you?

Complete medical history
Diseases/conditions
      High or low blood pressure
      Suicidal thoughts
      Life changing disease
      Broken bones, strains or sprains
      Systemic problems: Circulatory, endocrine, neurological, excretory, reproductive, digestive, muscular, skeletal
Surgeries
Hospitalizations
Injuries—details of falls, head injuries
Drugs:
      Prescribed
      Over the counter
      Recreational
Current medications and conditions

Allergies, asthma
Epilepsy
HIV positive
Active communicable diseases
Other specialists if currently under their care
Signed permission to consult
Family history of illness
    Physical
    Psychological
Sleep
    Number of hours and regime
    Dreams
    Quality i.e,. restful, fitful, insomnia cycle
    What time do you wake up?
Bowel movements and urination
BP
Cholesterol levels
Family history of diabetes or hypoglycemia
Current primary care physician
Precautions

What other holistic health therapies
Are you currently using—how effective?
Have used in the past—how effective?

Nonmedical remedies have taken and currently take
Were they prescribed? If so, by whom?
Homeopathic
Herbal
Essences

What are your eating habits?
How would you describe your overall diet?
Diet: how many servings of the following do you eat in a day?
    Water—how many cups per day
    Processed foods
    Organic
    Fruits vegetables
    Meats
    Fish chicken
    Carbohydrates—types
    Sugar
    Caffeine
    Tofu
How many meals a day do you eat?
Describe a typical breakfast
    Lunch
    Dinner
    Any snacking
What type of oils do you use?
Amount of food intake and times?

Drinking and smoking habits?

Work
Are you employed?
What type of work do you do?
How long have you worked there?
Describe your work environment.
Type of activity/responsibilities job requires?
Proximity of toxic substances?
How do you feel before you go to work?
How do you feel while you are at work?
How do you feel after you leave work?
How do you feel about your work in general?
If this weren't your job, what would you do?

Life-style questions
What is you home environment like?
  Where do you live?
  How many people live with you?
  Do you feel you have enough personal space?
  Are any people in your home suffering from medical/psychiatric illness?
  Are their any special needs individuals in your home?
  What are your living tasks and financial responsibilities?
Do you have pets?
  How long have you had them?
  What is your relationship with your pet like?
What do you do for leisure activities/recreation activities?
Do you have an avocation?
Do you have an art form in which you engage?
Do you listen to music—what type?
Do you watch TV regularly? If so, how long?
Do you use a computer—regularly-how long?
What's your favorite color?

Exercise
Any regular exercise routine?
Any aerobic exercise to increase heart rate?
Do you sweat?
What kind of shoes do you wear?

Psychological
Psychological history
  Family of origin history and world view
  How were you as a child—physical, psychological?
  Describe your relationship with parents and siblings.
  Early schools years
  Adolescence
  Earliest memory
Emotional and/ or physical trauma
How do you feel about taking on new challenges?
Presence of depression and depressive symptoms.

Presence of anxiety and anxious symptoms.
Presence of anger and angry symptoms.
Addictions
What are you afraid of?
Are you currently in psychotherapy?
    What kind
    With whom and permission to consult
Do you have a psychiatrist? If so, who and permission to consult.
Current relationships

Stress
Numerical stressor test: See Chapter 2
Do you have lots of stresses in your life?
If yes, list your stressors:
How do you deal with your stress?

Human energy/bioenergy
Describe your personal energy level
Do you feel you have too much, enough or not enough?
Are most of your interpersonal relationships:
    Balanced, giving and receiving?
    More giving than receiving?
    More receiving than giving?
Have you ever had or how often do you have intuitive or deja vue experiences?
Where in or around your body do think your energy is pooled or living?
Where is your energy center?
What do you do to feel safe and strong in new situations?
Do you experience heightened sensitivity to:
    Touch?
    Electronic equipment?
    Lighting?
    Individuals or crowds?
    Temperature?
    Colors?
    Places?
Have you ever had exposure to energy healing modalities:
    Acupuncture or shiatsu?
    Martial arts?
    Specific energy healing?
    Distance intentional healing?
    If so, for how long and level of effectiveness.

Social
Relationships, live alone, with someone
Animals
Significant intimate other
Children
Parents—living/ proximity/health status
How many times you have moved
Time of last move
What is your home life like?

Work colleague relationship
Unfinished relationships
Losses
How easy or difficult is it for you to make friends
How do you respond to criticism positive and negative?
Do you volunteer?

Spiritual
Part of a religious or spiritual belief or practice
Part of religious or spiritual communities who gather regularly-how often
Are you comfortable with your beliefs?
Do you have a spiritual leader, consultant, priest, minister, rabbi, and/or teacher with whom
    you can consult? If so, whom?

Observation
Body posture
Body movement
Personal hygiene
Body weight and proportion
Color and tone of skin
Intuitive observations
    Feelings, sensations, images from the somatic countertransference
    Energy fields and chakras
    High sense intuition received on behalf of client

Figure 11-1. Initial screening consultation questions.

program, the reality of any wellness program being a joint venture between client and practitioners as well as the signing of an informed consent document is relevant here. Such documents address confidentiality and its limits, release to discuss and consult with other health professionals including the client's physician or mental health therapist, and an understanding of what to expect given the type of program discussed. For example, the individual needs to be aware that appropriate touch may be used or that feelings may arise of which they may be unaware. Rules and limitations regarding cure vs. healing may also be specific to each clinician.

ADMINISTRATION AND SUPERVISION OF HOLISTIC HEALTH PRACTITIONERS

Holistic health practitioners must also be interviewed and screened. Often referral sources and administrators have sessions or take courses in order to get first-hand experience. Each practitioner should minimally have the practitioner level certificate, registry, license or degree. If there is no national or state ejudicating body over the particular practice, there may not be insurance available. At a center, each practitioner must have liability insurance and have a code of ethical practice by which they abide. Some forms of holistic health practice are beginning to be covered by insurance, making it easier for the client to afford the program.

SUPERVISION OF HOLISTIC HEALTH PRACTITIONERS AND PROFESSIONALS. Holistic health supervision is an interactional process between an experienced person (supervisor) who supervises a subordinate (supervisee) ". . . toward the supervisees acquiring appropriate professional behavior through an examination of the supervisee's professional activities" (Boylan, Malley, Scott, 1995, p. 67). There are several functions that a supervisor performs:

1. Direct clinical supervision entailing direct service training in holistic health practice
2. Administrative supervision entailing the overseeing of clinical assignments, relationship between the practitioner/therapist and the center including case presentations and inter staff communication, and the overseeing of all written material such as client or group assessments, treatment planning, and progress-noting,
3. Development of professionalism including the maintenance of standards of ethical practice.

Although there are many supervisory styles, it is important that the holistic health supervisor create a safe, caring, and empathic nonjudgmental environment in which the practitioner can discuss anxieties, vulnerabilities, and problems as they continue on their professional path. If the practitioner is only reporting successes and not the difficulties or questions they may have, more work needs to be done by the supervisor on creating a safe space. Reinforcing strengths and reframing weak areas as "growing edges" can create a competency-based positive attitude for both practitioner/therapist and supervisor.

DRAMA IN SUPERVISION. At times the practitioner's "inner critic" is projected on the supervisor and can be routed out through externalization in role-play. Role reversal can often bring out the "inner supervisor" in the practitioner. Having the practitioner role-play the client is often key while the supervisor becomes the practitioner/therapist. Another useful method is to use a "tag team" approach in group supervision to explore working with the difficult client, family, couple or group. The reflecting team model allows for practitioners to role-play a session while the rest of the supervision group observes and then comments among themselves at the end.

STAGES IN THE SUPERVISORY PROCESS OF A BEGINNING PRACTITIONER OR INTERN. Feldman and Kaslow (in Boylan, Malley, Scott, 1995) have identified six stages:

1. *Excitement and Anticipatory Anxiety:* awaiting the first client or group experience fears, without any reality to counteract them, can naturally attack the supervisee
2. *Dependency and Identification:* because of initial insecurity and newness to the program or center the supervisee often relays heavily on their supervisor which may take the form of idealization and pedestaling
3. *Activity and Continued Dependency:* the practitioner gradually takes over more responsibility in co-leading groups or in making interventions. It is no longer the client's fault that the supervisee just can't institute holistic health techniques
4. *Exuberance and Taking Charge:* the practitioner realizes that s/he is actually utilizing holistic health techniques to effect change and heal the client population
5. *Identity and Independence:* the practitioner has now moved to a level of professionalism, one in which they have begun to internalize the supervisor and have a sense of their own unique style, preference for theoretical approaches and techniques
6. *Calm and Collegiality:* the former supervisor becomes a peer.

Styles of Supervision

PHENOMENOLOGICAL APPROACH. This approach is the most nondirective. The supervisor reflects the supervisees' questions back to them and basically supports them through the stage of groping to find the answers within. This style assures that the practitioner/therapists are not just swallowing whole what the supervisor is suggesting and then parroting back but rather finding their own deeper knowing about the work.

PSYCHOTHERAPEUTIC APPROACH. Here the focus is upon the supervisees' dynamics including countertransference phenomena and thoughts, feelings, and fantasies regarding the holistic health processes with clients. Focus is placed upon any personal issues that are interfering with their ability to function as a practitioner/therapist. Videotaping or detailed process notes are required with detailed response by response commenting by both supervisor and supervisee. Areas of therapeutic context, derivative and symbolic material are discussed as well as the nature and stage of the transference. Typically psychodynamic, psychodramatic, object relational and other in depth models are employed.

SKILL BEHAVIOR APPROACH. Here the supervisor focuses on the specific attainment of competencies delineated by assessment, planning, treatment, and evaluation skills that are expected to be achieved. This approach looks to the practitioners' capacity to demonstrate the ability to utilize a wide range of holistic health paradigms and techniques appropriately and effectively.

Ideally practitioner/therapists benefit most when the supervisor is hired at the center and is an integral part of the system. Here there may be a possibility of engaging in an apprenticeship mentoring process that allows for them to first be a participant/observer, then gradually take over co-leading, then finally they assumes a leadership role with their own clients and groups. This model works best in groups such as mindfulness-based stress reduction programs.

ADMINISTRATORS AS EVALUATORS

An annual evaluation along with documentation of any areas of concern is a vital task for the administrator. Self-assessment, peer assessment, client evaluation and supervisor assessment have all been utilized as methods of evaluation.

The following are further delineated in the section on Areas of Holistic Health Competency (see Figure 11-2) and can be considered areas of evaluation:

1. Appropriate integration of holistic health theoretical approaches and techniques
2. The development and maintenance of interpersonal skills as a professional holistic health practitioner
3. The capacity to assess, derive goals, program or treatment plan, and evaluate outcome in holistic health
4. Relationship and helping skills
5. Quality of documentation including report writing
6. Application of individual, group and/or systems theory to holistic health process
7. Case conference, staff or psychoeducational presentations
8. The development of self-in-role as a holistic health professional

Areas of Holistic Health Competency

Listing of competency areas can allow for the administrator to clarify with the practitioner what is expected. The evaluative criteria are:

BELOW EXPECTATION. That is the expectation for where the practitioner should be at the time of the evaluation. If they are at the beginning of the professional career, for example, the evaluator should adjust their level of expectation accordingly.

At expectation: for their level of experience
Above expectation
Not yet demonstrated
Not applicable for holistic health practice competency

ETHICAL STANDARDS

The maintenance of standards of ethical practice is vital for each practitioner. Generic standards for holistic health practitioners should include:

• Do no harm
• Maintain the highest standards of professional and personal conduct
• Do not engage in dual relationships
• Only engage in holistic health practice of which they are professionally trained
• Does not misrepresent their competence
• Maintains confidentiality and is aware of appropriate breaches of confidentiality: duty to warn and danger to self or others
• Is aware of and abides by state and local laws
• Is ready to consult and seek the talents of other health care professionals when such consultation would be of benefit to the client
• Is up to date on research
• Engages in continuing professional education
• Collaborates with traditional health care providers where appropriate
• Encourages the client to participate in an integrative program including mindbody practices, diet, and exercise
• Is aware of precautions which may render a holistic health modality inappropriate
• Is aware of combination of prescribed traditional medications and any complimentary or alternative ingested recommendations
• Insure that the client isn't substituting alternative approaches where traditional medicine would be more effective
• Help the client make life-style changes that would support their health, healing and wellness program (AADP, 2000, Kuhn, 1999).

CONSULTATION

Integrative holistic health consultants are able to help organizations set up holistic health programs designed for the specific population(s), financial and physical space reality of the site. Some consultants pre-design programs and then market them to the appropriate systems, others are known for their ability to adapt to the requests of the settings. Consultation can include educational settings who want to develop course and curriculum material. The field of integrative holistic health is so young that there are few university programs that are offering degrees. Most of the training that is done at institutes, colleges, or universities focuses on one arena such as nutrition, holistic psychological counseling, or yoga. Graduate programs as well typically address one area.

Research consultation to document the efficacy of the growing number of alternative and complimentary techniques is also beginning to be in demand. Devices to measure bioenergy systems such as chi and chakras are just beginning to find their way into university medical centers.

CONCLUSION

There are many models and venues for integrative programs in holistic health. Visionaries, administrators, consultants, and practitioners need to be cognizant and literate in the various paradigms extant in the field in order to understand, refer, staff, market, and/or supervise the variety of practitioners and programs. Those, in particular, who are in a position of leadership must hold the philosophic vision not just in their mind but in their way of being. In this way the pro-

Holistic Health Practitioner Competency

Foundational Counseling
Applies understanding of human development
Demonstrates understanding of personality & psychic energy
Effectively applies understanding of psychopathology to client population
Applies understanding of group development and dynamics
Applies an understanding of group roles to group process
Able to put theories of group process into practice
Able to facilitate various types of groups (therapy, psychoeducational, mindbody, exercise, meditation, discussion, support, recovery, etc.)
Effectiveness as a leader with various client populations
Understanding and application of systems theories
Effective health counseling of_____population
Effective mindbody counseling of _____population

Interpersonal skills
Demonstrates emotional attunement and empathy
Demonstrates cognitive awareness
Maintains healthy boundaries
Demonstrates sensitivity to social/cultural issues
Shows comfort with authority relations
Shows positive regard for the client
Affirms strengths in client
Recognizes and works with the transference
Recognizes and works with the countertransference
Articulates ideas effectively
Gives and receives constructive feedback
Validates client experience
Utilizes counseling skills such as reflection, summarizing, reframing, interpreting and confronting appropriately
Can facilitate the expression of affect
Shows ability to be goal-directed

Assessment, treatment planning and/or goal setting
Explores nature of presenting request/problem
Gathers relevant information
Ability to make a case or program formulation using a theoretical perspective
Ability to assess risk (contracting re: harm to self or others)
Can set short and long-term goals with client(s)
Effectively responds to emergencies
Makes appropriate referrals
Utilizes center and community resources
Works collaboratively with other holistic health staff to develop and integrate program

Professional Role
Upholds standards of ethical practice of their holistic health practice and of the field
Demonstrates an understanding and adherence to legal guidelines
Demonstrates integrity, maturity and ability to handle personal issues
Attends to client's right to privacy and informed consent
Sets a frame for the session

Creates a safe space for the holistic health process
Informs clients about the potential use of touch and embodiment
Identifies oneself and responds as a professional
Develops collegial relationships
Prepares documentation and written assessments on time
Appropriately seeks and utilizes supervision
Demonstrates respect for self and client
Creates safe environment diminishing clients feelings of being exposed
Communicates with other holistic health staff

Integrative holistic health theory and application
Ability to establish a collaborative mindbody spiritually-based working staff and client
    relationship
Ability to translate goals into holistic health process
Ability to be creative and foster creativity in others
Ability to be flexible and adapt to the moment-to-moment process
Ability to be fully present and aid in other's connection to the moment
Applied understanding of the mind-body connection
Intuitive skills
Understanding and application of symbolism and symbolic themes
Psychoeducational skills
Understanding and facilitating the process of transformation
Use of cognitive approaches to limited thinking and core beliefs
Use of the creative arts
Use of imagery and guided visualization

Holistic health theory and application
Effective use of techniques within their modality
Effective use of holistic health practice with:
    Individuals
    Groups
    Larger systems/community/organizations/businesses
    Other_____

Effective use of holistic health with:
    Children
    Adolescents
    Adults
    Geriatrics

Effective use of holistic health with:
    Emotionally disturbed:
    Chronically ill
    Chronically stressed
    Chronic pain
    The anxious
    The depressed
    The traumatized
    The catastrophically ill
    The terminally ill
    The eating disordered

The physically ill
Surgical clients—pre and post op

Professionalism in Holistic Health
Ongoing commitment to inquiry into oneself and one's own issues
Ability to articulate what their particular holistic health practice is to clients and other
professionals
Ability to effectively utilize holistic health supervision
Ability to write professionally about the field
Capacity to develop new approaches and applications in holistic health
Research skills in holistic health

Figure 11-2. Holistic Health Practitioner Competency.

gram and/or center is held and influenced by the greater good. Additionally, other roles need to be filled if the center, program, and/or practice are truly integrative; for it is not sufficient that the philosophy or vision is integrative, all those that participate must feel an integral interrelated part as well. Supervising, collaborating, advising, conferencing, visioning, program developing, marketing and mutual referring are all part of integrative holistic health programs.

REFERENCES

Kuhn, M. (1999). *Complimentary therapies for health care providers.* Philadelphia: Lippincott Williams & Wilkins.

American Association of Drugless Practitioners. (2001). Code of Ethics. *www.aadp. net.*

Chapter 12

HOSPITAL AFFILIATED MINDBODY PROGRAMS

INTRODUCTION TO
THE PIONEERS

Benson, "The Relaxation Response" and the Mind/Body Medical Institute

IN THE SIXTIES, the link between the mind and body was undeniably affirmed from a variety of research sources. One of the most notable was the work carried out by Herbert Benson, M.D. regarding the influence of stress upon high blood pressure. Research at Harvard's Throndike Memorial Laboratory demonstrated that meditation techniques could reduce and control blood pressure. Joining with the California researchers, psychologist Robert Keith Wallace and physiologist Archie Wilson, who were studying transcendental meditation, a practice that had its devotees attending to the repetition of an assigned Sanskrit word for 20 minutes at a time, they were able to expand their sample population. They had catheters placed in the subjects' veins and arteries to record changes in physiologic functions as well as their brain waves. They were instructed to quiet themselves for 20 minutes, and begin meditating for 20 minutes followed by 20 minutes of returning to their normal way of thinking.

The results were astoundingly statistically significant. The subjects consumed 17 per- cent less oxygen during meditation even though they were relaxed before and after. There was a drop in the number of breaths taken, and in the amount of lactate in the blood which has been associated with affective state of tranquility and calm. The brain waves changed as well during meditation: more alpha, theta and delta waves were present (associated with rest and relaxation) and fewer of the beta waves associated with activity. Because these meditators already had low blood pressure, there was no significant drop in this factor.

From these studies Benson developed the now well-known concept of the "relaxation response." In 1988, Benson and his colleagues founded the Mind/Body Medical Institute at the New England Deaconess Hospital and Harvard Medical School. The Institute, devoted to research, training, and clinical work, was developed to study the relaxation response and to develop an integrative program for patients suffering from a variety of diseases and for those who wanted to maintain health and wellness. Individuals attend groups who suffer from high blood pressure, heart disease, cancer and chronic pain. The reduction of stress through meditation and other holistic modalities such as nutrition counseling, exercise, and cognitive psychotherapy can join with modern medicine to help heal patients.

Jon Kabat-Zinn and the Mindfulness-Based Stress Reduction Clinic

In 1979, Jon Kabat-Zinn, Ph.D., founded and directed the Stress Reduction and Relaxation Program and Clinic at the University of Massachusetts Medical Center and became the most influential leader in establishing mindbody meditation-based stress reduction programs. These programs now exist in hospitals and other organizational, social, educational and health systems in the United States, Canada, Europe, Asia and Latin America. He had come from years of engagement in the Buddhist discipline of mindfulness or *Vipassana* meditation, and believes strongly that only those who have had such a spiritual discipline of daily meditation are qualified to facilitate such a program. Kabat-Zinn, together with Saki Santorelli EdD, who established the Center for Mindfulness in Medicine, Health care and Society at the University of Massachusetts Medical School, have trained physicians, psychotherapists and other holistic health practitioners in this approach. The Center has four charges: the patient care stress reduction clinic, outreach to other systems in the community, education of medical students and health care professionals, and research designed to document the effects of the program.

MINDBODY MINDFULNESS-BASED STRESS REDUCTION PHILOSOPHY

The programs at BI-Deaconess and University of Massachusetts Medical Center now relocated to the medical school are outpatient experientially and psychoeducationally-based systematic client-centered complimentary medicine approaches which employ intensive training in meditation as their central focus. These programs in the form of courses inspire and train people to employ their mindbody resources to participate in their care and well being. Key principles include:

- Reframing the program "a challenge or adventure" rather than a "castor oil experience" that someone has to endure
- Delivering the clear message that this is not a passive process of the holistic health practitioner fixing the client, but rather one in which they are required to fully participate including homework beyond the time spent in the course. Additionally, that in order to continue the effects of the program, individuals need to *continue* to engage in the content of the program for life.
- This requires a life-style change in order for the possibility of the program to be successful.
- The suspension of time is vital whether it is the time allotted for meditation or the training itself. The experience of being fully present in the moment replaces the preoccupation with the clock.
- "An educational rather than a therapeutic orientation, which makes use of relatively large classes of participants in a time-limited course structure to provide a community of learning and practice and a critical mass to help in cultivating ongoing motivation, support, and feelings of acceptance and belonging" (Kabat-Zinn, 1999, p. 10).

Meditation

It is of interest that meditation and medicine come from the same Latin root *Medere* meaning to cure. There are many forms of meditation. It is generally considered an ancient form of mindbody and spiritual discipline that most of the world's religions have developed for the purpose of drawing the person into greater consciousness, grace and spiritual connection.

Neurophysiologically, it produces alpha waves that balance both hemispheres of the cortex creating an altered state. Within this state individuals not only experience Benson's relaxation response, lower blood pressure, heighten the immune system and the body's potential to heal, reduce pain, depression and anxiety; but additionally through heightened awareness and presence, can access states of bliss, sartori, and at-one-ment with the Source.

The are a variety of forms of meditation including:

• the catholic rosary which involves successively touching beads stranded together while repeatedly saying a prayer to the Virgin Mary,
• external object meditation in which the individual focuses upon a mandala, icon, or some natural visual image,
• the rotation of Buddhist prayer wheels,
• mantra meditation such as Transcendental meditation or the repetition of a phrase such as, "I am fully present in the moment . . . and there is only the moment," Hum Sah, "God is love," or "I surrender to thy will be done,"
• guided meditations in which an individual verbally facilitates a process for another,
• moving meditations such as yoga, mindfulness walking, nature walks, T'ai Chi and other martial arts, Dervish whirling, and repetitive rhythmic ritual dance and
• mindfulness samadhi practices of insight meditation in which an internal simple nonattached presence is the focus.

Mindfulness Meditation

Although these programs employ several of these forms, the primary discipline is based upon the use of mindfulness meditation as a daily practice. It requires an observing ego with boundaries that watches breath, sensation, and all the thoughts and feelings which can fill the busy beta wave mind with-

out becoming possessed, identified or attached. Kabat-Zinn says, "Mindfulness is a practical way of paying attention. Meditation is a way of being" (2001). The program begins progressively with more body-oriented forms of guided meditation shifting to longer and longer periods of the more disciplined formal sitting *Vipassana* meditation, gradually raising the barre of expectation, challenging the person to embodied presence.

Clients at University of Massachusetts Medical are told that "this is all there is" bringing them face to face with their expectations for the future and their reiteration of old scripts about the past. At the BI-Deaconess they are told the Buddhist tenant, "nothing is to be clung to as me or mine" (Borysenko, 2000). They are reminded that each individual has their own inner pharmacopoeia of neuropeptides that result in individuals making their own Valium. Participants are encouraged always to follow Rumi's directive and "look at the bandaged place, that's where the light enters you" (Santorelli, 2001).

FOLLOWING THE BREATH IN SITTING MEDITATION. Often called diaphragmatic breathing, yoga breathing or pranic breath is often encouraged as a first step in sitting meditation. Patients are encouraged to place their hands on their belly to notice the expansion when the diaphragm displaces abdominal viscera during inhalation and the natural pulling in which occurs in exhalation. Diaphragmatic breathing has been documented to calm even the most anxious of individuals. It is an obvious choice for attention during meditation; and since breath is always with living humans, it becomes one of the most universal foci for the mindful meditator.

MINDFUL MEDITATION MODALITIES AT THE UNIVERSITY OF MASSACHUSETTS MEDICAL SCHOOL MINDFULNESS-BASED STRESS REDUCTION PROGRAM

Mindfulness Sitting Meditation

Sitting upright in a chair or on a prayer cushion, the suggestion is made to bring the body into stillness and pay attention to breathing. The individual may for example, focus on the bulging and return of the abdomen, the expanding and relaxing of the lungs, or the sensation of the air flowing into and out of the body. When thoughts, feelings, other sensations or external phenomena distract the client, they are encouraged to notice without judgement or attachment and return attention to the breath. This form of "choiceless awareness" creates a deep stillness or *samadhi*. Often individuals complain that they "can't meditate" because they find their busy mind occupying much of the meditation. They are reminded that meditation is the entire process *including* the egressions of the busy mind.

Toward the end of a meditation, the mindfulness facilitator can offer exquisite archetypal poetry of Rumi, Eliot, Rilke and others that draws the already open meditator into an expanded experience of undifferentiated grace.

Body Scan

The body scan is a form of guided meditation which directs the supine or seated patient to sequentially attend to different parts of the body. Unlike similar guided body visualizations, its purpose is not to relax, but to bring conscious attention to the present moment focusing inner seeing on one body part at a time. For some it is the first time they have actually focused this amount of attention to their body parts that weren't screaming out with pain without judgement. Letting go of sensation, thoughts, and feelings about the regions of the body.

Specific to the UMMC program, the body scan becomes the first formal meditation homework. The voice of the facilitator is given to the client on tape thereby continuing to hold them through tone and imagistic content as they venture forth on their own during these first days in between the classes. For those with chronic pain, attending to the body may have been something they have attempted to avoid at all costs. Others with post-traumatic stress may have numb or blank spots. Noticing without judging whether there is sensation or not is part of the process. Others with physical pain are encouraged to initially place themselves in as comfortable a position as possible and then attend to the painful area(s) in the same way they did those that held no discomfort. Precisely noting the exact sensation without judgement or invoking prior emotional or cognitive interpretation regarding the distressed area allows the client to both be open to the sensations and let them go as they move to another region in the body scan.

Kabat-Zinn refers to this technique as a "zone purifier": "The moving zone of your attention harvests tension and pain as it passes through various regions and carries them to the top of your head, where, with the aid of your breathing you allow them to discharge out of your body leaving it purified" (2001) (1990, p. 88).

Yoga Meditation

Yoga meditation or stretching entailing yoga asanas are part of both programs. Done with the awareness of the physical limitations and precautions, yoga builds on the body scan through encouraging individuals to move into various postures, lengthening in inhalation and stretching during exhalation. Meditative attention is brought throughout the yoga process. When individuals notice sensation without judgement such as, "I can't hold this position a second longer," they often find that they are able to work the asana longer.

Walking Meditation

Walking meditation entails attending to the physical experience of walking. Drawing attention inward, gaze is focused directly in front where the next step would be located. There is no destination other than fully present mindfulness. Suggestions are made to walk in a specific track either back and forth or in a circle. The process of walking naturally slows down to a pace that heightens mindfulness as there is no hurry. Like following the breath meditation, attending to one aspect of walking such as the body rebalancing itself or the sequentially moving muscle groups slows down the busy mind's ability to distract itself.

Informal Meditation

In addition to the above formal meditations, individuals are instructed to bring meditation into their daily lives. Noticing pleasant and unpleasant events, utilizing cognitive constructs and Buddhist nonattachment, participants begin to understand that limiting thoughts, attitudes and beliefs can subtly but profoundly influence their quality of life. Patients are shown that optimism, confidence, an understanding that everything passes and an ability to find meaning and restore balance produces stress-hardy self-actualizing individuals.

Eating Meditation

Eating meditation or mindfulness driving, walking, and interpersonal communications help to bridge the gap into bringing these practices into daily life thereby developing a seamless continuity of presence into all life.

THE MINDFULNESS-BASED STRESS REDUCTION (MBSR) PROGRAM AT UNIVERSITY OF MASSACHUSETTS MEDICAL SCHOOL

1. The client/patient may be self, doctor, therapist, or mandated referred. They all undergo an intake in which the key principles of the program are discussed. The potential client's readiness is ascertained and a pretraining assessment is administered.
2. Participation in 8 weekly classes from 2 1/2 to 3 hours in duration along with the completion of homework assignments.

- Each class introduces and or deepens and expands the clients' formal and informal mindfulness meditation practices.
- Didactic presentations–discussions that serve to educate the participants on the mindbody paradigms and the effects of a mindfulness practice
- Class discussion includes confidentiality, self-responsibility, and a shame and fix it free environment. The role of the facilitator is one that embodies the practice in the nonjudgmental, attuned compassionate acceptance, and supports with a nonattachment to outcome attitude, each participant's authority of their own experience.
- Homework assignments of formal and informal practices as well as a variety of cognitive awareness exercises.

3. An all-day silent nonverbal communication retreat during the 6th week of the program comprised of sitting, walking, yoga, and eating meditation watching whatever comes up accepting how things are. Included in this day is a "crazy walking" meditation in which entails changes of tempo and gesticulated affective expression. Body contact occurs when the participants are

facilitated to move backward toward the center of the meditation room with their eyes closed until they form a clump.

At 3 individuals are encouraged to share for an hour; followed by a final 15 minutes of sitting meditation.

4. Individual exit interview and post-training assessment.

MODALITIES OF THE MIND/BODY MEDICAL INSTITUTE AND CLINIC AT BETH ISRAEL-DEACONESS MEDICAL CENTER

Benson's discoveries of the Era II interrelationship between mind and body are foundational to the institute and clinic's premise that the treatment of illness is best supported if attention is paid to mindbody interactions. Thus, along with Era I medicine treatment through drugs and surgery, era II is encouraged by providing the following:

Developing the Relaxation Response

Training in various exercises to elicit the relaxation response include:
- progressive muscle relaxation,
- diaphragmatic breathing,
- mindfulness meditation,
- informal day to day mindful exercises,
- use of guided imagery.

Exercise

Physical activity is needed to be healthy, to rejuvenate the body, and harmonize the mind/body/soul. Thus, respecting the limitations of physical conditions, the following is recommended:
- Aerobic exercise such as: brisk walking, jogging, bicycling, swimming, skiing or dancing, 3–5 times a week for 20–60 minutes

- Strength training: free weights, weight machines, calisthenics, etc., 2–3 times per week; 1–2 sets of 8–12 rounds
- Stretching, balancing and moving meditation through yoga

Nutrition

What is ingested affects how individuals feel, how much energy they have, as well as their capacity to stay healthy. Mindfulness eating allows for the appreciation of flavor, slowing down intake and increasing greater satisfaction of smaller portions of food.

The following researched diet is recommended:
- The ingestion of five servings of fruits and vegetables a day
- The consumption of whole grains and legumes which have been shown to fight off cancer, heart disease and diabetes
- Decreasing saturated and hydrogenated fats aids in reduction of body weight and lower cholesterol
- The ingestion of good cholesterol such as olives, peanuts, and fish oils which support the immune system
- Limiting proportions of starches, sugars, and fats.

Stress Management, Beliefs and the Power of the Mind

The way individuals think, what they believe and how they habitually respond to situations produce and maintain chronic stress. Through cognitive behavioral counseling individuals can:
- Recognize self-defeating thoughts and limited irrational beliefs
- Identify the negative statements and resultant behaviors
- Change automatic thinking through cognitive restructuring
- Reframing thoughts through positive affirming ways of viewing life

THE PROGRAM AT THE MIND/BODY MEDICAL INSTITUTE AND CLINIC AT BETH ISRAEL-DEACONESS MEDICAL CENTER

The MBMI mission is "dedicated to the study of mind/body interactions," including the relaxation response. The institute will use its expertise to enhance the recognition and understanding of the mindbody medicine's role in the practice of medicine, health care and other appropriate settings (www. mbmi.org). The programs are specific to various clinical populations and are designed to reduce stress, promote positive attitudes, prevent some diseases and decrease symptoms and improve quality of life.

ROLE OF THE MINDFULNESS HOLISTIC HEALTH FACILITATOR

Qualifications

It is expected that providers have minimally completed a training program in mindfulness-based stress reduction such as the Harvard University course taught by professionals such as Dr. Ann Webster or the residential 5-7 day intensives given by Kabat-Zinn and Santorelli. An ongoing daily meditation practice which has been active for the past three years, three years of yoga experience and two years of teaching stress reduction and yoga or body-oriented therapies or disciplines with groups. Zinn also recommends minimally two cloistered, silent meditation retreats of at least 5 days in duration.

Abilities

Knowledgeable in group development and process with a variety of populations, the holistic health practitioner needs to be able to create a sense of trust and safety in a nonattached caring compassionate interpersonal style. Emotional maturity and professionalism that adheres to group counseling ethical standards is foundational. Additionally the ability to readily translate concepts of mindbody stress reduction and meditation into understandable accessible languaging is key as well (Kabat-Zinn & Santorelli, 1999).

Practitioner-in-Role

"This work is sacred and our responsibility to it is sacred. It is the transmission of dharma" (Kabat-Zinn, 2001).

The role of the facilitator is neither to give advice, fix nor to judge, but to discuss in general about ideas with respect to the client's needs. Each individual's strength and coping skills are honored and affirmed. Supporting the tenant that the questioning is more important than the responses, help the clients experience that "the best way to get somewhere is not to try as there is no vehicle and no road" (Kabat-Zinn, 2001).

Since the processing is also the practice, enter the water with them whether it is meditation, yoga, or walking meditation, it will help support the understanding of their experience in the room. The use of present participles such as "sitting in stillness . . .", "attending without attachment . . .", "notching the waves in between the stillness . . ." helps the clients stay in "being presence" and allows for the experience to flow like a dancer with seamless transitions.

Creator of a Sacred Container

It is the role of the facilitator to foster an empathic holding environment, a temenos, a holding vessel and openness for grace to enter. Within this space the individuals wholeness rather than their disease is honored. Within this space community can be built where everyone's humanity is honored.

Borysenko (2000) asserts that the staff

must also provide a relationally connected container. If the program is an integral part of the hospital, than hospital staff need to be encouraged to go through a training.

The first vessel is the being of the facilitator. The capacity to embody stillness, attuned listening, acceptance, compassion and genuine humanity. Thus, a profound commitment to the process is vital. If someone does not show, the practitioner will need to call, ask how they are, and give them the homework. Holding a lifeline to them that neither attempts to sell nor to be attached to outcome. Normalizing and reframing participants experience help them feel comfortable to continue.

CLIENT POPULATION

Patients first come because of chronic pain, anxiety, stress or a debilitating disease. They learn through the experience of mindfulness meditation, exercise, nutrition, stress management and altering beliefs to be able to diminish the experience of pain, to reduce anxiety and stress and to be able to cope with life-threatening or chronic disease. After all this is why they have entered these programs. But what they are learning is a way of being. Although not presented as such, these programs are about their whole life, about who they are and more profoundly, about their spiritual-mystical connection. True facilitators of this approach such as Kabat-Zinn, Santorelli, Borysenko and others are gentle shaman tricksters who help individuals begin a journey the destination of which they may be initially entirely unaware. Without attachment to outcome or judgement and serenely holding presence, the holistic health mindful practitioner keeps expanding the possibility of consciousness.

Chronic Pain and Chronic Fatigue

Individuals with chronic pain are encouraged to notice sensations without attaching to judgement or outcome. The individual is encouraged to relabel the pain as sensation. Letting go of afflicting thoughts reduces suffering. Dividing the physical sensations from the attitudes about the sensations has resulted in diminished cognitive awareness of pain. At the mindbody clinic Borysenko suggested that individuals look for and notice the sensations of discomfort and then find a place in the body that has more pleasurable sensations. The group is then instructed to allow the pleasure sensations to move and expand into the entire body filling each cell (Borysenko, 2000).

More actively, imagistic approaches have also been used at the mindbody clinic by envisioning the problem and then visualizing an antidote, changing the color of the pain or its shape or anatomically and physiologically reversing or healing that which causes the pain.

At UMASS vipassana meditation encourages individuals to "look at the bigger picture." As individuals expand their consciousness, the symptoms become smaller in proportion. At the Mindbody Institute patients are supported to help reduce symptoms and increase quality of life through techniques which elicit the relaxation response, life activity management, self care and nurturance, the increase of effective communication with caregivers, and exercise and nutrition counseling.

Kabat-Zinn, Lipworth, et al. (in Kabat-Zinn & Santorelli, 1999) conducted a 4-year follow-up study of 225 patients who had completed the MBSR program. Reductions in the negative body image scale (BPPA) and the number of medical symptoms (MSCL) and global psychology symptomology (GSI) were maintained over the four years. Although a pain scale, the (PRI) reverted to original scores, a retrospective measure of overall improvement (OA) maintained post-training levels. In another study by Kabat-Zinn, Lipworth, et al., (1984) (in Kabat-Zinn & Santorelli, 1999) in which a control group was utilized, statistically significant reductions were reported in pain, negative body image, symptoms, mood, anxiety and depression as well as a reduction in analgesics.

Chronic Anxiety

Individuals in generalized anxiety live in chronic stress. Fundamental to their anxiety is a survival fear. Type A, polyphasic behavior are often produced by cognitive distortions such as awfulizing, dichotomous thinking, and imagining the worst case scenario. "When we live in the fantasies of the mind rather than the reality of the moment, then the breath follows the fantasy" (Borysenko, 2000). Diaphragmatic breathing during mindfulness meditation while concentrating on exhalation reduces anxiety. Every time an obsessive fear-driven thought enters, the client is instructed to notice it, perhaps identify the type of limited or distorted thinking and return to the breath. Meditation is about not taking thoughts more seriously than physical reality. Thoughts are only thoughts.

The use of the guided meditation of the creation of a visualized safe place has also proven to be effected with this population as well as chronic pain patients.

Miller, Fletcher, and Kabat-Zinn (in Kabat-Zinn & Santorelli, 1999) conducted a three-year follow-up study of the MBSR program with anxiety disorders utilizing the Hamilton Beck Anxiety and Depression scores. Repeated analysis showed maintenance of statistically significant gains.

Chronic Depression

Nongenetically determined depression has as its root a sense of helplessness. Having a meditation practice not only gives hope but also provides them with a tool to observe without getting caught in feelings of powerlessness and despair. Noticing where the depression is in the body, helps the client gain needed ego distance from the symptoms. Separating the thoughts from the feelings and sensations allows for healthy mind-

ful nonattachment.

Depression can be caused by retroflexed anger turned inward, complicated bereavement when an individual is unable to let go and mourn a loss, or interpersonal anxt filled with guilt, blame and/or resentment. Cognitive homework and its processing can help individuals identify the emotions, choose to let it go, reframe or take action, practice forgiveness, and mindfully let go of attachment. Clients learn that they cannot control external events, but they can control their response (Borysenko, 1998).

Cancer and HIV/AIDS

Focused intention on the shrinking of the cancer reduces the sense of powerlessness and improves the production of T-cells. "With every breath the cancer shrinks" (Borysenko, 1988). Learning to cope with these and other life-threatening diseases may help improve quality of life and aid in healing. The MBMI (Mindbody Medical Institute) 11-week Mindbody cancer and HIV AIDS programs entails stress management, relaxation response techniques, goal setting and meaning making, cognitive restructuring, nutrition, yoga, journal writing, group support, and humor. All of these modalities focus on the person as a whole rather than the disease or its symptoms.

Cardiac Wellness

The MBMI has a life-style modification 13-week (1-3 hour) program-entailing interaction with RNs, dieticians and exercise specialists and involvement in a stress management program.

School and Job Health and other Venues for Stress Reduction Programs

These mindfulness-based programs have also been used in a variety of venues from prisons, to schools, to corporations to reduce stress. It is always advisable to have those at the administrative and managerial top of the hierarchy participate as the effect trickles down rather than up the system.

MBMI has Corporate Wellness and Workforce Wellness programs addressing stress management and resiliency, relaxation, diet, exercise, and improved communication and management skills. Additionally, there are K-12 and College Programs for students, staff and teachers which entail stress awareness, relaxation techniques, and coping skills strategies for primary and secondary school and goal setting, yoga, visualizations, mindfulness and cognitive strategies in the College Network Program.

Benson, Wilcher et al., (2000) sighted a positive correlation between exposure to a relaxation response curriculum and academic achievement.

CONCLUSION

Mindbody stress reduction programs such as UMASS Medical School's Mindfulness-Based Stress Reduction Program and Beth Israel-Deaconess Medical Center's Mind/Body Medical Institute and Clinic focus upon the whole person, helping to break the cycles of stress, the limiting and distorted beliefs, and disabling coping behaviors. They transform them into mindful beings capable of positive attitudes and healthy behaviors.

REFERENCES

Borysenko, J. (2000). Omega Institute: Weekend workshop.

Borysenko, J. (1988). *Minding the body, mending the mind.* New York: Bantam Books.

Benson, H., Wlcher, M., Greenberg, B., Higgins, E., Ennis, M., Zuttermeister, P. C., Myers, P., Freidman, R. (2000). Academic performance among middle school students after exposure to a relaxation response curriculum. *Journal of Research and Development in Education,* Vol. 33: No. 3, Spring.

Benson, H. & Klipper, M. (1976). *The relaxation response.* New York: Avon.

Benson, H. (1993). The relaxation response, in Goleman, D. and Gurin, J. *Mindbody medicine.* New York: Consumer Reports Books pp. 233–257.

Kabat-Zinn, J. (1990). *Full catastrophe living.* New York: Dell Publishing.

Kabat-Zinn, J. and Santorelli, S. (2001). *Mindfulness-based stress reduction professional training.* Santa Cruz, Mount Madonna, CA: Omega Institute. Feb-March.

Kabat-Zinn, J. (1993). *Mindfulness meditation: Health benefits of an ancient Buddhist practice,* in Goleman, D. and Gurin, J. Mindbody medicine. New York: Consumer Reports Books, pp. 259–275.

Kabat-Zinn, J. & Santorelli, S. (1999). *Mindfulness-based stress reduction professional training: Resource manual.* Worcester, MA: Center for Mindfulness in Medicine, Health Care and Society.

Santorelli, S. (1999). *Heal thy self: Lessons on Mindfulness meditation.* New York: Random House.

Further Information and Training:
Mind/Body Medical Clinic at Beth Israel–
Deaconess Medical Center
110 Francis Street
Suite 1A
Boston, MA 02215
Tel: 617-632-9530
Email: *mbclinic@caregroup.harvard.edu*
Web:www.mbmi.org

Center for Mindfulness in Medicine, Health
Care and Society
University of Massachusetts Medical School
And U Mass Memorial Health Care
Shaw building
55 Lake Ave North
Worcester, MA 01655
508-856-5849

Chapter 13

SOLUTIONS CENTER FOR PERSONAL GROWTH, INC. AND THE IMAGINATION PROCESS

WENDYNE LIMBER

INTRODUCTION

I AM HONORED AND EXCITED to have the opportunity to write this chapter during this most moving, inspiring and profound evolutionary time in history. Healing and transformation has been my passion in life and I now present and support this model. Imagination is an integrated whole healing process model which takes into account the many fascinating aspects of the human being and being alive–body, mind, spirit, emotions; past, present and future; consciousness and unconsciousness; left brain, right brain; old and new; psyche and spirit; traditional and nontraditional; east and west. I have learned that I must seek to know the big picture, the bigger story, in order to heal and transform my life or help any other person do the same. How individuals think, feel, eat, move, meditate, work, communicate, and dream has developed their personality and will create the future. Each of these domains must be evaluated and worked with for a whole healing and transformation.

GENESIS

Dare I say that the beginning of this process was deep within my own psyche returned to me in a vision? Yes, I saw the work I must do in 1987, long after the foundations had been laid by the many theorists, counselors, teachers, writers, psychotherapists, thinkers, physicians and metaphysicians. I sought after my own healing, traveling the world through books, education and workshops of all kinds, physical, mental, and spiritual. I laughed and wept, moved and breathed, meditated, studied and became still. The answers were inside me. I noticed I had healed and transformed. This was a process, a passage. Every aspect of my being must be addressed through a series of actions, changes and functions to bring about my desired result. It would take time.

There were no coincidences. My body, my vocation, my relationships, my experiences were all a segment of the process of the whole, painful and joyful. Every part of my personality took on the shape of my feelings, beliefs and thoughts, conforming to the structure and systems blueprinted in my psyche. I had created the past, present and future. I seemed to attract to me experiences that matched my state of being, thinking, and feeling. Could it be so?

I was inspired by my studies in family systems, developmental psychology, life cycles and the healthy or dysfunctional navigation of such. Erickson (1963), in his psychosocial theory, informed me of stages a child must master in order to progress toward independence and wholeness. John Bradshaw (1990) presented the precious and wounded inner child and dysfunctional family to the recovery community, which definitely created a portal for my own reclaiming of self. I was influenced by Maslow's hierarchy of needs and attentive to Freud's (1988) presentation of the unconscious. Joseph Campbell (1991) inspired me with myth and symbol. I was fascinated with Jung's work (CW), which connected me with the unconscious archetypal themes, myths and depth psychology. I loved and personally participated in Gestalt group work with a therapist who loved Fritz Perls. This quest lead me to the study of spiritual and transpersonal psychology with Jacquelyn Small (1991), directing me toward the works of Stanislav Grof (1990), perinatal psychology, birth trauma, womb work and a world of sensory and transpersonal enlightenment. Deepak Chopra, MD (1990) awakened my inquisitive mind to energy, information and quantum physics as well as the Indian medical system, Ayurveda. Dr. Gabriel Cousens (1986) intrigued me with his incredible system of spiritual nutrition and conscious eating. These disciplines allowed me to think, feel and create in new dimensions. Later, the study of psychoneuroimmunology through the work of Candace Pert (1997), Era III Medicine and Larry Dossey (1989), and age old concepts of the body maps and chakra system allowed me to integrate the mind/body connection

in a bold and major way for myself and my private practice I had developed in the meantime as a Marriage and Family Therapist.

It seems that the more open I became, the more information came to me. Albert Einstein seemed to follow me around in those days, with a book, a picture or quote everywhere I turned. Expanding my horizons, I was introduced to the richness of ritual and ceremony from Shamanism and Eastern healing systems combining all of these together with the creative expressive arts, drama therapy, music, sound, movement, dance and writing. This was the genesis of what would become Imagination . . . a healing and transformational process, a complete and wholly integrated process for the healing of the human being. It would include the past, present and future, integrating old and new psychology, Eastern and Western healing systems, body, mind, and spirit taking into account the mystery of life, and the whole memory of the soul. I began to see how it was all connected and that all aspects of the human being must be addressed. Imagination was born!

Today, I am teaching this holistic and integrated Imagination healing and transformational model to students who have chosen to work and study with me through Soul Studies Institute, Inc., an outgrowth of Solutions Center for Personal Growth, Inc. in Stuart, Florida. Our mission: we are guiding and loving people to their highest potential and being using the expressive therapeutic arts and education. Students working in independent degree programs will earn an MA Degree in Transpersonal Transformational Creative Arts Therapy and will be certified in this Imagination Model. Student interns, who eventually assist in the Imagination process as part of their fieldwork experience, also have gone through this process as part of the training program.

The Evolution of Solutions

I am thinking back about the last 10 years for me at Solutions Center for Personal Growth, Inc. In 1989, I decided to open my own business, interested in risk taking, going to the edge of reality, taking people to new places of being, experiencing pain and joy to break through the old and transform into the next. In my effort to heal and transform my own self, Solutions Center for Personal Growth, Inc. and the Imagination process manifested.

I had wanted to leave the old place, express my personal best, be my own boss, because there was so much I wanted to do. Other people, old bosses, thought my ideas were too "far out." This way, I could do what I wanted to. If we wanted to yell and scream and march around the room singing the Italian National Anthem, or crawl and cry and feed each other singing nursery rhymes, it would all be ok. Because I decide!

So, I took the risk to quit. I found a quaint little office on Seminole Street with one large room, a small room and a bathroom. It was in downtown Stuart, Florida, on the water, a perfect location, and a building I had always loved. I must have it! After finding it for rent one Friday afternoon, I told the landlord who lived next door that I would "take it." I had no money. By Monday morning I would need first, last and a deposit, around $1200. I told no one about this. After all, was I being realistic? On Sunday afternoon two different people, unknown to each other, called me saying, "God told me to give you $1000." By Monday morning I had the money and I was even able to have power and a telephone. It was a sign. I was on the right track.

I remember my friends painting and repainting that first office. And I remember when two men carried the secretary desk up the stairs for me. They placed it in the perfect spot and we began to wipe off the dust. In the bottom drawer we found a 20-year-old newspaper on which was printed two advertisements for two separate businesses in town. Incredibly, the ads had been taken out by the two men who had at this moment lovingly volunteered to carry this desk upstairs, unknown to each other. It was another sign that I was on the right path.

I turned 40 that year. The clients lined up a city block holding balloons for me in celebration. I was touched and surprised. I was helping people take risks to express their pain and joy, going beyond the traditional. I was loving people well and it was working. We were attacking co-dependency, addiction and repressed feelings from our lives. We were learning to sing and dance together too.

Today, 12 years later, Solutions Center for Personal Growth, Inc. is a holistic health center. In addition to the Imagination process, a variety of CAM modalities are offered including Yoga, Music Together, Integrative Bodywork, Imagine Transpersonal Breathing, Reiki, Awakening the Artist Within, Rhythms of Energy Dance, Soul Writing, Therapetee Theater, African Drumming, Live Foods Consultation, Meditation, Mind Body Workshops, Money Grows On Trees, and Sound Therapy. Students enrolled in Soul Studies Institute, Inc., holistic health practitioners and volunteers have joined the Solutions team in an effort to offer the community an integrative holistic healing system. Solutions Center for Personal Growth, Inc. is thought of as a sacred and powerful energy field in which to heal, transform and co-create life.

FRAME OF REFERENCE

Imagination is based on the theory that people are constantly moving toward and desiring wholeness, health, intimate relationship, love, peace, joy, magic and connection to the divine, that there is a natural unfolding and evolution toward wholeness and balance. It is my belief that one's effective attainment of these values and states of being, doing, and feeling are initially dependent upon a healthy navigation of the developmental stages of growth and the healing and transformation of all soul wounds. The soul brings all memory and emotionally inherited passion and pain to the womb. Experiences from the womb, birth and early childhood form a blueprint or imprint in the psyche that individuals continue to match or reenact until which time, this imprint is healed or transformed. One's original imprint is unconscious until it becomes conscious. Pivotal to the Imagination model views, is the tapping into unconscious stored material in the body/mind. The unconscious mind is manifested in the body and life of each individual. As the body and mind are one, illness and issues of health are directly related to and dependent upon the unconscious or conscious imprints in the psyche. Upon healing and transformation, the individual has the ability and power to create a desired future of unlimited possibilities, to reprogram the mind and transcend this early blueprint, as well as move toward a greater human experience, connecting with a greater divine purpose, and commitment to mindful transformational practices.

People who embark on such a healing journey open their heart where it has been closed, attain physical and mental health, which heretofore was in question or serious trouble, and connect and acquire a spiritual belief system, which, individuals can depend upon to move through life's experiences.

Imagination is a whole and integrated system based on theory and practice which includes core concepts in the areas of health and healing, consciousness, family systems, spiritual emergency, psychoneuroimmunology, psychospiritual integration, group process, and principles of quantum physics. In general, these core concepts and frames of reference include the mind, body and spiritual aspects of the self.

BASIC CONCEPTS

Health, Healing and Transformation

Health is freedom from disease or abnormality. It is soundness, a condition of optimal well-being (The American Heritage Dictionary of the English Lauguage, 3rd Edition). Excellent health is about vitality, wholeness, fitness, goodness and celebration. Maslow's concept of self-actualization, or the capacity to expand into higher states of consciousness while unfolding life purpose, is key. Maslow's model is simple and profound to me. In his hierarchy of needs, he states that one cannot achieve these states of being, optimum health or self–actualization, until one's physical, safety and security, love and belongingness, and self-esteem needs are met first, in the order given.

Healing and restoring to wholeness is a process involving transformation. Each individual can transform, transfigure, recover, evolve, be influenced, affected, and reborn. Evolving toward health and wholeness, a person ultimately moves toward higher potential and possibilities. Through transpersonal psychotherapy and psychospiritual group process, the Imagination process invites participants on a holistic healing journey:

> You are about to enter a sacred process resulting in a transformation of your life, your body, your mind and your spirit. You will go deep into the lost places of your soul as you remember your own true essence. You will remember how to love, and this will create peace. You will see and discover the truths you have really always known. Our process utilizes the expressive creative arts: writing, transformational theater, music, sound, movement, dance, art, breathwork, psycho-spiritual group process, body work, and expression. (Limber, 1997, p. ii)

Transpersonal Psychotherapy is defined as the process through which individuals transform their identity from a limited history based sense of self to an experience of their soul essence. From the experience of soul, individuals can access a relationship to the numinous and their unique life purpose. (Lewis, 2000, p. 260)

The Imagination process assists individuals in discovering the original blueprint designing their lives and further draws participants into a healing process, which corrects and reverses any faulty thought or negative mind-body programming. Participants in the Imagination process learn how they may be miscreating their lives, unconsciously attracting life experiences into the original plan, with all its characters and themes. Clients have the opportunity to reexperience and reframe past pain, which gives one the power to write new outcomes, hence to design a new kind of future. The very physical cells of the human being can be transformed, even transmuted in an alchemical dance.

Family Systems and Object Relations

Family Systems theory, therapy and techniques have been a part of the organizational structure, belief system and evolution of the Imagination process. Family systems theory in general teaches that the family represents a complex relationship in which causality is circular and multidimensional (Goldenberg & Goldenberg, 2000). Early family relationships directly affect thoughts, feelings, actions and ways of being. Ways of being turn into major beliefs, patterns, and finally complex interpersonally triggered systems. Systems become creations reenacted over and over.

Object Relations theory teaches that the infant's primary need for attachment to a caring person is monumental, that an individual who did not receive this in a healthy, loving way does not internalize a good enough caregiver. They continually seek for

this primary and so needed bonding through other relationships (Scharf & Scharf, 1987). Eric Erickson's work in psychosocial development instructs that each developmental stage results from an interpersonal crisis, primarily with parents, but also with peers and schoolteachers. The crisis is a time of heightened vulnerability and increased potential, with the resolution of each stage creating the next crisis. Erikson believes that the resolution of each crisis produces coping and adaptations producing ego strength (Erikson, 1963). A child acquires the ego strengths of hope (infant–trust vs. mistrust); willpower (toddler–autonomy vs. shame and doubt); purpose (preschooler–initiative vs. guilt and doubt); and competence (school age–industry vs. inferiority). John Bradshaw's approach supports this hypothesis using transactional analysis–identification of the "inner child"–a combination of Freud's id and self psychology's self, he focuses upon the potential wounding of the precious and wonderful inner child. The original "wonder child" had wonder, optimism, naiveté, dependence, emotions, resilience, free play, uniqueness, and love. Through physical, mental, emotional and sexual abuse the wonder child becomes spiritually wounded and full of toxic shame. Reclaiming the inner child involves going back through the developmental stages and finishing unfinished business. The most important first step is to help the wounded child grieve its unmet developmental dependency needs (Bradshaw, 1990).

Murray Bowen, family systems theorist presents a Transgenerational model based on natural systems. He describes human behavior as the result of an evolutionary process and as one type of living system. According to Bowen, the human family is seen as appearing as the result of an evolutionary process in nature. In particular, the theory concerns itself with a special kind of natural system–the family's emotional system (Kerr & Bowen, 1988). Imagination theory maintains that these emotional patterns and systems are indeed transgenerational, moving through time and on into the next generation until they are healed and transformed by whomever becomes the identified healer (patient) of the family.

Structural family therapy has described the dysfunctional family as a family that has failed to fulfill its function of nurturing the growth of its members (Colapinto, 1991). Dysfunction suggests that the covert rules that govern family transactions have become (perhaps temporarily) inoperative and require renegotiation (Goldenberg & Goldenberg, 2000). Family systems offer many important concepts with which to work and understand in the healing process: family of origin, functional or dysfunctional family system, boundaries, shame, abandonment, family rules, family trance, communication, fair fighting, feedback loops, developmental tasks, transgenerational, triangulation, and recovery. The Imagination process teaches these concepts as part of the process.

The Imagination process honors the inner child and offers opportunities for healthy reenactment of one's developmental dependency and attachment needs; to grieve the loss of a healthy and nurturing family of origin and an opportunity to design and live by new functional rules. Therapists and group participants become a new family to trust and believe. Through experiential group process, healthy communication, insight and risk taking, one can heal and transform negative belief systems, family of origin pain and trauma. People are given the opportunity to reenact and reexperience developmental stages with healthy caretakers and family members through transference and countertransference. Attention is given to the inner infant, inner child and inner-teenager present inside each one, encoded in memories of the cells. Communication becomes overt and functional. A person has an opportunity to become conscious of old systems and ways of being, proactively designing and committing to new patterns and behaviors. Reclaiming childhood and mourning what was absent are components of the Imagi-

nation process. Grief work left undone becomes neurosis. As Jung said, "all our neurosis are substitutes for legitimate suffering" (Jung, 1963).

Consciousness

Consciousness, as viewed in the Imagination model, is seen as awareness, a knowing. A core concept of the Imagination model is that people have been unconscious—not aware of why and how they may be having painful or dysfunctional experiences in their present life; that there is truly a reason, a core issue, a core imprint which is unconscious and is a result of their soul memory, womb and birth experience, early childhood and any other trauma held in the body. An end result or goal of the Imagination process is that individuals become conscious of all the aspects of their being. This entails the bringing forward into consciousness what has been unconscious; revealing the patterns, thoughts, memories and feelings which have been imprinted in the soul and reintegrating what was split off. Transformation to fully self-actualizing individuals naturally follows.

Jung

Imagination theory is aligned with a Jungian view of consciousness. Jungian analysis involves the conscious revelation of the content and meaning of the unconscious, through the interpretation of symbolic products of the unconscious mind. The interpretation of symbols includes the examination of dreams, fantasies, drawings, religious phenomena, hallucinations, sculpture, myths, and early memories becomes part of the process. In Jung's scheme, all human behavior is both purposive and prospective—that is directed toward the future (Bankart, 1997). The psyche is seen as a self-regulating system whose function is purposive, with an internally imposed direction toward a life of fuller awareness (Kaufman, 1989). Imagination recognizes that Jung's theory is based on the demands and transformations of human energy systems. The following concepts explored by Jung are applicable: a collective unconscious which he called the region of the mind that contains a universal source of mental energy and the psychology of archetypes–universal human symbols passed in the DNA from one generation to the next, from the earliest forms of organic life to the child being born at this very minute. Every human being possesses an intuitive, instinctive knowledge of these archetypes (Bankart, 1997).

The Imagination process is an alchemical process parallel to Jung's alchemical stages. (1)The beginning of the alchemical therapeutic process is likened to chaos and the formless mass of soul, spirit and body. Later, a separation where soul and spirit separate from the body or mental identity experienced as a symbolic death takes place. (2) This is followed by a state of pregnant, receptive, creative waiting. In this phase the Imagination therapy rooms and processes serve as a container and place for an individual to turn inward. (3) In the third phase, the soul and spirit join the oneness of the universe, as the Imagination participant becomes conscious of negative aspects. (4) In the final phase, opposites become united in the sacred marriage, in which illumination occurs, filled with insight and understanding. When the process is complete, the attention returns to the outer world transformed (Harris, 1996).

Grof

The work and research of Stanislav Grof MD, in the field of human consciousness, has had great influence upon the creation, theory and techniques of the Imagination model. Grof, who systematically studied consciousness for over 30 years, views consciousness and the human psyche as expressions and reflections of a cosmic intelligence that permeates the entire universe and all of existence. These fields of consciousness are without limits, transcending time, space, matter and linear causality. From *The Holotropic Mind*, Grof, states:

As a result of my observation of thousands of people experiencing non-ordinary states of consciousness, I am convinced that our individual consciousness connects us directly not only with our immediate environment and with various periods of our own past, but also with events that are far beyond our physical senses, extending into other historical times, into nature, and into the cosmos. (Grof, 1992, p. 18)

Grof has given us a cartography of the unconscious aspects of the human psyche wherein he has mapped out various types and levels of experience that have become available in certain special states of mind and that seem to be normal expressions of the psyche.

Besides the traditional (1) biographical level containing material related to our infancy, childhood, and later life, this landscape of the inner space includes two additional domains, (2) The perinatal level of the psyche, which, as its name indicates is related to experiences associated with the trauma of biological birth, and (3) the transpersonal level, which reaches far beyond the ordinary limits of our body and ego. This level represents a direct connection between our individual psyches, the Jungian collective unconscious, and the universe at large. (Grof, 1992, p. 20)

The key experiential approach used and taught by Grof to induce nonordinary states of consciousness and gain access to the unconscious and superconscious psyche is Holotropic Breathwork which will be discussed in greater depth in the therapeutic process portion of this chapter.

Of particular interest and importance to the Imagination process is Grof's work with womb and birth trauma, the perinatal level of the psyche. Grof describes Birth Matrix I,

II, III and IV, which begin with intrauterine experiences, cosmic unity, good or bad womb, expulsion from the womb, the death-rebirth struggle, the agony and ecstasy of birth, and the mystery of the journey, to name a few stages of experiences. Grof also discovered and explains the COEX system– memories of emotional and physical experiences are stored in the psyche not as isolated bits and pieces but in the form of complex constellations, which he calls COEX systems (for "systems of condensed experience").

> Each COEX system consists of emotionally charged memories from different periods of one's life, the common denominator that brings them together is that they share the same emotional quality of physical sensation. Each COEX may have many layers, each permeated by its central theme, sensations, and emotional qualities. Each COEX has a theme that characterizes it. For example, a single COEX constellation can contain all major memories of events that were humiliating, degrading or shameful. Rejection and emotional deprivation leading to our distrust of other people is another very common COEX motif. Each COEX constellation appears to be superimposed over and anchored into a very particular aspect of the birth experience. The birth experience contains the elementary themes for every conceivable COEX system. In addition, to these perinatal components, typical COEX systems can have even deeper roots. They can reach farther into prenatal life and into the realm of transpersonal phenomena such as past life experiences, archetypes of the "collective unconscious," and identification with other life forms and universal processes. (Grof, 1992, pp. 24, 25)

Grof explains that his work and research with COEX systems has convinced him that they serve to organize not only the individual unconscious, but the entire human psyche itself. The Imagination model incorporates the work of perinatal psychology into its theory and practice. Participants become aware of their birth trauma, and womb experiences, and set out to reverse and positively

reexperience birth. This view and study of consciousness supports the idea that womb and birth experiences create a blueprint, which the human being will continue to recreate until which time the blueprint or COEX is transformed or dismantled in some way.

The Imagination process seeks to transform negative belief systems and programmed thoughts and feelings into healthy awareness. One is able to make new decisions about old ideas; become conscious of old paradigms of thinking and shift into the light of consciousness, energetically correcting and creating new reframes and responses to negative memories which have been buried inside the body/mind complex. It is written in the Phase I Imagination workbook, *I Am the Honored Guest at Your Healing.*

> Memories and experiences are encoded in every cell of the body as the body, mind and soul interprets your experiences from conception to adulthood. Therefore, what happened in your family is significant. It is for this reason that we begin from the beginning, searching deep inside for the lost parts of ourselves. The inner child is that part of ourselves that was vulnerable, feeling, naive, loving, creative and wonderful. The inner child is the body in a sense, the basic earth bound, dependent part of ourselves, as well as the part of us with imagination. To imagine is to create, and if you want to create new patterns and new joy in your life, you must clear out the past once and for all. It is a matter of science and energy. You do not have enough energy to create what you want now, if energy is stored in the body from the past pain of your life. If this part of ourselves was wounded, we must go back and get our little child for healing. (Limber, 1997)

Work in nonordinary states of consciousness allows experiences with all soul memory. Many who open the psyche and soul through work in altered states have come to believe in the existence of past lives, that patterns and systems which continue to "show up" may be emotionally inherited or due to abuse, past behaviors and death in former lives. In this way, Imagination participants are healing at the level of soul, clearing "karma," a Buddhist term defined as "the total effect of a person's actions and conduct during the successive phases of the person's existence, regarded as determining the person's destiny" (*The American Heritage Dictionary of the English Language*, third edition).

Spiritual Emergency

The Imagination process involves evaluation and assessment using a very thorough Life and Family History and the development of a Plan of Intention or treatment plan. This usually takes 2 or 3 hour-long sessions with client and therapist prior to the group process work. The therapist notes a DSM-IV psychological diagnosis as part of the system requirements. There is also always an awareness of the principle of "spiritual emergency." Spiritual emergency refers to the dramatic and intense experiences or unusual states of mind that one may experience on the healing path, which normally would be treated as a mental illness by traditional psychology. According to Christina and Stanislav Grof in their book, *Spiritual Emergency*,

> Some of the dramatic experiences and unusual states of mind that traditional psychiatry diagnoses and treats, as mental diseases are actually crises of personal transformation, or "spiritual emergencies." Episodes of this kind have been described in sacred literature of all ages as a result of meditative practices and as signposts of the mystical path. When these states of mind are properly understood and treated supportively rather than suppressed by standard psychiatric routines, they can be healing and have very beneficial effects on the people who experience them. The positive potential is expressed in the term spiritual emergency, which is a play on words, suggesting both a crisis and an opportunity of

rising to a new level of awareness, "spiritual emergence." Throughout the ages, visionary states have played an extremely important role. From ecstatic trances of shamans, or medicine men and women, to revelations of the founders of the great religions, prophets, saints and spiritual teachers, such experiences have been sources of religious enthusiasm, remarkable healing, and an artistic inspiration. All ancient and pre-industrial cultures placed high value on nonordinary states of consciousness as an important means of learning about the hidden aspects of the world and of connecting with the spiritual dimensions of existence. (Grof, 1989, p. x, xi)

Imagination theory honors nonordinary states of consciousness, unusual and visionary states of mind as an ordinary part of the healing and transformation process. In addition, such states are viewed as important processes and ways for participants to discover the hidden parts of themselves as well as personal openings and connections to the spiritual dimension. In perceiving such states as natural and important parts of the process, participants are encouraged to allow these states to take their natural course versus attempting to suppress these conditions with medical or other strategies. Student interns are trained to understand the difference between states of spiritual emergency and psychosis, honoring the balance between traditional and spiritual approaches to healing and transformation.

The Body/Mind Connection and Psychoneuroimmunology

Theory, research and work in the field of mind/body and psychoneuroimmunology is an integral part of the Imagination process for two reasons: (1) Physical illness may result from and be a part of the healing and transformation process and (2) a person may come to the Imagination process with the intention of healing a present illness or physical state.

Drs. Elmer and Alyce Green (with Walters, 1969), proposed a rational for mind-body regulation. It was their suggestion that perception (or imagery) elicits mental and emotional responses that generate chemical responses in the limbic system, thus activating the pituitary and bring about physiological responses. These physiological responses are then responded to, in turn, completing a cybernetic feedback loop. Candace Pert (1997), a biochemist, was one of the first researchers to discover that in order for opiates and other psychotropic drugs to work, there must be receptor sites in the brain. These receptor sites were also found to be scattered throughout the body, as well. Pert, who believed in the beginning of her work that emotions were in the head or brain, now documents that they are in the body as well-forming an incredible information/communication network (Pert, 1997). Pert and others have shown evidence that one's imagery can change the functioning and chemistry of the body, that changing one's thoughts, beliefs or images can change one's emotional response to the world.

Psychoneuroimmunology (PNI), coined by Dr. Robert Ader (1981) is the study of the connection between the mind/emotions, the central nervous system, the autonomic nervous system, and the immune system. The research in this field is fascinating as in the studies of multiple personalities by Nicholas Hall, Ph.D., who documented with blood samples that changes can occur in six seconds when a different "mind" or "alter" takes over the body. Dr. Diedre Brigham (1994), in *Imagery for Getting Well*, describes a personal communication with Dr. Hall: "one of his most interesting examples was his finding a full-blown diabetic subpersonality while others, alters of the same person, evidenced perfectly normal blood sugar levels" (Brigham, 1994, p. 5). In another case study, a multiple personality, Jill, came in for a therapy session with the flu, nose running, and laryngitis–a wheezing mess. During the session, the therapist asks to speak to Jane,

another of the personalities. In the six or so seconds it took for the transition, Jane appeared–with none of the symptoms Jill was manifesting. The therapist/author reports, "in that six seconds not only had a "world image" changed, but a body had also changed, significantly. I realized this amazing "ability" which emerged from a condition usually thought of as pathological was potentially available to anyone willing to change basic images or attitudes" (Brigham, 1994, p. 5).

Ernest Rossi, author of *The Psychobiology of Mind Body Healing* (1986), incorporated Pert's work and suggests that the neuropeptide and the communication system formed by the receptor sites is the psychobiological basis of therapeutic hypnosis and mind-body healing. Rossi says that how we believe and how we project our beliefs in images affects our being, right down to the cellular and genetic level. Rossi suggested later that in the mind-brain connection, the neural networks of the brain-dependent memory and feeling-toned complexes of the mind's words, images, etc.–encode from the information substances (hormones, neruopeptides) received from all cells of the body (Rossi, 1990). Drs. Jeanne Achterberg and Frank Lawlis (1980, 1984) did an intense study of the relationship among imagery, beliefs, attitudes and stress and the progression and remission of cancer and other life-threatening conditions discovering statistically sound relationships. James Pennebaker (1990) studied the relationship between the ability to share one's feelings and the physical health of those who are able to do this. He found that "confessional writing" could lead to significant changes in the immune system and better health in general–that inhibiting feelings creates stress for the immune system. Larry Dossey (1989) introduced us to ERA III Medicine and transpersonal healing along with Jon Kabat-Zinn (1990) who reminded us of the practice of "mindfulness" to the healing process.

Carolyn Myss, recognized as a medical intuitive, and a pioneer in the field of energy medicine, teaches about the human being's bioenergetic spiritual framework. Eastern religions teach that the human body contains seven energy centers. Each of these energy centers contains a universal spiritual life-lesson that we must learn as we evolve into higher consciousness (Myss, 1996). It is believed by Myss and others in the field of energy and vibrational medicine that physical dysfunctions may occur in any of these chakras which include certain corresponding organs and systems when one does not successfully master developmental mental and emotional issues or life lessons.

The Imagination process honors greatly these core theories and research from psychoneuroimmunology, with the awareness that "every voluntary behavior is preceded by an image of what will occur, no matter how brief or elusive to our consciousness this image may be" (Brigham 1990, p. 32). Imagination teaches that one can choose the direction of the mind providing images that will speak directly to the body. In the healing and transformation process, some kind of transcendent consciousness or awareness occurs first as in an epiphany, then the healing of the body, mind or emotions follows. As one becomes conscious and experiences an uncovering of meaning, the pieces of the puzzle come together. Physical illness as a result of the healing and transformation process is viewed as "part of the process," a detoxification of emotional pain, a cleansing of the energetic blockages in each chakra or energy center in the body. Imagination is a process of reversing conditioned responses so to eliminate fear. These processes affect the body, for a full healing of body, mind and spirit.

Psychospiritual Integration and Transpersonal Psychology

The Imagination model is a transpersonal psychological model integrating one's psyche with the spiritual nature of Self. With healing, transformation, health and consciousness, one is merging the psyche and the spirit—hence the term, psychospiritual integration. According to one of my greatest teachers, Jacquelyn Small, psyche is the root of the word "psychology," and it means soul, or spirit, something psychologists seem to forget. The psyche is huge, our total self. Transpersonal Psychology is attempting to bring back a respect for the wholeness of the Self. Its goal is to move forward along the trajectory of our unfolding lives, to help us manifest the theme "from fragmentation to wholeness" so that we can actualize our full potential. It is the first psychology (because it includes the work of Carl Jung) that explains the client's process as being a hero's or heroine's journey, an inner awakening or pilgrimage back to our spiritual source. This journey has been known throughout history by many names: The Tao, The Way of the Christ, enlightenment, the shamanic journey, kundalini awakening, the middle path, the Royal Road, the path of Initiation, the hero's journey, or simple 'going home,' to name only a few (Small, 1991, p. 30).

The Imagination process is the hero journey, described so profoundly by Joseph Campbell—"the goal of the hero trip down to the jewel point is to find those levels in the psyche that open, open, open, and finally open to the mystery of the Self being Buddha consciousness or the Christ" (Osbon, 1991, p. 23).

Quantum Physics and Universal Law

In addition to core concepts mentioned above, imagination aligns closely with theory from quantum physics which states that we are energy and information, and that energy and information can be focused through our intentional thought to create the future. Deepak Chopra, M.D., in Quantum Healing, reports:

From a famous mathematical formula,

knows as Bell's theorem, Quantum physics teaches us that the reality of the universe is non-local; all objects and events in the cosmos are inter-connected with one another and respond to one another's changes of state. Physicists now accept inter-connectedness as a ruling principle, along with many forms of symmetry that extend across the universe. Contemporary theorists such as British physicist, David Bohm, has had to suppose that there is an "invisible field" that holds all of reality together, a field that possesses the property of knowing what is happening everywhere at once. The invisible field sounds very much like the underlying intelligence in DNA, and both behave very much like the mind. The mind has the property of holding all our ideas in place, in a silent reservoir so to speak, where they are precisely organized into concepts and categories. (Chopra, 1990)

Chopra says that consciousness remains 95 percent the same from day to day, and it is this consciousness (or imagery) that is the blueprint for what happens to the body, mind and spirit. He asserts that molecules do not produce thought; rather, thought produces molecules (Brigham, 1990). In other words, an individual's present state of consciousness and words are a blueprint for the body, for diseases or health. From this work the concept of the art of co-creation, learning to create with the power of thought is posited. The art and skill of this knowing is that as all energy is connected, it can be moved with an individual's thought and feeling vibration, so to create and attract what is desired. Imagination teaches the art and skill of co-creation, pointing out that clients are creating all the time by their thoughts and feelings in an unconscious way.

Imagination participants are told, "Each person has the ability and the power to create the future. We are co-creators with the universe. You have been creating your life now unconsciously by the way you believe, think and feel. These processes begin to make your life and your process conscious. In this way, there are no limits to what one can create; all things are possible as we begin to speak a language of power" (Limber, 1997).

Vibrational Medicine

Dr. Gabriel Cousens, in an introduction to the book, *Vibrational Medicine*, by Richard Gerber, M.D. reports at the conclusion of this book that "we as human organisms, are a series of interacting multidimensional subtle-energy systems, and that if these energy systems become imbalanced there may be resulting pathological symptoms which manifest on the physical/emotional/mental/spiritual planes. These imbalances can be healed by rebalancing the subtle energy templates with the right frequency of vibrational medicine."

According to Gerber, "The Einsteinian paradigm as applied to vibrational medicine sees human beings as networks of complex energy fields that interface with physical/cellular systems. The recognition that all matter is energy forms the foundation for understanding how human beings can be considered dynamic energetic systems. Through his famous equation, $E=mc^2$, Albert Einstein proved to scientists that energy and matter are dual expressions of the same universal substance. That universal energy is a primal energy or vibration of which we are all composed. Therefore, attempting to heal the body through the manipulation of this basic vibrational or energetic level of substance can be thought of as vibrational medicine" (Gerber, 1988, pp. 39–40).

Likewise, the Imagination process model, through the transpersonal transformation creative arts therapies attempts to heal the body, mind, emotions and spirit through the manipulation of this basic or energetic level of substance, and we call it Imagination.

TRANSPERSONAL TRANSFORMATIONAL AND CREATIVE ARTS THERAPIES AND PRACTICES AT SOLUTIONS, CENTER FOR PERSONAL GROWTH, INC.

Understanding the importance of energy, DNA shifts, psychoneuroimmunology, body/mind biochemistry and the relationship of these to health, healing and transformation, the Imagination model, at Solutions, incorporates techniques and practices which span and integrate a variety of paradigms. Such therapies include the creative arts therapies utilizing art, music, sound, writing, drama, movement and dance; meditation and breathwork; yoga; exercise; nutrition, especially live foods; body work; and other physical therapies such as herbs, homeopathic remedies, Ayurveda, Chinese Medicine and more. Each of the expressive therapies or transformational practices are whole systems in their own right, and are woven together in the integrated healing model, known as Imagination. Participants discover their pain and blockages within the body, release and express this energy in an individual unique expression during weekly and weekend intensive group sessions committing also to daily transformational practices.

SUMMARY

These core concepts are integrated then into a 21-week program at Solutions Center for Personal Growth, Inc. Simply stated, Imagination holds that as a whole, humanity desires health and healing, self-actualization, peace, success, abundance and loving relationship. Some have achieved this self-actualized and joyful state of being, and others have not. Imagination teaches that human beings have unconsciously created and attracted experiences and people into their lives who energetically match the original blueprint, or COEX system. This blueprint is a physical, mental, emotional and spiritual imprint originating from soul memory, womb, birth, early childhood and/or dysfunctional family of origin system experiences. These experiences continue to be re-enacted until the enactor wants to stop the repetition. Within this consciousness, the individual can move toward wholeness, healing and transformation, dismantling systems, which no longer serve. Becoming conscious in a healing and transformational process may involve bringing painful memories and perhaps traumatic experiences from the psyche and soul memory, into the present waking reality. Here, an individual's true essence or spirit begins to emerge. In such a process, a person can experience a state of spiritual emergency, incur intense and dramatic feelings, visions, experiences and pain, which are part of the process and not to be confused with psychosis. In addition, persons on the healing path, especially those with an intention of healing the whole Self, may experience physical illness as a part of emotional detoxification of core issues held deep within the body. Psychoneuroimmunology teaches that chronic or acute physical illness is part of a process, which when activated toward healing can result in a detoxification or cleansing of the negative and painful thoughts and feelings, which have affected every cell in the body.

With awareness of these principles of healing, clients are ready to heal and transform through psychospiritual group process and transpersonal psychotherapy, merging their psyches with the spiritual aspect of Self. The hero's journey can take each participant to that point where the whole self awakens. Once awakened, nothing is impossible! Imagination participants learn the art of co-creation through the teachings from quantum physics and begin to affirm energetic intentions that not only affect their mind/body but, the cosmos as well creating interconnectedness which is desired. Finally, a client at Solutions is introduced to the bigger picture of the life process, becoming aware of the mysteries of the universe, the Shift of the Ages, the questions and opportunities known and unknown. Participants discover, express, release and transform through the transpersonal transformation creative arts and other vibrational practices, which are part of the integrated Imagination model.

PARTICIPANTS' ORIENTATION TO THE IMAGINATION PROCESS AT SOLUTIONS

The following is included in the Imagination Orientation package at Solutions Center for Personal Growth, Inc:

This We Believe.

This work is based on the following ideas, principles and universal laws:

1. All things are possible! It is possible to open your mind to all the possibilities this life can hold.
2. The planet earth is in an evolutionary process; therefore, human beings are in an evolutionary process. In our work, we are merging the psyche and the spirit– hence the term, psychospiritual integration.
3. You have a conscious evolutionary choice. You can consciously change your perception of yourself, others, your life, and your work and discover your true essence. You can know and live your purpose.
4. Each person has the ability and the power to create the future. We are co-creators with the universe. You have been creating your life now unconsciously by the way you believe, think and feel. The Imagination processes will begin to make your life and your process conscious.
5. All your experiences and your pain are part of something BIGGER for your learning and unfoldment and is a gift. You can use your mind, body and spirit to step into all the unlimited potential that exists. As one learns this and heals the past, the victim consciousness is reversed and you begin to attract new

healthy experiences, people, and abundance into your life.

6. The universe, including our bodies, is composed of energy and information. The body is a metaphor of the mind and emotions from all time, and a record of your experiences that have been imprinted. Trauma and negative imprinting can be reversed through the healing process of release and expression. Releasing stored energy for detoxification of the body, mind and emotional fields is important for healing.
7. All is well. All is perfect. Everything is happening for a reason. There are no coincidences. Each person will awaken to his/her own true essence and will remember why they are here on the planet earth in their own perfect time. Therefore, there is no need for fear, tension and control. Love will help you heal and transform.

THE IMAGINATION PROCESS MODEL

Imagination is a 21-week process, divided into 3, 7-week phases. The phases are numbered: I, II, and III. A client may enter into the process at the beginning of any phase, as healing is nonlinear. Each phase has a beginning and an ending, a primary focus, goals and objectives.

Each phase has a name: Phase I: Imagination, Phase II: Inspiration, and Phase III: Intuition. Jacquelyn Small identifies imagination, inspiration and intuition as the three soul powers, "when we access our soul powers, we move on to relationships with "high callings" that enable us to fully develop our creativity" (Small, 1991).

There are definite stages in each phase:
- (1) beginning with a bonding stage,
- (2) a discovery stage–which is a moving and stirring up of energy held in the body;
- (3) a release and expression stage;
- (4) an integration illumination stage;

- (5) which then gives individuals' access to the transpersonal where they go beyond all they have known.

As there are 21 weeks of the process, offered weekly or in Imagination Weekend Experiences, 21 unique and structured therapeutic experiences have been designed for the healing and transformational work. Group sessions are experiential, psychoeducational and usually contain access to nonordinary states of consciousness that may include visualization, meditation, ecstatic dancing, moving or breathwork. Sessions utilize music, lighting, and creation of safe space and may include expressive therapies of drama, art, movement, writing, sound or transformational theatre. Ritual and ceremony is employed at the beginning and ending of each group session, however, what happens in-between is always a surprise. Imagination promises to take the participant "out of control," as a part of the healing, allowing participants to experience and practice new ways of perceiving and being, giving themselves permission to trust and allow, let go and let the process work.

THE SOLUTION'S CENTER EXPERIENCE

Pre-Imagination Assessment and Evaluation

When individuals are referred to Solutions, they undergo an extensive evaluation and assessment using a thorough Life and Family History. They are screened and those who have stable egos co-develop a Plan of Intention or treatment plan with the Solutions holistic practitioner. This usually takes two or three hour-long sessions with the therapist and may involve several other individual sessions if needed. Upon completion of the 30-page history, the therapist reads and co-creates a Plan of Intention which addresses:

- Family of origin pain,
- Birth trauma,
- Repression of feelings,
- Physical issues,
- Losses,
- Abuse, and
- Addiction.

This is one of the most important aspects of the process, as the Plan of Intention has several usages. The plan is a bonding tool for the therapist and client, as the therapist goes over all the material within the Life History and has spent time designing an individualized plan. Secondly, the intention set forth in the plan creates an organizing field for the energy that is released in the work to follow.

Individual Therapy Sessions

Participants take part in individual therapy sessions approximately every other week in addition to the group work to process the material which has usually come forward from the unconscious. This is very important as a way to work through spiritual emergency.

The transpersonal psychotherapist must be trained and able to handle a variety of unusual experiences as participants open to the deep recesses of the human psyche. Psychic openings may include spiritual, mystical, religious, occult, magical and paranormal experiences such as transformational crisis, the reliving of birth memory, past life experiences, shamanic crisis, the awakening of kundalini, peak experiences, psychological renewal, communications with spirit guides, "channeling," near-death experiences, and possession states (Grof, 1986).

Most every client sooner or later must work through "the dark night of the soul," feeling vulnerable, anxious and fearful, as the inner child and all soul memory is invited into the sacred space to heal. The therapist serves as a guide through the work, holding the energy and safe space.

Safe and Sacred Space

Solutions Center is considered sacred space. When individual's walk through the door, they have entered a temenos of transformation. Before each phase begins, student interns present the rules and guidelines for the group process in order to recreate a safe and sacred space for the work to take place. The room becomes the "womb" and must be respected as such; therefore food, drinks, shoes, side talking, and running out are discouraged. Confidentiality, being on time, completing assignments, and practicing rigorous honesty is encouraged. Each participant gets a list of the following rules in the Imagination Orientation package and these guidelines are discussed during the first session of every phase or weekend intensive:

Program Guidelines for Creating a Safe and Sacred Space

- Be on time and attend every session. We commit to do our best to begin and end on time. If, for any reason or emergency you cannot attend a session, please call the office and let us know. Remember that the times you do not feel like coming are the times you most need to be here. We invite you to perceive any obstacles in your way as part of your process and life patterns.
- Participate in activities, experiences and projects. Your work is accelerated when you commit to participate! Be accountable to the group and any partner you have the opportunity to work with. You will get out of the process what you put into it.
- Complete the daily assignments in your Imagination workbook every day. We will use your assignment work during the group each week. Bring any assignments which have a star to the group session.
- Stay in the session/room during the group work. Often times intense feelings may surface and it is important not to leave to go to the bathroom or get water, etc. This is a natural defense mechanism to pain and fear; so, please COMMIT TO STAY IN THE SESSION. Bathroom breaks will be given. In addition, please ask for tissues if you need them. Likewise, please do not give other people tissues when they are crying unless they ask for one. In this way, we allow each other to cry, express and release pain and address our own unconscious discomfort and emotions which may become triggered.
- Drink or eat before or after the session. Drinking 8 glasses of water each day is great during this process, as you are detoxifying your body, mind and emotions. You are encouraged to bring a closed water bottle with you to the session. Water helps to cleanse the system.
- Be free from any mind-altering substances during the entire process. Alcohol and drugs will cover up that which you are here to bring up and heal! Please let us know if you have a problem stopping the use of mind-altering substances.
- Maintain CONFIDENTIALITY at all times. "Who you see here, what you hear here, when you leave here," let it stay here. Please do not talk about others unless they are present; become conscious of your communication patterns. In addition, please do not discuss what happens in the sessions, as this may influence someone else who might like to come to Imagination feeling they could not ever "do what we do."
- Practice Rigorous honesty WITH YOURSELF AND OTHERS; THE TRUTH REALLY WILL BRING YOU FREEDOM!
- Be aware that emotional/spiritual intimacy may be mistaken for sexual feelings/attraction. This is normal when people begin to open up and feel. Relationships with other group members may distract you from your process and is discouraged. If this happens to you, talk about these feelings with your therapist. It is a normal part of the process.
- Do not make any major decisions during

the process. Afterwards, go for it! Change your whole life. As you keep your dreams in your mind, so they will come to pass.

Expressive Model and Energy Cheering

Energy cheering is a process for honoring each person in the process. It consists of moving energy, clapping, noisemaking and celebrating that a person has spoken and is here doing the work. Energy cheering happens after each person speaks in opening introductions. The Imagination model is a fully expressive and energized model resonating to all frequency vibrations for the purpose of moving energy. There are times of extreme release, loud noises, evocative music and movement as well as moments of silence, mindfulness, innerretreat and quiet.

Workbooks and Daily Transformational Exercises

Workbooks are another integral aspect of the Imagination model. A workbook for each phase contains 49 days of work, one teaching for each day of the process, plus templates for the 7 daily transformational practices:

---

7 Daily Transformational Practices

1. writing the daily intention,
2. affirmations to give energy to intention,
3. expression of feelings using the feelings formula,
4. meditation exercise
5. contemplation of the universal law,
6. live foods commitment, and
7. exercise commitment.

I Am the Honored Guest at Your Healing (Limber, 1997), introduces the reader/writer to the inner child, teaching concepts and giving daily assignments, which assist in the process of remembering and releasing. The act of writing is also a therapy in itself, allowing a releasing and commitment to the information. *Journey Into Power* (Limber, 1997), corresponds to Phase II–Inspiration, challenging the Imagination participant to speak a language of power; to learn the art of co-creation so to let go of old energy blockages, and create future joy. Phase III, Intuition, is accompanied by *The Journey Deepens* (Limber, 1997). This workbook outlines the universal spiritual truths and introduces the journeyer to the shadow aspect of the psyche. Imagination participants are asked to complete the teaching and assignments each day of the process, to allow the workbook to become part of the process. Workbooks include extra pages for journaling and drawing for full expression of the individual.

Phase I–Imagination (The Body): Goals, Objectives and Focus

Phase I is the reclaiming of the inner child, birth and womb experiences and full consciousness of family of origin pain. The inner child is invited to come into this waking consciousness through meditation and visualization with the help of a stuffed animal, favorite book, and pictures of the individual as infant and child. Participants begin to remember that which has been locked inside. They draw, paint, write with subdominant hand, and get to play as children.

Experiences include exercises that build trust and test boundaries, open the heart for those who have been abused and live in fear. Participants begin to risk a new family of affiliation. Stage I recovery principles include "surrendering to pain, trust and telling your secrets, affiliation needs, group support, first order change, experiencing emotions, collapsing grandiosity, giving up denial, self-acceptance, values restored, externalization of shame, rigorous honesty and yin/yang balance" (Bradshaw, 1988, p. 204).

Participants are presented with exercises, which "stir up" the energy of anger and give themselves permission to express anger and pain that is to "have a voice." This is a purposeful process of discovering and releasing feelings which have been stored in the body, to give voice to that which has been sleeping somewhere in the body creating the "same old patterns and experiences over and over again." The inner children who have feared expression and felt unworthy, guilty, scared and shamed, begin to dance their dance, sing their song, feel and love again. Finally, this phase of work moves into a forgiveness stage wherein the inner child is ready to be nurtured by a new caring adult, the higher self, and let go of the past. Forgiveness is viewed in this model as a liberation of the self from longsuffering; taking one's power back; a letting go of stored energy in the form of anger and resentment. It is not condoning abusive behavior of caretakers and parents or letting someone "off the hook." The goal of this phase is compassion.

"You find the jewel and it draws you off. The purpose of the journey is compassion. When you have come past the pairs of opposites, you have reached compassion. The goal is to bring the jewel back to the world, to join to the two things together" (Osbon, 1991, p. 24).

Phase II–Inspiration–(The Mind): Goals, Objectives and Focus

This phase of the Imagination model focuses on how the mind became programmed from internal experiences encoded in the psyche. Inspiration introduces the student to the art and skill of designing one's life, creating the future, letting go and reversing negative mind programs, thus disorganizing and breaking apart the COEX system in operation.

The phase begins with "What Do You Want?" and "Why Don't You Have What You Want?" type of exercises. Students learn concepts about energy, information, and other views of the world from quantum physics. Structured experiences assist the student in discovering hidden negative messages in the psyche and making energetic declarations about reversing those messages, thus creating and coming to a new language of power. With a new language of power, students are coached to do chasm jumping, which is an exercise in stretching beyond the limits one has created for the self. Chasm jumping, through the use of transformational theater, is the final project and piece of work the student completes, having in some way, gone beyond what he/she has done before. The student gains confidence and self-esteem building, pushing the envelope through the zone of comfort, thus creating an incredible healing and transformation.

Phase III–Intuition (The Spirit): Goals, Objectives and Focus

The Intuition phase focuses on the spiritual aspect of healing and transformation; introduces the universal spiritual truths and invites participants to discover and integrate the shadow. Jacquelyn Small, quoting Carl Jung, says, "at the very core of our humanness exists a dualism—the shadow and the light. Before we can manifest our light and become that winged bird, we must first come to know and accept our shadow. He called it the "skeleton in the cupboard." Jacquelyn continues, "the shadow is our Holy Grail; its sacred purpose is to bring all our unconscious, denied feelings into conscious awareness. It makes such a fool of us with its antics that it forces us to get real and deal with the parts of ourselves we're trying to skip over. The shadow is our antiself or negative ego, and it serves as the polar opposite of our positive ego as we learn to discriminate between our truth and untruth." Jung said it is an "apprentice" as opposed to the "masterpiece," which is the Self" (Small, 1991, pp. 41–42).

Clients who engage in the Intuition phase explore the shadow side of self as they recognize the disowned and despised part of the psyche along with the hurt, self-destructive patterns and feelings of being "not good enough." The shadow, which will never stay hidden anyway, is invited out of the basement into this waking reality needing only to be accepted, integrated and honored. Intuition is a deep phase as it invites the secrets of the soul into the healing space. Students dance, create masks, costumes, drawings, music and sounds as they embody and hear the shadow's voice.

In addition to shadow work, the universal spiritual truths are presented and taught as new ways to perceive, think, feel and be. Universal laws are those spiritual teachings, which appear to be collective across all religions, philosophies and schools of thought. Many spiritual leaders and teachers present these truths in many formats, from business consultants such as Dr. Stephen Covey in the 7 Habits of Highly Effective People, who explains paradigm shifts, proactivity and synergy, to Deepak Chopra's 7 Spiritual Laws of Success (1994) (see Chapter 9).

THERAPEUTIC TECHNIQUES

Now the question! How in the world does Imagination at Solutions:
- heal the past, addressing soul memory, womb, birth, family of origin experiences, the unconscious blueprint, and COEX systems;
- focus on the present, reversing negative mind programs, understanding quantum physics, learning, speaking and writing a new Language of Power; and
- create the future by integrating the shadow and practicing the universal spiritual laws, not to mention meditating, eating healthy live foods, exercising, expressing feelings, writing intention and affirmation and contemplating the universe?

The expressive therapeutic techniques along with components of the process as discussed earlier (assessment and evaluation, safe and sacred space, workbooks, individual therapy sessions), come together in an integrated approach, which addresses the whole self, the body, mind, emotions and spirit. The integration of these theories, techniques and process is the holistic integrative model: Imagination.

Expressive therapeutic exercises, or the creative arts, are chosen for each exercise to achieve desired outcomes. Drama therapy, sound therapy, art therapy, movement and dance, writing, journaling, chasm jumping, communication techniques, family systems therapy techniques, cognitive-behavioral methods, live foods and nutritional therapy, exercise, yoga, meditation and integrative breathwork are all tools in the therapeutic process. The model is experiential and psychoeducational.

According to Lewis, in *Creative Transformation: The Healing Power of the Arts*, "The dance between the conscious and unconscious is choreographed in the magical place of the imaginal realm. Creative arts therapists have long known that transformation toward wholeness can only happen through experience within this symbolic realm. The containers are the expressive arts media, the patient's body, the therapist's body as vessel for the somatic countertransference, and the bi-personal field between patient and therapist or within a group. These containers hold this liminal space within which healing can occur" (Lewis, 1993, p. 5).

Experiential

The Imagination model has a major experiential component in that the work is active as participants experience the process in the now. They learn to identify and express feelings, release and let go of pain, which has been buried deep in the body and psyche. Sessions are designed to evoke a depth journey into the psyche for each participant. All experiences are processed and interpreted. Insight or feedback is provided by the therapist and group members, viewing the experience in the now as a symbol and/or metaphor of a recuring pattern or theme with which to be reckoned. At the end of every session, participants report an awareness from the session and a commitment for the week. The client is perceived as the expert of his/her own process with the right to accept or reject interpretive analysis.

Psychoeducational

The teaching of basic skills and concepts is woven throughout the model; teaching moments include mini-lectures on subjects such as: dysfunctional family rules and roles, COEX systems, map of the consciousness, energy or chakra systems in the body, the feelings formula, fair fighting, and principles from psychoneuroimmunology and quantum physics. Therapists and practitioners in intern training also teach through storytelling and personal disclosure when appropriate.

Cognitive Behavioral Strategies

Imagination uses cognitive behavioral strategies, such as cognitive restructuring and reframing to allow a participant to shift existing paradigms of thought. These strategies are used especially during Phase II: Inspiration, when the client is being introduced to his/her own negative schemas and thought processes along with a plan of action for reversing imprints, which no longer serve a purpose. The client's new paradigm is reinforced through group encouragement, feedback and other energy processes. Similar to Zen Buddhism, participants are taught to discipline the mind, to conserve energy, allowing the imagination to work in a positive way. The client moves from a beginner's mind to the advanced student, able to become the observer of the experience, and a master of the universal spiritual laws. This place of mindfulness allows the participant to move on to higher levels of consciousness, awareness, clarity, and spirituality, becoming one with the sacred.

Drama Therapy

The Imagination model is a dramatic therapeutic adventure. The 21 structured choreographed sessions are a series of sequential therapeutic activities requiring specific lighting, music, sound and movement in a perfected experiential encounter. Individuals actively participate in each series of 7 sequential group processes with the entire group or subgroup (known as family group). Each session has a specific goal, focus and design, yet moves and honors the energy in the room and so "goes with the flow" of what is needed in any individual circumstance which may arise. Imagination utilizes many different drama therapy techniques combined and integrated together in its own unique design.

Drama therapy is a profession and an action method which is utilized clinically and psychoeducationally. Clinical Drama Therapy is an embodied action method in which a client, the drama therapist(s) and/or group members engage in improvisational play or the enactment of habitual scenes or roles from an individual's life, dreams or fantasies. For many, clinical drama therapy is a depth approach that utilizes the unconscious and in some cases the transference and countertransference relationships while entering into the realm of imagination of the client (Lewis, 2000, p. 442).

Techniques from the field of drama therapy which are employed in Imagination include authentic sound, movement and drama, improvisation and role playing, family sculpting, interactive theater, psychodrama, sand play, opening and closing ritual, free play, guided shamanic journeys and visualizations, mask making, replay, role rehearsal, monologue, soliloquy, theater games, therapeutic and transformational theater (Lewis, 2000). These techniques are woven together with other creative therapeutic techniques creating the masterpiece: Imagination.

Sound Therapy

In Imagination, participants including facilitators sing, chant, use mantras, tone, warm up the voice, create new names in song and sound, use heartbeat recordings, play musical instruments, especially drumming and rattling, use repetitive sounds with ritual techniques and employ evocative instrumental music for many of the processes. There is a healing power in music and the human voice, which have been used throughout history as natural therapies for healing. According to Olivia Dewhurst-Maddock, "healing mantras, chants, and incantations have very ancient and obscure origins. Egyptian medical papyri from 2,600 years ago refer to incantations as cures for infertility, rheumatic pain, and insect bites. In about 324 BC, the music of the lyre restored Alexander the Great to sanity. The Old Testament records that David played his harp and lifted King Saul's depression. The Essenes and Therapeutai used sacred words for healing. And, in Hellenistic culture, flute playing eased the pain of sciatica and gout. Knowledge of sounds, rhythms, and chants was an essential ingredient in the healing powers of the shaman, the medicine man or woman, and the druidic priest-doctors of Celtic cultures. The power of music to evoke emotional response has been a recurring theme of poetic celebration, and the life-blood of performance. Music can bypass the mind's logical and analytical filters, to make direct contact with profound feelings and passions deep in the memory and imagination. This in turn, produces physical reactions" (Dewhurst-Maddock, 1993, pp. 11–12).

Specific music is used for each of the 21 psychospiritual group experiences, mediations, visualizations and integrative breathwork sessions. Each piece of music is chosen for its vibrational quality and healing effects. Research by sound therapists and biologists has demonstrated the effects of sound vibrations on living cells. Specific sound frequencies that relate to parts of the body have been identified (Maddock, 1993). The Imagination model works with sound and music, matching music to different parts of the body for release in the corresponding body area or chakras.

In *Music and Miracles*, Patricia Warming reports Jung as writing in 1950,

Music certainly has to do with the collective unconscious . . . this is evident in Wagner, for example. Music expresses, in some way, the movement of the feelings (or emotional values) that cling to the unconscious processes. The nature of what happens in the collective unconscious is archetypal, and archetypes always have a numinous quality that expresses itself in emotional stress. Music expresses in sounds what fantasies and visions express in visual images (Warming, 1992, p. 233).

Art Therapy

Art is another creative arts therapy utilized in the Imagination model. Participants may be painting, drawing, creating a fear sculpture or quietly completing a breathwork through a mandala piece. There are art projects in the Imagination workbooks to complete, extra drawing pages, and art projects to render during the sessions. Participants are painting for the process–the healing and transformation; accessing yet another doorway into an experience with the true self, once again releasing and energizing the soul. "When you paint for process you listen to the magic of the inner voices, you follow the basic human urge to experiment with the new, the unknown, the mysterious, the hidden. Creation is a response. To create is to move into the unknown–to move into the mystery of yourself, to have feeling, to awaken buried perceptions, to be alive and free without worrying about the result" (Cassou & Cubley, 1995, p. 5).

The Imagination painting processes and experiences allow participants to journey to the innate creativity inside. When the body/mind expresses, one becomes free, takes risks, and uses color for vibratory healing. Every color has a vibration and is rich with meaning, corresponding to different vibratory frequencies in the emotional, mental, physical and spiritual body. The soul speaks through the hands and the paintbrushes engaging and revealing the psyche. Paintings become symbols and metaphors for the healing and transformation process. Every part of every work of art is purposeful and part of the process.

Movement and Dance Therapy

The Imagination process utilizes movement and dance in an effort to free the body, heal past wounds protected by body armor, and open to the passion of the soul in the creation of a new future. We dance ecstatically, move, march, play, do the copycat dance, slip and slide, mill around, become animals or engage the angry walking process. Some use dance to chasm jump (stretch their limits) or for final transformational theater presentations as an initiation rite. According to Gabriel Roth, "your body is the ground metaphor of your life, the expression of your existence. It is your Bible, your encyclopedia, and your life story. Everything that happens to you is stored and reflected in your body. Your body knows, your body tells. So the body is where the dancing path to wholeness must begin. Only when you truly inhabit your body can you begin the healing journey" (Roth, 1989, p. 29–30).

Dancing and moving heals. Dance for healing is about moving. With every movement, you embody the creative fire. There, with the dance, your body has a life of its own. Within every one of us is a dancer. Dance heals by spiraling us down inside ourselves to a center where tensions are released and there is freedom and spaciousness. To dance is to harness the fire inside your belly that moves you. Dance is a vehicle for emotional expression, an opportunity to embody emotions. In dance, you are truly embodied, translating thought and emotion into movement. When you get cells moving, neurotransmitters flow, endorphins flow. You express any fluidity you are capable of. Whatever is tense is let go. The body itself leads you to where it wants to be naturally. It is this deeper place of being where you (Samuels & Lane, 1998).

Writing and Poetry Therapy

Writing is a therapeutic component of the Imagination model. This encompasses journaling, prose, poetry, song writing, monologue and more. There are writing assignments every day of the process contained within the workbooks including a place to write intention, affirmation, and feelings. Writing gives the client a way to express feelings, commit to words, open awareness and expression. The writing process begins when the client writes the original Life and Family History. This is a 30-page piece of writing in which the writer must answer questions about his childhood, grandparents, parents, losses, addictions, health, dreams, money, education, birth process, fears, feelings, wishes, obstacles, relationships, life traumas and belief systems. Once individuals commit to writing their life histories, the process is engaged.

Workbook assignments may be anything from nondominate handwriting by the inner child, a goodbye letter to mom or dad or a poem written by the "shadow." I believe what John Fox writes about in *Poetic Medicine*, is true for all healing writing assignments.

> Poetry is a natural medicine, it is like a homeopathic tincture derived from the stuff of life itself–your experience. Poems distill experience into the essentials. Our personal experiences touch the common ground we share with others. The exciting part of this process is that poetry used in this healing way helps people integrate the disparate, even fragmented parts of their life. Poetic essences of sound, metaphor, image, feeling and rhythm act as remedies that can elegantly strengthen our whole system–physical, mental and spiritual. (Fox, 1997, p. 3)

Writing is a form of therapy and art as the writer is able to release feelings, heal wounds, process grief, commit to new ways of being, set healthy goals, and externalize experiences. Everyone has a story to tell, a poem to write, a song to sing. Our healing becomes art as we capture our own soul and true essence in the writing process.

Breathwork

Participants come to Solutions Center for Personal Growth, Inc. one day a week for 21 weeks and include one weekend per month for an intensive Imagination Weekend Experience and/or a Breathworkshop.

The breathwork, a deep breathing com-bined with evocative music, is an integral part of the Imagination work, allowing individuals access to the depth levels of consciousness–the sensory, biographical, perinatal and transpersonal bands of consciousness as written about by Dr. Stanislav Grof in *The Holotropic Mind* (1990). Grof says,

> This seemingly simple process, combining breathing, evocative music, and other forms of sound, body work, and artistic expression, has an extraordinary potential for opening the way for exploring the entire spectrum of the inner world. In work with non-ordinary states, significant biographical material from our earliest years frequently starts coming to the surface in the first few sessions. Not only do people gain access to memories of their childhood and infancy, they often vividly connect with their births and their lives within the womb and begin venturing into a realm of experience even beyond these. (Grof, 1990)

Healthy Life Force Nutrition, Exercise, Yoga and Meditation

As part of a whole process, the Imagination model at Solutions goes beyond the therapy room, group process and individual sessions encouraging participants to commit to live foods, seasonal fasting, exercise, yoga and meditation as ingredients in the healing and transformation process. What individuals take into the body, how they move or do not move, is part of an integrated whole. Ingestion and movement are absolutely necessary for holistic health. Becoming conscious and mindful of the physical condition is equally as important as healing the past. In fact, a person's body is the past manifested. "Your biography becomes your biology," said Caroline Myss (1997). We are called to detoxify and cleanse our bodies and begin to honor our bodies as we are so doing with our minds and emotions. Hence, the work at Solutions is a bio/psycho/spiritual/integration process.

CONSCIOUS EATING. Dr. Gabriel Cousens,

a teacher in the field of conscious eating, live foods and spiritual nutrition writes, "Our relationship to food is a primary means of survival, which enables us to relate to others and learn the lessons we need to learn while on this earth. What we eat is both the cause and the effect of our awareness. It reflects our ongoing harmony with ourselves, the world, the universal laws, and all of creation. Individualizing one's diet at the most refined level is eating to further enhance communion with the Divine. The art of conscious eating lies in creating an individualized diet that reflects and supports one's realization of the highest state of awareness and that is appropriate for the functions in the world of one's everyday life" (Cousens, 2000, p. 6).

A healthy eating and exercise plan is developed for each client, which supports these energies to activate and increase energy potential for the awakening of the spiritual energy. If an individual is addicted to alcohol, cigarettes, drugs or any kind of substance, including sugar, white flour products or caffeine, the Imagination process is affected. Food is a vibratory energy system with life force. Simply, when individuals ingest live foods as part of the daily diet, they are cleansing the system of blockages, which correspond to emotional blockages. Every organ in the body corresponds to an emotional issue. Every illness has an emotional counterpart. Working on the physical is a way of working on the emotional and mental aspects of the Self, as body and mind are not separated. As the body is the manifestation of an individual's beliefs, thoughts, feelings, behaviors and life patterns; the body cells, tissues and organs are seeded with information and memories from all time, including the past, present and future. As individuals bring more life force into their bodies, they are more clear and able to access this information. As the toxins leave, so might sadness and pain.

SPIRITUAL FASTING. Solutions also offers opportunities for spiritual fasting. According to Cousens, "Spiritual fasting is conducive to rest and rejuvenation on every level of mind, body, and spirit. It allows our physical bodies to turn to the assimilation of Divine or cosmic energy rather than biochemical energy. Because fasting accelerates purification of the body, it enhances the movement of all levels of energy in the body, including the spiritualizing energy. Fasting has a powerful effect on the body as well as the spirit. It allows the vital force within to rebuild and recharge. Overall mind-body organization is increased with fasting. It is this curative force, which throws off the accumulated toxins, clears the dead cells, and rebalance and rejuvenates the body (Cousens, 2000, p. 229-231).

YOGA. Yoga is also recommended and offered at our holistic healing center, Solutions Center for Personal Growth, Inc. Yogic teachings focus on the union of the individual with the universal. Yogic practices encourage the development of physical self-regulation and autonomic self-control through prescribed exercises. This enhanced voluntary control over physiological states and processes is believed to be the key to self-realization. Yoga is based on a view of the self-similar to that held by Carl Jung–an eternal, unchanging essence that is the common inheritance of all the people (Bankart, 1997, p. 473).

The yogic practices of meditation, postures, breathing, concentration and control of vital energy greatly enhance the Imagination process as participants are actively promoting the integration of the physical, social, emotional, and spiritual ways of being. According to Frager and Fadiman (1984), "The discipline of Yoga must include a complete reformation of consciousness. Otherwise the subconscious tendencies eventually will seek to actualize themselves, sprouting suddenly like dormant sides. Through meditation, self-analysis, and other powerful inner disciplines, it is possible to "roast" such seeds, to destroy their potential for further activity; that is through fundamental inner change we can grow free of the influence of the past" (Frager & Fadiman, 1984, p. 411).

MEDITATION. Meditation is another pre-scribed practice of the Imagination model. Participants are asked to mediate every day and learn different types of meditation through the workbooks and group practices. "Meditation, which is at the heart of yoga, is known as the royal path toward self-realization, or God consciousness. Through our purified or disciplined consciousness, we can discover our immortal substance, our true identity–the ego transcending Self" (Feuerstein & Bodian, 1993). Imagination teaches meditation so the student will learn to calm the mind, let go and be open to the world and to love.

EXERCISE. Daily aerobic exercise, which might include walking, running, dancing, or any exercise, which brings more oxygen into the body, is also a part of the process. As the healing process is about bringing light to the darkness, making conscious that which has been unconscious, so oxygen acts as the light, or life force of breath. Any activity, which requires the breath, is a healing and transformational practice. As for the emotional effects of aerobic exercise, Brigham reports in *Imagery for Getting Well*, "Research tells us that aerobic exercise: is a natural outlet for tension, anxiety and aggression; increases the release of endorphins, has a calming effect on the mind, contributes to better sleep, increases stimulation of the right hemisphere of the brain, allowing for greater creativity, particularly during the exercise, builds self-esteem, confidence and a sense of joy in being in charge of your life, an enhanced ability to enjoy the senses, an awareness of physical well-being, a feeling of independence, and self-responsibility, allows one to turn inward, to be in touch with what it feels like inside oneself, to be connected with one's body and with the miracle of life and being and finally can be used as a meditation connecting one with others, the planet and the universe (Brigham, 1994, p. 162–163).

Integrative Bodywork and Massage

Brigham describes therapeutic touch: "Therapeutic touch (TT) is a technique whereby energy is transmitted from one person to another for the purpose of healing. In a sense, it goes beyond merely relieving pain or helping lungs to clear. It brings everything together. In my mind, TT is tapping into the wholeness and unity of the universe and becoming attuned to the energies of the universe, in which lies true healing of the body, mind and spirit" (Brigham, 1994, p. 251). Integrative bodywork is offered at Solutions as an integral aspect of the Imagination process, the whole program. Bodyworkers, who are licensed massage therapists, practice massage, Reiki, Cranial-Sacral therapy and Emotional Release work. Each unique type of hands-on work begins with an intention and focus for healing, cleansing, relaxation, and release of any energy blockages in the body. Brigham continues, "People are energy fields. The energy field is the fundamental unit of a living system, and as Einstein indicates, the physical is just one manifestation of that energy. TT assumes that sickness or pain is merely an imbalance or blockages in the energy field, and that people are open systems engaged in continuous interaction with the environment. Therefore, when one person utilizes his or her intent to heal another, the energy transfer takes place, stimulating healing in the other person" (1994, p. 252).

ROLE OF THE THERAPIST

The therapist is the mentor, teacher, counselor, guide, shaman, healer and magician. The therapist is active and wise, listening to her own inner voice to direct each scene in the production, the group process, allowing the work to "go with the flow" when needed, perhaps diverting from the original plan, although moving always toward the goal. The therapist is an integrator, knowing from whence each theory originated; yet has added her own unique personality to the design. She knows how to create safe and sacred space. People feel safe with her because she remembers how to love.

The therapist has done her own personal work, and is ever moving in her own process of healing and transformation. The therapist is a role model, living the spiritual law and is a human being as well, with strengths and weaknesses that she tells about when appropriate. She is a storyteller, and surely has a story to tell. How else would she be directing this play, writing the lyrics and melody, putting it all together in this grand design, this tapestry of music, light, sound, love and compassion, healing and transformation into the imagination.

POPULATIONS SERVED

I say quite often, when speaking about Imagination at Solutions Center for Personal Growth, Inc. that just about anyone off the street would benefit from this model of personal growth, healing, transformation and spiritual awakening. Anyone in need of healing past trauma and abuse will definitely benefit from this holistic healing approach, as well as those with subtle negative programming from rigid and perfectionistic families, who do not always know "what is wrong with them." Imagination especially appeals to those who are wondering what to do next in their life, for those who are seeking their mission and purpose and for individuals who are ready to make major life changes. Couples come to the program often and have excellent results as each does his and her own healing process as well as learn communication skills for practicing loving kindness.

The model has worked well for clients with depression or other mood disorders, PTSD or any other kind of disorder where pain and trauma has been repressed with a resulting phobia, anxiety or panic disorder. Oftentimes, people come with physical illness or complaints, and they too benefit from this model, becoming aware of the physical manifestation of their emotional core issues. Most every client I have ever treated has eventually been able to go off of antidepressant and anxiety reducing medications at the end of their program. Imagination has been used in coordination with addiction treatment programs as part of an intensive outpatient process, where the client is also attending addiction group or 12-step programs. The Imagination model is offered to all age groups, including children and teens.

SUMMARY

Imagination at Solutions Center for Personal Growth, Inc. is an integrated holistic healing model, which takes into account the many aspects of the human being–being alive–body, mind, and spirit. The Imagination components, processes, therapies, techniques and theories are interdependent, and create a whole and complete healing process. The Imagination model works with energy and vibration, past, present and future, incorporating experiences that release the old and bring in the new. Everything a person thinks, feels, believes and practices becomes part of the process. Life takes on new meaning once Imagination is engaged. I have been the honored guest at many healings, experiencing those who desire to heal and transform their lives, live in greatness and love. There is an incredible perfection in this process, and I am honored to be the teacher of this work.

CASE EXAMPLES

Dave came into the Solutions Center one day in a business suit with slick-backed hair driving a high-priced car. He said he hated his job and all the pressure of his life. After one 7-week phase and a breathwork session he quit his job and began to roam the beach for a short time. Soon he began picking up beach artifacts and making jewelry. Today he has an abundant business selling his jewelry all over the world.

Mary called Solutions one afternoon, drunk, suicidal and feeling guilty about everything in her life. She hated herself and was ready to end it all. During the Imagination process, she was regressed to a time in the womb where she saw that she had a twin brother. The twin brother died at birth and Mary realized she had felt guilty all of her life for being alive. Mary asked her 80-year-old mother if this was true—had she indeed had a twin brother who died. "Yes," her mother said, "we never wanted you to know."

Josephine came into Solutions Center reporting that she saw visions and heard scary voices all of her life. She was fearful of taking showers and leaving the house. During one particular Imagination process, she began to have memories of someone being murdered in a bathroom with the shower water running. Josephine went into spiritual emergency, thinking she was "going crazy" as the information became more and more real and vivid; she stayed with the process, breathed, and continued to allow the information to come forth as her body and the therapist's body became a container for this information buried deep in her soul memory. Josephine reported the information as it came up, crying, feeling scared yet in a safe place to do the work. Since that day, Josephine is able to take showers and leave her home without fear. She immediately went to sign up for college courses so to become a therapist to help others through the same kind of mysterious experiences.

Martha and Joe came into Solutions Center because they were having trouble communicating in their marriage. Martha felt as though she was caretaking Joe, who was always sick. As both Martha and Joe participated in the Imagination process, each one became aware of the childhood roles they played—Martha had been the caretaker of the family and Joe had been the responsible little boy. He was needless and wantless, no one ever took care of him. In their marriage, Joe was ill all the time needing permission to not be so responsible and desiring someone to take care of him. As they both did their own personal work, the marriage communication became better and stronger. Each became responsible for their feelings and took responsibility for their behaviors. Today, they are very excited and happy about their deep and loving communication.

Olivia was a 15-year-old teenager who got caught cheating on a test and took an overdose of Advil, ending up at the hospital. Her parents discovered she had also had sex and tried alcohol and drugs, as this information was on the hospital record. After the 21-week Imagination process, Olivia was able to believe in herself, let go of peer pressure and give herself permission to be real. Today she leads other teenagers into the program and has decided to abstain from drugs and alcohol.

Michael was fearful of swimming, almost drowning many times in his life and experienced depression and panic attacks in addition to self-mutilation behaviors. During the Imagination process and several breathwork sessions, Michael became aware that his umbilical cord had been wrapped around his neck in the womb. Additionally in an altered state, Michael had a memory of his father kicking his mother's stomach while he was in the womb. Michael's first imprint was one full of anxiety, panic and abuse. This pattern continued to be reenacted until Michael healed his birth and womb experience through 21 weeks of the Imagination process. Since that time, Michael has had no more near-drowning experiences, does not hurt himself anymore, created a healthy family and reports feeling happy, free and safe.

Susie was married to a person who was very controlling, did not want her to work, and made all the money decisions in the house. Susie, who was very fearful of her husband, came to Solutions often having lied about where she was. After 21 weeks of Imagination, Susie reclaimed her wounded inner child who had been beaten and controlled by her father for 12 years. As she completed the process, she also divorced her husband and began to paint wooden bowls. Today, she has a prosperous painting business, selling painted bowls and furniture, expressing her joy and teaching other women to express.

The stories go on and on. Every day, the people come to Solutions Center and into the process and leave transformed. Participants transform their fears and insecurities into power, discover true mission and purpose, begin new careers, new relationships, are willing and eager to create a life with no limits and connect to something greater outside of themselves–the universe, the divine. We move through time and space together into the mystery of this universe. We open our hearts to love and we love ourselves happy, joyous and free.

EPILOGUE

In all my years of work there is one thing
  that I have loved the most,
the healing secret, if you will:
that one who risks to speak the truth,
to go inside the depths of one's own psyche
and make known the pain, the joy,
in pure expression
brings healing and transformation to the
  journey.
In this way, the dance between
consciousness and unconsciousness

takes on the story told,
our past, our dreams, our love of life.
We are the players in our play.
And when we seek to tell our story,
change our script
and dance our dance,
we honor our own soul.
We write, we paint, we sculpt, we dance, we
  move, we sound, we sing, we touch.
We act the parts of all our selves inside,
the ones we love,
the ones we have disowned.
So then we see just who has been
living "me."
We can express our history,
our childhood,
and see in color, light and sound
just where we've been.
The expression is the journey.
So in our work, we build the sacred space,
the sacred bridge–
the womb in which our new intentions
lay to be ignited by the energy of arts–
our masterpiece unfolds.
Our wounds will heal here,
as we trust the process of it all.
We enter the symbolic and imaginal realm
as we call in our artist Self.
And here, our imagination has a chance!
We use our body, mind and soul
to navigate the layers of our own
rhythms of energy.
Our bodies are involved as well.
We move them in the consciousness of what-
  ever is coming up for us.
We are closed, or we are open.
Our bodies tell the secrets as they move.
Creative arts allow us to embody all our
  parts, our selves, our pain and feelings.
There is a transformative power in expres-
  sion,
which goes beyond the therapist's chair in
  quiet talk.
The talk must one day cease,
and movement must begin to take its place.
In this expression we dare to reenact
Whatever holds us in our pain and patterns.
There is a melody, which sings our song,

and if it is not written yet, we write.
We dare to write, explore the themes of our
own lives
that have occurred at each level of our
growth.
There is a reexperiencing, a reclaiming of
our wholeness,
When we bring the story from the depth of
our body memories–
The crevices and shadows of our existence,
into the light of this reality.
My passion–expression!
For there were days,
I sat in my own corner twirling hair,
my inner child still locked inside.
There was that moment when some helper
said,
"come and tell your story,
dance your dance, laugh with me."
There was the call–the awakening–a whole
part of my consciousness
I had not even touched!
The years have gone by quickly now.
I have evolved.
I have become the Expressive Therapeutic
Artist.
I have written the opera of my life!
You think you cannot paint, or write, or sing,
or dance.
Your fears and shame sit in your heart and
soul
and wait for you to invite them out to play,
to become real, to be exposed.
Your patterns keep you prisoner–
as they play old drama over and over and
over.
There is a way to set them free–
to be, spontaneous again,
to heal, and know that all is perfect.
There is a reason for it all.
The universe is changing every day and we
are one
together walking through our journey
toward the meaning and the purpose.

REFERENCES

Bradshaw, J. (1988). *Bradshaw On: The Family: a revolutionary way of self-discovery.* Deerfield Beach, FL: Health Communications, Inc.

Brigham, D. D. (1994). *Imagery for getting well.* New York, NY: W.W. Norton & Company, Inc.

Campbell, D. (1992). *Music and miracles.* Wheaton, IL: The Theosophical Publishing House.

Cassou, M., & Cubley, S. (1995). *Life, paint and passion, reclaiming the magic of spontaneous expression.* New York, NY: G. P. Putnam's Sons.

Cousens, G. (1986). *Spiritual nutrition and the rainbow diet.* San Rafael, CA: Cassandra Press.

Cousens, G. (2000). *Conscious eating.* Berkeley, CA: North Atlantic Books.

Dewhurst. Maddock, O. (1993). *Sound therapy, heal yourself with music and voice.* New York, NY: Fireside, Simon & Schuster Inc.

Fox, J. (1997). *Poetic medicine.* New York: Jeremy P. Tarcher/Putnam.

Frager, R., & Fadiman, J. (1984). *Personality and Personal growth.* (2nd Ed.). New York: Harper & Row.

Gerber, R.. (1988). *Vibrational Medicine.* Sante Fe, NM: Bear and Company.

Grof, S., & Grof, C. (Eds.). (1989). *Spiritual emergency, when personal transformation becomes a crisis.* New York, NY: Jeremy P. Tarcher/Putnam.

Grof, S. (1992). *The Holotropic Mind: the three levels of human consciousness and how they shape our lives.* New York, NY: HarperCollins.

Lewis, P., & Johnson, D. (Eds.), (2000). *Current approaches in drama therapy.* Springfield IL: Charles C Thomas.

Lewis, P. (1993). *Creative transformation, The healing power of the arts.* Wilmette, IL: Chiron Publications.

Limber, W. (1997). *I am the honored guest at your healing.* Stuart, FL: Solutions Center for Personal Growth, Inc.

Osbon, D. K. (Ed.). (1991). *A Joseph Campbell companion, reflections on the art of living.* New York, NY: HarperCollins.

Roth, G. (1989). *Maps to ecstasy, teachings of an urban shaman.* Novato, CA: Nataraj Publishing.

Small, J. (1991). *Awakening In Time, the journey from codependence to co-creation.* New York, NY: Bantam Books.

BIBLIOGRAPHY

Achterberg. J., & Lawlis, G.F. (1980). *Bridges of the bodymind.* Champaign: IPAT.

Achterberg, J., & Lawlis, G.F. (1984). *Imagery and disease.* Champaign: IPAT.

Ader, R. (Ed.). (1981). *Psychoneuroimmunology.* New York: Academic Press.

Bankart, C. P. (1997). *Talking cures A history of western and eastern psychotherapies.* Pacific Grove, CA: Brooks/Cole.

Bradshaw, J. (1990). *The Homecoming, reclaiming and championing your inner child.* New York, NY: Bantam Books.

Colapinto, J. (1991). Structural family therapy. In A.S. Gurman & D. P. Kniskern (Eds.), *Handbook of family therapy* (Vol II). New York: Brunner/Mazel.

Corey, G. (1991). *Theory and practice of counseling and psychotherapy.* Pacific Grove, CA: Brooks/Cole.

Chopra, D. (1989). *Quantum Healing, exploring the frontiers of mind/body medicine.* New York, NY: Bantam Books.

Chopra, D. (1994). *The seven spiritual laws of success.* San Rafael, CA: Amber-Allen Publishing and New World Library.

Covey, S. R. (1990). *The seven habits of highly effective people.* New York: Simon & Schuster.

DeLaszlo, V. S. (Ed.). (1990). *The Basic writings of C. G. Jung.* New York: Princeton University Press.

Dossey, L. (1989). *Recovering the soul.* New York: Bantam.

Erikson, E. (1963). *Childhood and society.* New York, NY: W.W. Norton and Company.

Feurstein, G., & Bodian, S., (Eds.). (1993). *Living Yoga, a comprehensive guide for daily life.* New York, NY: G. P. Putnam's Sons.

Goldenberg, I., & Goldenberg, H. (2000). *Family Therapy, An Overview,* fifth edition. Belmont, CA: Wadsworth/Thompson Learning.

Green, E. E. & Green, A. M., & Walters, E. D. (1969). Feedback techniques for deep relaxation. *Psychophysiology, 6:*371–377.

Harris, A. S. (1996). *Living with Paradox, An introduction to Jungian psychology.* Pacific Grove, CA: Brooks/Cole.

Jennings, S. & Minde, A. (1993). *Art therapy & drama therapy, masks of the soul.* London: Jessica Kingsley Publishing, LTD.

Jung, C. G. (1963). *Memories, dreams, reflections.* New York: Random House, Inc.

Kabat-Zinn, J. (1990). *Full catastrophe living.* New York: Bantam.

Kaufmann, Y. (1989). Analytical psychotherapy. In R. J. Corsini & D. Wedding (Eds.), *Current Psychotherapies* (4th ed). Itasca, IL: F. E. Peacock.

Kerr, M. E., & Bowen, M. (1988). *Family evaluation: An approach based on Bowen theory.* New York: Norton.

Murphy, M. (1992). *The future of the body.* New York, NY: G.P. Putnam's Sons.

Myss, C. (1996). *Anatomy of the spirit.* New York: Crown Publishers.

Pennebaker, J. W. (1990). *Opening Up: The healing power of confidence in others.* New York: Avon.

Pert, C. B. (1997). *Molecules of emotion.* New York, NY: Scribner.

Rosenblatt, Paul C. (1994). *Metaphors of family systems theory, toward new constructions.* New York, NY: The Guilford Press.

Rossi, E.L. (1986). *The psychobiology of mind-body healing.* New York: Norton.

Rossi, E. L. (1990). From mind to molecule: More than a metaphor. In J.K. Zeig & S. Gilligan (Eds.), *Brief Therapy: Myths, methods and metaphors.* New York: Brunner/Mazel.

Samuels, M. & Lane, M. R. (1998). *Creative healing.* New York, NY: HarperCollins Publishers.

Small, J. (1992). *Transformers: The artists of self-creation.* Martina Del Ray, California: DeVorss & Company.

FURTHER TRAINING

Soul Studies Institute, Inc., an outgrowth of Solutions Center for Personal Growth, Inc. offers training and certification in this integrated and holistic healing model, Imagination, under the supervision of Wendyne Limber, MA., LMFT. In addition, Soul Studies Institute, Inc. has joined The Institute for Healing and Wellness, Inc., and Omega Theater in Boston, to offer training toward an MA degree in

Transpersonal Transformational Creative Arts Therapy through Lesley University's Independent Degree Program. We are offering classes, mentorship, advising, supervision, internships and practica in addition to Imagination Certification and a Certificate in Transpersonal Drama Therapy which fulfills Alternate Route Academic requirements towards RDT (Registered Drama Therapist) credentialing with the National Association for Drama Therapy (NADT.)

Solutions Center for Personal Growth, Inc.
865 N. Federal Highway
Stuart, Florida 34994
Phone: 561-692-3679
Email: solution@treco.net
www.solutionscenterforpersonalgrowth.com
www.soulstudies.com

Chapter 14

SADDLEBROOK: A WELLNESS CENTER BLUEPRINT

NICK HALL WITH AL MARTINEZ-FONTS, JR.

INTRODUCTION

Setting

THE SADDLEBROOK WELLNESS CENTER is situated on 480 acres of private, natural Florida countryside. The unique walking village enables guests to have access to all amenities without the need for transportation. This includes four restaurants from poolside casual to resort elegant. A special spa menu featuring carefully selected healthy options is also available. A lounge that features entertainment, live music and dancing is an option for those seeking a social context in which to recover. Other recovery options include two 18-hole championship golf courses and 45 tennis courts including all Grand Slam playing surfaces. Bike trails, lake fishing, canoe trips on the nearby Hillsborough River and four swimming pools provide additional options to meet whatever preference a client seeks.

Core Components of the Wellness Program

The core components of the Wellness programs are the executive challenge course, spa, and fitness center. Initiatives at the 5-acre low and high ropes challenge course enable clients to step outside their normal comfort zone in a safe yet emotionally challenging environment. Most importantly are the stress-recovery strategies that are taught in conjunction with these protocols. This is done at debriefing locations situated throughout the course. Next, the client is taught to recover from the physical consequences of stress. They can set their own pace in the 3,300 square foot fitness center and 3,000 square foot outdoor activity pavilion where state of the art exercise equipment and trainers insure that specific objectives are met.

Ultimately, it is recovery that matters. Most people do not need less stress. They need more recovery. For those who seek passive ways to unwind, the European-style luxury spa features massage therapy, hydrotherapy, herbal and seaweed body wraps, moor mud treatments, and aromatherapy seven days a week. Other amenities include saunas, whirlpools, steam rooms, herbal tea bars, and even a unique couple's massage room. The program is all about options. One size does not fit all and so guests are encouraged to choose those combinations of activities that best meet their needs. If they are not sure what's best, counseling is available to help them make the best choice.

PHILOSOPHY

The Saddlebrook Resort Wellness Center programs are predicated upon science, but tempered with pragmatism. There are times when some healthy guidelines simply cannot be followed. Especially when the client is logging 100,000 miles per year in airplanes and may not have time for anything other than fast food. In these situations, the program is tailored to fit the person's lifestyle. That includes a discussion of healthy options that might be available when ordering fast food. Regardless of how it's structured, each program begins with the end. "What do you want to accomplish?" is always the first question posed to a prospective client, followed immediately by, "Why?" The latter often takes people by surprise. They assume good mental and physical health are worthwhile objectives requiring no further justification. For some, that may be sufficient motivation. For others, it may not. Not all people need to be healthy in order to enjoy a high quality of life. Highly successful executives earning six or seven digit salaries are sometimes overweight, smoke cigarettes and reward themselves with liberal amounts of alcohol. That lifestyle may be acceptable. If a person sits behind a desk analyzing financial reports and then derives pleasure from watching television or reading, they will not require the same degree of health being sought by a client whose work entails physical activity and who's pleasure is found on a tennis court. The decision to participate in any wellness program should always be predicated upon meeting a basic need that is valued by the individual. Finally, there must be a long-term objective that wellness will facilitate. It might be continuing to enjoy athletic pursuits in later decades or being at a grandchild's wedding. Saddlebrook programs seek to identify a personal motivator that is essential for compliance. That process begins with a review of basic human drives and then a discussion with the client as to which is/are the most important.

Researchers at Ohio State University have formulated a list of 15 basic desires that drive human behavior (Reiss & Havercamp, 1998):

Food	Vengeance
Sex	Citizenship
Honor	Physical Exercise
Order	Learning
Social Contact	Time with Family
Prestige	Avoidance of Rejection
Power	Avoidance of Pain
Independence	

While these appear to be universal drives shared by all, their intensity and the impact each has upon the choices people make varies from person to person. Past experiences, beliefs, and individual values will dictate whether a person plays the game of life to win or to avoid losing, whether honor and prestige are paramount, or the avoidance of rejection. The prospective client is asked to reflect upon what they most value and then select the top three. If they are not sure, the Meyers-Briggs Type Indicator or similar instrument may be used to help in assessing their preferences and tendencies. The next step is to identify the appropriate strategy to achieve the desired endpoint in a manner consistent with their primary motivator. This increases the probability of compliance with the prescribed wellness protocol.

The amount of anything is a function of two variables–production and degradation. Regardless of whether the objective is wealth or health, the amount always will be determined by the relative amounts of those things leading to its creation and those resulting in it's destruction. Stress is universally recognized, and scientifically documented, as one of the greatest impediments to optimal mental and physical health. Therefore, regardless of the ultimate objective, the Saddlebrook wellness programs always incorporate protocols designed to assist people to rapidly and appropriately recover from inevitable stressors.

In addition, there is a place for wellness within organizations. Corporations are responsible to their shareholders to maintain optimal productivity that is directly related to the health of their employees. There are other unique considerations when considering wellness within an organization. Optimal leadership and managerial skills, the ability to function as a team, effective interpersonal skills, and the ability to communicate are all signs of a healthy organization. Ultimately, the concern is with the health within and between multiple systems. This chapter will describe the manner by which this integration has been accomplished at the highly successful wellness center at Saddlebrook Resort near Tampa, Florida. The client can choose a variety of options ranging from the boot camp-like Executive Challenge Course to the soothing ministrations of massage therapists in the European style spa. Each option plays a significant role in the creation of both individual and corporate wellness.

The success of any program is contingent upon the marketing effort undertaken to promote it. Virtually all avenues are pursued. Saddlebrook Resort's web site (Saddlebrook resort.com) includes a prominent display and description of the available services which attracts considerable business, especially from corporations. Collateral material is also distributed to meeting planners via direct mailings or placement of advertisements in meeting planner's periodicals. Editors and writers are occasionally invited to visit as guests of the resort. These visits, along with press releases whenever new components are added, have resulted in many articles in meeting periodicals, travel trade and consumer magazines, as well as newspapers. Information is also disseminated through the hosting of familiarization lunches with members of the local Chamber of Commerce and the Tampa Bay Convention Bureau. These representatives are then able to disseminate the information to organizations considering Saddlebrook as a meeting site.

INDIVIDUAL WELLNESS

It is supposed to be the happiest day of her life. She's about to be married, yet her head is pounding as she focuses upon all the things which can go wrong. The cause of her headache is clearly stress which is the fast track to illness, not wellness. Sources of stress must first be identified and dealt with before embarking upon a wellness program. Otherwise, every movement towards attaining the desired goal will be delayed if not directly counteracted. Family, finances and work are usually the primary sources of stress for young adults. As people get older, they may be replaced with social isolation and medical problems. Do stress management programs available through wellness centers help those already suffering from a stress-related illness? The answer provided by scientists at Duke University is clearly "yes." A study of people diagnosed with heart disease revealed that learning to recognize and control responses to stress can reduce the likelihood of suffering heart attacks by up to 74 percent (Blumenthal et al., 1997). Because of the pivotal role it plays during the pursuit of wellness, the subject of stress will be dealt with in some detail before describing the approaches used to best recover.

STRESS RECOVERY

A very practical definition of stress was put forward by Richard Lazarus when he stated, "It seems wise to use stress as a generic term for the whole area of problems that includes the stimuli producing stress reactions, the reactions themselves, and the various intervening processes. It defines a large, complex, amorphous, interdisciplinary area of interest and study" (Lazarus, 1966). It is not a helpful definition because it is too broad. However, it does address all the important variables which a person has to take into account when using the word "stress." Each client defines the word in a very specific and highly personalized way. Hence, the need for the broadest of definitions. Everyone manifests a stress response that may differ from one individual to another. Some people, when confronted with a major stressor, may experience a very rapid increase in heart rate, perhaps even to the point of experiencing tachycardia. For other individuals, their stomach might turn into knots with a major impact on their gastrointestinal system. Yet others may experience headaches or muscle tension. All these symptoms have a tendency to occur, but different individuals will have a predominance of one type of symptom or another.

Furthermore, the type of response a person has is the one they will likely manifest regardless of the stressor. If a supervisor at work has just given their subordinate a letter informing him that his services are no longer needed, the subordinate is likely to experience a stress response. And whatever the type of response, it's the same he'll experience if cut off while driving down the interstate. Hence, if a person can learn to recover from one type of stressor, chances are he'll be better able to cope with others. This is how stress recovery is taught at the Saddlebrook Wellness Center. Stress is induced under controlled conditions which, in turn, enables the client to learn firsthand how to recover. Ultimately, a person has to experience stress in order to practice recovery skills.

Biological Basis of Stress and Recovery

Every wellness program begins with a description of the biological basis for what is experienced. The information is valuable because it helps the client predict what may happen next. In the context of stress, the client is given a brief overview of stress physiology (Hall, 2001). There are just two chemical reactions in the context of stress that are important. Those dealing with *anabolism*,

which is a chemical term used to describe building processes, verses *catabolism*, which describes the breaking down of products. During the stress response, there is a shift from anabolic to catabolic processes, and the reason is quite logical. Why build for the future if there isn't going to be a future? For the same reason that a person would not build a summer cottage on the seaside when a hurricane was bearing down on the lot, the body is not going to waste valuable time and resources on reproduction and other construction projects when the future is uncertain. In the short term, halting unessential building projects will not be harmful. For a period of days, even weeks, the changes actually can be very beneficial. Problems occur when a person switches from anabolic to catabolic processes over an extended period of months or years. That is when stress-related illness can result and it's the aspect of stress that's emphasized at Saddlebrook.

The stress response can also be viewed as a series of chemical reactions designed to provide energy—a process for extracting glucose and other energy substrates from storage. Glucose is not the only substrate. Other things might be needed as well, but glucose is one of the primary substrates, especially for the muscles and the central nervous system. However, converting glucose from stored energy sources and then putting what isn't required back into storage is very wasteful. About 30 percent of the usable energy is lost, which is why many people coping with chronic stress suffer from fatigue. Once fatigue sets in compliance with any wellness program is going to be limited. Therefore, the wellness protocols emphasize strategies for obtaining optimal amounts of the deep, restful stage of sleep referred to as delta or slow wave sleep. This can be accomplished through a combination of diet, exercise and temperature regulation. Only after this stage of sleep will a client awaken refreshed and able to mentally and physically engage in a wellness program.

Somatic Versus Psychogenic Basis of Stress and Wellness

There are many ways of categorizing the stress response. Somatic stressors result in physical injury to the body. Chemical changes occur within the body, the tissue is repaired, and unless damage is very severe, things will return to some sort of a homeostatic balance. It is the psychogenic stressors that cause problems. The anticipation of something that is perceived to be injurious to the body (even though it is not) can result in physiological changes. This is a bit misleading because a somatic stressor clearly will impact psychological health. Likewise, a psychogenic stressor will affect a number of nervous system pathways that are capable of impacting the body. What follows is a listing of some of the potential ways a person might respond when faced with uncertainty or a threat. These are reviewed with the client in order to assess whether the focus should be upon the options for physical recovery from stress or emotional recovery (Sapolski, 1998) (see Figure 14-1).

Active Recovery from Emotional Stress: "Cross-stressing"

At Saddlebrook Resort, we have created a program that's designed to deal with what is probably the greatest impediment to personal growth and corporate success: the fear of failure. The initial focus is upon the issue of fear. Clients are taken out of their comfort zone and away from all the things that provide security. They are taken into a wooded executive challenge course where there are no walls displaying certificates of achievement. There's no place for the coat and tie that convey power and authority in the workplace. It's a place where the expensive gold watch or reserve of cash are of no value. That alone enables some people to push their personal comfort envelope and learn to deal with the mild fear of being in a novel environment. Of course, everyone is having

fun during the process. They are problem solving and enjoying themselves. There's no reason learning a valuable lesson cannot also be fun. And sometimes this serves as a useful diversion, or what is referred to as "emotional interference." The friendly exchanges as people enter this unfamiliar territory serves to counterbalance their uncertainty.

In this new environment, the old familiar beliefs are easier to let go of as a new group with a different purpose and different dynamics begins to form. A team evolves that now requires different skills to function effectively. This is the first critical step to change–getting rid of the old beliefs. Otherwise, the person will always use the default beliefs since under stress a person will tend to revert to the more familiar ways of responding. In this new environment, the ability to predict has now vanished . . . especially when the training course comes into view. The ropes course resembles a militia camp with ropes suspended from trees, cable bridges and a rock-climbing wall. Some people greet this new environment and the uncertainty it brings with excitement and even elation. Others are clearly uncomfortable being away from their normal routine. In their own way, each person is dealing with change on their own terms. We have created an environment where they can learn to overcome fear safely. The new manager with rock climbing experience overcomes his nervousness of speaking to the owner of the company when it becomes clear to the group that his skills are now going to be a tremendous asset. The CEO learns to deal with the discomfort of being in a subservient position and having little to offer in this new setting. No one is ever pressured into crossing out of his or her comfort zone. But if they want to explore, one small step at a time, what it's like to experience a fear response and then recover from it, they can do it safely, in a wonderfully supportive environment, and on their terms. That evening, they view film clips of the day's activities and discuss the day's objectives.

Physical Symptoms of Stress		
Tension headaches	Problems swallowing	Frequent urination
Frowning	Frequent colds or bouts	Constipation
Trembling of lips or	with flu	Nervous diarrhea
hands	Hives	Decreased sexual desire
Muscle tension	Rashes	Difficulty reaching
Neck aches	Chills or goose bumps	orgasm
Back pain	Heartburn	Appetite change
Jaw pain	Stomach cramps	Fatigue
Increased sensitivity to	Nausea	Insomnia or hypersomnia
light and sound	Difficulty breathing	Weight change
Lightheadedness, faint-	Restlessness	Digestive upset
ness, or dizziness	Heart and chest pain	Pounding heart
Ringing in ears	Night sweats	Shortness of breath
Enlarged pupils	Sweaty hands	Rapid heart beat
Blushing	Cold hands and feet	Autoimmune symptoms
Dry mouth	Flatulence or belching	Increased perspiration

Mental Symptoms of Stress		
Anxiety	Disorganization	Low productivity
Guilt	Indecisiveness	Negative attitude
Increased anger	Feeling overwhelmed	Defensiveness
Frustration	Discontentment	Suspiciousness
Moodiness	Suicidal thoughts	Whirling mind
Depression	Fear closeness to people	Lacking creativity
Nightmares	Loneliness	Boredom
Trouble learning	Dulled senses	Spacing out
Forgetfulness	Poor concentration	Confusion

Behavioral Symptoms of Stress		
Inattention to grooming	Overreaction	Mood swings
Increased tardiness	Prone to minor accidents	Bad temper
Serious appearance	Perfectionism	Crying spells
Unusual behavior	Reduced productivity	Stuttering
Nervous habits	Fast or mumbled speech	Nervous laughing
Rushing around or pacing	Unusual risk-taking	Excessive worrying
Increased alcohol use	Gritting of teeth	Easily discouraged
Increased tobacco use	Lying or making excuses	Procrastination
Gambling	Social withdrawal	Nail-biting
Overspending	Self pity	
Edginess	Strained communication	

Figure 14-1. Physical, Mental and Behavioral Symptoms of Stress.

Effective communication, leadership and trust are some of the more common team building themes that also happen to be the key ingredients of corporate wellness.

When it's over, the participants are better equipped to deal with the fears of change. They have learned to accept change and to cope with uncertainty on their terms so when they experience similar challenges in the workplace or in their personal lives, they know what to expect emotionally and physically. Its called "Cross-Stressing." Having learned to recover from one form of emotional challenge, it becomes easier to recover from others.

Active Recovery from Physical Stress

The mind is an important part of the equation, but equally important is training physical recovery (Loehr, 1993). Every cell within the cardiovascular system, the respiratory system, and even the immune system has the ability to learn to withstand stress. It is well documented that if the concentration of a chemical increases within the body, there will be a corresponding adjustment in the ability of the receptor to attract the chemical. It's one of the ways the body adapts to change. By bathing the body's cells in stress hormones, the cells learn to recover, and then, when another stressor arises, those cells are better able to adapt.

The best form of stress to train physical recovery is exercise, yet very few people take advantage of this powerful tool. Some studies suggest that the average person spends two and a half-hours a day watching television, yet only 15 minutes per day exercising. Many people do not exercise at all. Never in the course of history have people been more inactive, and never have we been more susceptible to so many stress-related diseases. Physical activity of any kind will help prevent coronary arterial disease, colon cancer, breast cancer, and obesity. If performed in a specific manner, it can also enable a person to recover rapidly from stress.

Exercise is a form of stress. It's not in the same category as losing a job or loved one because the person is in control. Nonetheless, there are enough shared features that exercise can be used as a means by which to condition the body to rapidly recover. They are:

• Increased heart rate
• Increased respiration rate
• A switch from anabolism to catabolism
• Decreased salivation
• Inhibition of digestion

When people learn to adapt to one form of stress, they are able to better cope with most other forms. It's like learning to drive a car. No two automobiles are exactly the same, yet having learned to drive one model; a person can readily apply her basic driving skills to all others. She may have to search for the light switch, or hood release button, but the essential components are about where they would be expected. The same applies to stress. Once a person learns to respond to one form of stress, she will have the basic skills to respond to most all other types. Exercise is the form of stress that's used for this part of the wellness training.

ASSESSMENT

Prior to beginning the exercise-based stress recovery programs, the client receives a comprehensive fitness evaluation that includes measures of strength, cardiovascular fitness, flexibility, resting and maximum heart rate, heart rate recovery, and body fat composition. Trainers then customize a program for improving fitness safely and effectively.

A key measure is the determination of maximum heart rate, which is the number of beats per minute (BPM) that cannot be exceeded despite increasing the intensity of exercise. If the heart were a car, it would be the highest number on the speedometer. The engine might be capable of going faster, but the needle on the gauge can't go past its limit. There are several ways clients are instructed to determine their maximum BPM. The best is to take a stress test. Under a doctor's supervision, they exercise to the point where heart rate levels off. Even though they may run faster, their heart fails to increase after the maximum is reached. This method will enable a person to identify their precise maximum under medical supervision.

Some very fit individuals will test themselves using a heart rate monitor. This should be discouraged. Pushing the heart to its maximum may unmask a latent heart condition. For this reason, this approach is not recommended. A less accurate but better alternative to pushing the limit uses a simple mathematical formula. The holistic health practitioner subtracts the client's age from 220. This very simple calculation is not very accurate. It assumes that all men and women of the same age are basically the same, and fails to take into account medical problems, genetics, or the type of exercise. A person who is very fit may have a measured maximum heart rate considerably higher than the value calculated using the formula. Furthermore, many athletes discover that their maximum heart rate for bicycling is quite different than for running. Swimming may yield yet another value. Despite its inherent flaws, the client will at least have a starting point.

Next, the heart rate equivalent of high, medium, and low stress zones is calculated. These are based upon some of the same guidelines athletes use to determine their aerobic and anaerobic zones. Aerobic means oxygen is being used. Anaerobic is without oxygen. If a person exercises at an intensity that results in shortness of breath, chances are his body will not have enough oxygen to maintain aerobic-based pathways to generate energy. That's when a person shifts to anaerobic pathways to produce the energy required to keep pace with the physical demands being placed upon the body. This is very important if the objective is to lose weight. That's because oxygen is needed for fat to be converted into energy. If a workout is too intense, fat will be spared while energy is derived from stored glycogen–a process that does not require oxygen.

The **Low Stress Zone** is where a person should start if they have not exercised before, or if the individual is recovering from an injury. When in this zone, heart rate will be between 50 and 60 percent of the maximum.

In the **Moderate Stress Zone**, physical activity will help increase a person's endurance for the stress of exercise. The heart will beat at a faster rate because it will be bathed in larger amounts of adrenaline and other stress-related chemicals. The number of beats per minute will be between 60 and 70 percent of the maximum. At the same time, the body will become accustomed to this change so when similar events occur under circumstances outside the person's control, the body will be able to recover more efficiently. Breathing is rapid, but the client is still able to obtain enough oxygen to maintain aerobic metabolism.

The **High Stress Zone** is the zone within which the body will learn to recover from an even greater amount of stress. When in this zone, heart rate will be between 80 and 90 percent of the maximum, and the average person will not be able to take in enough oxygen to sustain some of the more common processes for obtaining energy. The body will switch to anaerobic metabolism.

At this point, the client has all the information needed to train stress recovery which is the key to wellness. It's important to realize that stress causes harm when the intensity of the stressor overwhelms a person's capacity to recover. Exercise is a form of stress, but one the client has total control over. She determines the start time, the intensity, as well as the end of the regimen. Consequently, she is subjecting her body to many of the same physiological events that occur during uncontrollable stress, but without the harmful consequences. That's why exercise is used at Saddlebrook to induce a form of stress that trains recovery.

Clients are instructed to spend approximately 80 percent of their time exercising within the moderate stress zone. The remaining time should be spent oscillating between the low and high stress zones creating a wave-like pattern of heart rate change. When heart rate reaches 90 percent of the maximum, the person should slow down until it gradually descends to 60 percent. Then they should repeat the cycle, perhaps reaching 85 percent. Then, heart rate should be slowed until it reaches about 65 percent. In doing this, the person is incorporating a universal principle into the workout. *For every action, there is an equal and opposite reaction* (Dishman et al., 2000). Or, for every episode of stress (increased heart rate), there needs to occur an equal amount of recovery (a decline in heart rate). It really doesn't matter what form of exercise the client chooses. What is important is that they do something they enjoy. However, it is important to recognize that some exercise regimens enable you to attain a higher heart rate than do others.

The fitness program at Saddlebrook provides several options: There is a half-mile course designed to enable a person to either warm up or cool down. The cardiovascular equipment includes advanced stair-climbers, treadmills, stationary bikes and a Sky Walker for a maximum number of cardiovascular workouts. Cybex equipment and free weights are available for resistance weight training. However, virtually any exercise equipment or aerobic activity could be used.

MODALITIES

Massage and Wellness

Touch has long been regarded as a healing modality (see Field, 1998 for review).

Humans rub sore and tender spots while animals lick the abrasion. A symbolic form of this behavior is a mother kissing her child's wound in order to make it better. It makes sense that touch would play an important role in the induction and maintenance of good health considering the skin is one of the largest organ systems of the body and is constantly at the interface of the environment. Furthermore, massage is able to induce a state of relaxation that serves to counter the adverse effects of generalized stress and to reduce anxiety and depression in those suffering from chronic fatigue syndrome, in adolescent mothers, and in those who are HIV positive. This may explain the correlation between massage and elevated Natural Killer Cell activity and T-cell levels in those diagnosed with HIV.

Some massage therapists assert that massage may stimulate the movement of immune system cells within the lymphatic channel (Elkins et al., 1953). It is argued that by engaging in a form of deep massage, a person would be able to stimulate the migration of lymphocytes. This is not an unreasonable claim. It is essential that lymphocytes constantly move around the body in order to seek out pathogens. They move through the circulatory system as well as within the lymphatic channels. The lymphatic channels can be looked upon as being like a series of garden hoses that link the lymph nodes and the spleen. Lymph nodes and the white pulp of the spleen are filters where pathogens accumulate and where they come into contact with disease-fighting lymphocytes. But the lymphatics, in contrast to the circulatory system, have no heart. There is no equivalent pump. What enables the cells to move, albeit very sluggishly, from one lymph node to another is the peristaltic movement of muscles surrounding the lymphatic channels. An argument is made that by recreating that peristaltic movement through massage, one can facilitate lymphocyte trafficking. Regardless of whether the effects are direct or indirect, massage certainly has been found to have positive effects in treating a variety of immunologic illnesses such as asthma, chronic fatigue syndrome, pediatric dermatitis, and HIV. For that reason, the Saddlebrook Spa offers the following options:

- Aromatherapy massage for stress relief
- Reflexology foot therapy
- Sports massage for muscle soreness
- Neuromuscular therapy for pain relief
- Shiatsu massage to rebalance chi in the body
- Swedish massage for relaxation
- Underwater lymphatic massage

Aromatherapy and Wellness

Evidence suggests that the sense of smell is a means by which to manipulate emotions. Proof of this claim is not available, although when considering how olfaction is mediated within the brain, it is certainly feasible. Most of the sensory systems course through the brain via a labyrinth of structures and pathways. For example, the sense of hearing as well as vision wind their way through the sensory apparatus, arriving initially within a structure called the thalamus. From this relay site, the information is transmitted to so-called "higher brain centers" where it is processed in ways that enable a person to make the appropriate decision about what is happening in the environment. Eventually, all of the information arrives in the amygdala, the brain's emotional computer. The sense of smell is different. Olfactory information is able to short-circuit many of the higher brain areas and plunge directly into the emotional brain. Some of the information goes into the part that controls the autonomic nervous system as well as many of the hormonal pathways that are activated during stress. This very well may explain the well-documented association between the sense of smell and those behaviors that are linked with emotions. They would include sex as well as aggression. Many species actually recognize each other, as well as each others

emotional state, on the basis of smell alone.

It is the study of reproductive pheromones, which provides the most convincing argument that aromas can impact health. Pheromones are molecules emitted into the environment by a number of species. They communicate information from one member of that specie to another. Fish, rats, dogs, and even humans rely upon them. Some evoke the emotion of fear, others anger, but those that have been most extensively studied are those that elicit the emotions associated with arousal of the reproductive system. The most convincing documentation that pheromones function in this manner in human society is to be found in those situations where women live together. Women who live in college dormitories have been found to have synchronized menstrual cycles. The same is true of women who live on the same floor in prisons. In addition, men and women each produce chemicals which serve as an attractant for the member of the opposite gender. A short chain fatty acid called copulin has been identified in the vaginal secretions of a variety of female primates with the amount of copulin increasing as estrogen rises. When men are exposed to a large number of odors, they will exhibit preference for secretions containing copulin. In addition to men being attracted to copulin, which is found at highest concentrations at the time of ovulation, women are attracted to a chemical called exaltalide. It is a macrocyclic ketone which children, men, and post-menopausal women have a very difficult time detecting unless they are given estrogen. Studies have revealed that not only will exposure to exaltalide affect the judgment of women when evaluating the written and interviewed descriptions of male job candidates, but they will selectively seek out and sit on chairs which contain a trace amount of this chemical. This is the basis of the perfume industry. People wear fragrances primarily for the purpose of making themselves attractive to members of the opposite sex.

The observations made in the context of

reproductive pheromone research clearly reveal that trace amounts of chemicals can make their way into key areas of the brain and arouse not only the endocrine physiology that is paramount for reproduction to occur, but also libido and other behavioral manifestations of procreation. Is it really that farfetched to propose that other types of odors might not arouse other physiological systems, including those that influence health? This is the basis of aromatherapy. It is predicated upon the belief that essential oils found in plants are capable of imparting fragrances that are capable of impacting not only emotions but also mental and physical well being. For example, the fragrance associated with lavender is believed to be relaxing and serve as a gentle sedative. Rosemary, on the other hand, is thought to have the opposite effect and serve to stimulate. While rose oil is said to calm the emotion of anger. Claims are made about many other fragrances as well.

There are three forms of aromatherapy. *Holistic aromatherapy* is the first and incorporates the use of essential oils, often in the context of massage. The second form is *medical aromatherapy* during which specific fragrances are prescribed in order to counter various maladies. Finally, *aesthetic aromatherapy* involves the use of oils and fragrances to treat skin problems such as stretch marks. It's also used to induce a state of relaxation. While the use of aromatherapy dates back 5,000 years to the days of the early Egyptians, the form of aromatherapy practiced in Western society dates to sixteenth century Germany. A large number of claims are made regarding the use of aromatherapy. Conditions ranging from arthritis and allergies to anger and depression are thought to be impacted by different aromas. Whether these claimed benefits are really due to something associated with the chemical configuration of the odor-inducing molecule or simply the evocation of memory is hard to discern. Many people do associate fragrances with certain situations or people,

and it may be the memory of that circumstance which is actually evoking the emotional state. Of course, the same odor may evoke completely different states depending upon the nature of one's memory.

At least one study conducted in mice under well-controlled laboratory conditions has revealed that, when animals are exposed to a stressor, they produce a type of pheromone that is capable of inhibiting the immune system of other mice. This includes a reduction in the proliferation of antibody producing cells as well as the proliferation of T-cells that coordinate so many aspects of the immune system. It was concluded that the most likely mechanism was activation of brain circuitry that gives rise to elevated stress chemicals. These are the same chemicals that are capable, at high concentrations, of suppressing the immune system. For this reason, essential oils with aromatic properties are incorporated into not only the wellness center's massage protocols, but a variety of balneotherapy aroma baths for stress relief, detoxification or pain relief depending upon the desired outcome.

The Immune System, Wellness and Herbalism

Many clients equate wellness with optimal immunity. There is no question that it is the most important component of the healing system within the body. However, the widely accepted belief, "more is better" can be very dangerous advice when dealing with this entity. That's because the immune system is a double-edged sword. Too little may lead to infections, but too much is what characterizes people with autoimmune disease (Hall, Anderson, & O'Grady, 1994). The immune system is engaged in a form of friendly fire, attacking the body's own healthy tissue. The philosophy at Saddlebrook is that a person strives for immunologic balance. What follows is a discussion of some of the most commonly asked about interventions along with the information provided to clients who seek an herbal component to their wellness program.

Echinacea has been found in many investigations to stimulate cytokine release from macrophages, the cells that destroy viruses and bacteria. Extremely small amounts stimulate a significant increase in the production of IL-1, TNF-alpha, IL-6 and IL-10 that help to regulate various aspects of the immune system. Natural Killer cell activity also can be enhanced when Echinacea is administered to both healthy volunteers as well as those with depressed immunity. The clinical relevance of such in vitro studies is difficult to assess, however, since some of the cytokines stimulated by Echinacea can suppress others. For example, IL-10 can negate the effects of the other cytokines which might explain why the plant is able to reduce the severity of cytokine-induced symptoms, but its inability to prevent the common cold (Tragni et al., 1988).

The average person would be concerned primarily with an alleviation of symptoms and, therefore, might erroneously attribute a remedy to impacting immunity when, in fact, it is exerting a direct effect upon either the expression of symptoms or the proliferation of a pathogen. This may explain the popularity of Echinacea. By increasing IL-10, it may alleviate symptoms by blocking other cytokines while having minimal impact upon those immune system pathways that might be required to eliminate a virus. While a number of studies have demonstrated that Echinacea can modulate measures of the immune system, it is not clear which of the eight species is most effective, nor which part of the plant is optimal. Neither is much known about the appropriate dose to administer. Compounding the problem even further is the fact that commercial preparations often contain multiple herbs as well as zinc.

Nutrition and Wellness

Clients at Saddlebrook also have access to nutrition counseling. As a nation, Americans have become obsessed with fat, both the amount they carry on their bodies and the amount they consume. And well they should be. Dietary fat has been linked with obesity, cancer, and heart disease. In 1980, one out of four people was obese. Now, it's one out of three and getting worse. The rates of breast, colon and prostate cancers are on the rise, and heart disease is the no. 1 killer of both men and women. All of these diseases are directly linked to fat consumption.

Despite the constant bombardment of information through the media, health-care providers, and even food labels, Americans are heavier than ever before. Since people claim to be eating less fat, why does this paradox exist? Probably it exists for a variety of reasons. The average person doesn't have a clue about what they are actually consuming, in part, because food labels are misleading. Fat content may be expressed as a total percentage of the food, as a percentage of the daily minimum requirement, or in grams, all of which require an educated analytical ability held by few people other than dietitians and nutritionists. Much of the available information received is terribly confusing. For example, not all fat is the same. Monounsaturated and polyunsaturated fats are less harmful to the arteries than highly saturated fats found in meat, dairy products and coconut oil. In order to predict the impact of the fat noted on the food label, it's important to be aware of what type of fat it actually is.

Compounding the issue is that while polyunsaturated fats found in corn, sunflower and other oils are less harmful than saturated fats, polyunsaturated fats are not nearly as effective in lowering the so-called 'bad cholesterol' as are the monounsaturated fats in olive and canola oils. In fact, there is evidence that monounsaturated fats not only reduce the bad cholesterol, they also augment levels of the good cholesterol by helping transport artery clogging factors from the bloodstream. Even the term "fat free" does not mean that. FDA regulations dictate that for a product to make such a claim, it only must contain less than one-half gram of fat per serving. "Reduced fat" means the product contains 25 percent less fat than its regular version. The term "low fat," with the exception of milk, means that the product has no more than three grams of fat per serving. Milk labeling really adds to the confusion. When a person sees "2 percent Lowfat" on the milk label, he's likely to assume that means it has a 2 percent fat content. In fact, 2 percent milk derives about 36 percent of its calories from fat. That's better than the 50 percent of calories from fat in whole milk, but its certainly a far cry from the perception implied by the large print on the label. So people should be wary of labeling claims, and careful to read all the fine print.

As confusing as the fat issue is, the solution is simple. People should consume no more than 20 percent of their calories as fat, no matter what its source. Even the beef industry endorses no more than a three and a half-ounce serving of meat per meal. How can the correct portion be gauged in practical terms? It's about the same size as a deck of cards. As important as it is to limit dietary intake of fats, some research indicates that by adulthood, it may be too late to alter any link to correlated cancers. Two variables have been correlated with breast cancer– increased height and age of menstruation onset, both of which are determined in part by the intake of dietary fat. It's important to instill healthy nutritional habits early and keep dietary fat intake at the recommended 20 percent level for children above the age of two. The best way for parents to do this is by setting a good example through their own eating habits. Extra fat is called for, though,

during the initial phase of growth.

When it comes to adding vitamin and mineral supplements to the diet, clients are instructed to do so wisely. It is far better to receive the proper nutrients through whole foods. Research has yet to prove supplements in capsule form work in the same protective manner that natural sources provide. Certain of these supplements, when present in larger amounts than are necessary, are simply flushed from the body by the kidneys, while others can build up to toxic levels. As a society, Americans are known to have the most expensive urine in the world. In the United States, people spend an average of $13.30 per person on vitamins each year. Germans spend $9.81; the French $7.40; in Britain, it's $6.01, and in Spain, only 48¢. And there's no conclusive evidence that links the amount spent with the health and wellness of a population (see Balch & Balch, 1997 for review).

A very important component of the wellness center's programs is providing instruction so clients can evaluate what is best for them. To accomplish this, they will need a heart rate monitor, a watch, and access to either a stationery bicycle or treadmill with an odometer attached. The routine will always be the same. They should warm up until their heart rate reaches 75 percent of the maximum. This is in the moderate stress range. Then, they should note the time, and maintain that heart rate as closely as possible for exactly five minutes. Two variables are then measured: (1) the distance traveled during the five minute test, and (2) the time it takes for the heart rate to return to 50 percent of the maximum. The client should make every attempt to keep the conditions exactly the same each time they take this test. This is especially important with respect to the warm up and cool down phase of the regimen.

First, this test should be taken after individuals have eaten their favorite but not necessarily healthy meal. Then they should adhere to the food guidelines suggested in this section, if they are different. As a result of eating healthier foods and smaller portions, the entire body should function at a greater level of efficiency. At the same heart rate, the client will be able to cover a greater distance and their heart will recover faster. It's also an effective way to check out the claims made by those selling supplements. In this instance, the supplement is evaluated in the same manner. Because exercise is a form of stress, the client is testing the effects of specific foods upon the ability to perform and recover against a backdrop of physiological stress. This is beneficial because what works during exercise will also serve the person well in the corporate boardroom, negotiating with a teenager, or dealing with the myriad of daily stressors that are simply unavoidable. The test is not perfect. Each time the person experiences this brief workout, there will be a modest training effect which might confound the measures. So instruct the client to vary the sequence, and then repeat certain dietary regimens to control for circadian, monthly, or seasonal effects. Clients are often amazed to discover what a profound impact foods can have upon their body. In all likelihood, they will see a greater magnitude of effect with increasing amounts of stress.

ALCOHOL AND WELLNESS

A lot of media attention has been given lately to the connection between alcohol and the reduction of coronary arterial disease. At first, the theory was that the alcohol itself flushed out the arteries, but research now shows that the effective element are chemicals called flavonoids which are found in red wine and dark beer. Red wine provides more flavonoids than white because the skins, seeds and stems are left in during the winemaking process, and it's these components of the grape, which contain the highest concentration. A similar accumulation of flavonoids occurs in the processing of dark

beer—the longer the hops, barley and malt are left in the liquid, the more flavonoids are present.

This is neither a license nor recommendation to increase consumption of alcoholic beverages. Consuming more than two ounces of alcohol a day has serious, detrimental effects on the brain and liver. The benefits of flavonoids in the diet can be obtained from a variety of other sources such as grape juice that has about one-third the anticlotting capability of red wine. Broccoli, onions, apples and garlic, plus the skins of fruit and green and black teas also contain large concentrations of flavonoids. Nonetheless, the association between wine consumption and wellness may well be due to its chemical composition.

WELLNESS IN A CORPORATE SETTING

Stress and wellness programs, which typically incorporate exercise, nutrition, and stress-management components, have been the subject of a growing number of scientific evaluations. From these evaluations, it has become increasingly evident that health and wellness programs can facilitate the attainment of multiple business objectives, including enhanced productivity, a stronger corporate image, and improved economic well-being. Studies have revealed a beneficial effect of health and wellness programs on absenteeism, job performance, turnover, job strain, and employee attitudes such as commitment, morale, and job satisfaction. For example, participants in Johnson and Johnson's Live for Life health and wellness program showed a significantly lower absenteeism rate, relative to their peers, over a three-year period. The Live for Life program was also shown to favorably change employee attitudes toward the company including commitment to the organization, perception of job competence, and feelings about supervision, working conditions, job security, pay, and fringe benefits. Similarly, an evaluation of Fitness Systems' health and wellness program found that employees who followed the program regularly evidenced increased productivity and working effectiveness. This included a decreased rate of absenteeism ranging from 2.5 to 8.6 days per employee per year. Furthermore, studies of hospital employees and NASA executives have shown health and wellness programs to reduce participants' experience of strains including anxiety and muscle tension. Research also suggests that health and wellness programs, by reducing strains, have a favorable indirect influence on counterproductive behaviors including theft, on-the-job violence, alcohol misuse, medical malpractice, and serious on-the-job mistakes. One such study found that emotional and physical exhaustion on the job was significantly related to employee theft among hospital workers. Therefore, helping workers to deal with stress may reduce the tendencies of theft-tolerant employees to act out their frustrations in dishonest or counterproductive ways (see Pritchard & Potter, 1990 for review).

A corporation's image may also be enhanced. Surveys of corporate executives suggest that the presence of health and wellness programs reflect a healthy environment that can be a key factor in the recruitment and retention of employees as well as the attraction of investors. Executives from major companies such as Central States Health and Life Company of Omaha and Tenneco, Inc. have reported finding health and wellness programs to be an enormous recruiting tool which "can aid in attracting high-level upbeat employees" and which can "create a sense of bonding among employees." Yet despite all these clear benefits, wellness may not always be cost-effective.

There are compelling arguments against wellness within a corporate setting. From a purely economic standpoint, wellness may not be advantageous since having healthy employees may not save money. A study conducted by Dutch scientists has revealed that spending money to prevent and treat heart disease and stroke may not be cost-effective. That's because they increase life span and extension of medical services later in life. It was determined that the lifetime health care costs of Dutch men and women in 1988 was approximately $92,000 and $132,000 respectively. Part of the reason for the increased costs for women was their longer life expectancy (80 vs. 73.5 years). Heart disease accounted for 19 percent of the deaths yet only 2.7 percent of the lifetime health care costs. On the other hand, mental disorders were responsible for only 0.6 percent of all deaths yet consumed 26 percent of the health care budget. A similar conclusion was drawn after a tobacco-funded study that revealed that the death of smokers from tobacco-related disease saved the Czech Republic an estimated $30 million in 1999. The costs of health care and lost productivity were more than offset by the savings through welfare, housing and pensions for the elderly (Associated Press report of a study conducted by Arthur D Little International, July, 18, 2001).

Savings will result only from the elimination of nonfatal chronic conditions such as musculoskeletal diseases and mental disorders thus contradicting the conventional wisdom that wellness can reduce health care costs. It depends upon the type of illness being countered by the wellness program. The primary objective of wellness is to prevent suffering and improve the quality of life, not save money. Saving money is, however, the bottom line for corporations. The promotion of wellness must therefore be based upon humanitarian arguments, not necessarily financial. Clearly there are benefits which may indirectly benefit the economic climate of an organization.

CONCLUSION

In conclusion, participating in any wellness program should always be predicated upon meeting a basic need that is valued by the individual as well as focusing on a long-term objective that wellness would facilitate. Saddlebrook programs seek to identify a personal motivator that can drive the individual through stress-producing experiences. Prior to beginning the exercise-based stress recovery programs, the client receives a comprehensive fitness evaluation. Through individually tailored programs which entail full embodied experience in stressful exercise and enactment-based scenarios, clients become able to cross-stress their responses. This allows them to be better equipped to deal with the fears of uncertainty on their terms so when they experience similar stressors in their life, they know what to expect emotionally and physically. Having learned to recover from one form of emotional challenge, it becomes easier to recover from others.

REFERENCES

Balch, J. F. & Balch, P. A. (1997). *Prescription for nutritional healing.* New York: Avery Publishing Group

Blumenthal, J. A., Jiang, W., Babyak, M. A. et al. (1997). Stress management and exercise training in cardiac patients with myocardial ischemia. *Archives of Internal Medicine,* 157:2213.

Dishman, R.K., Nakamura, Y., Garcia, M.E., Thompson, R.W., Dunn, A.L., Blair, S.N. (2000). Heart rate variability, trait anxiety and perceived stress among physically fit men and women. *Int J Psychophysiol* 37(2):121–33.

Elkins, E.C., Herrick, J.F., & Grindlay, J.H. (1953). Effects of various procedures on the flow of lymph. *Archives of Physical Medicine,* 34: 31.

Field, T. (1998). Massage Research. In *Alternative medicine: Implications for clinical practice.* Harvard Medical School Department of Continuing Education, Cambridge, MA.

Hall, N.R. (2001). *Winning the Stress Challenge.* Institute for Health and Human Performance.

Hall, N.R., Altman, F., & Blumenthal, S. (Eds.) (1994). *Mind-Body Interactions and Disease.* National Institutes of Health.

Hall, N.R., Anderson, J., & O'Grady, M.P. (1994). Stress and Immunity in Humans: Modifying Variables. In: (Glaser, R., ed.) *Handbook of stress.* San Diego: Academic Press.

Lazarus, R.S. (1966). *Psychological stress and the coping process.* New York: McGraw-Hill.

Loehr, J.E. (1993). *Toughness Training for Life.* New York, NY: Dutton.

Pritchard, R. E. & Potter, G. C. (1990). *A Guide to Corporate Health and Wellness Programs.* Homeward, IL: Dow Jones-Irwin.

Sapolsky, R. M. (1998). *Why zebras don't get ulcers: A guide to stress, stress-related diseases, and coping.* New York, NY: W.H. Freeman.

Reiss, S. & Havercamp, S. M. (1998). Toward a comprehensive assessment of fundamental motivation: Factor structure of the Reiss profiles. *Psychological Assessment, 10.*97.

Tragni, E., Galli, C.L., Tubaro, A., Del Negro, P., & Della Loggia, R. (1988). Anti-inflammatory activity of Echinacea angustifolia fractions separated on the basis of molecular weight. *Pharmacological Research Communications, 20* Suppl 5:87.

Chapter 15

THE WELLSPACE MODEL
FOR DELIVERY OF COMPLEMENTARY AND
ALTERNATIVE MEDICAL SERVICES

OLIVIA L. CHEEVER

INTRODUCTION

WELLSPACE FRESH POND opened in Cambridge, Massachusetts in July 1998 with the intention of providing Complementary and Alternative Medical (CAM) health care services for the community. Since then, this Center has employed naturopaths, chiropractors, acupuncturists, massage therapists, somatic/movement educators, registered dieticians, and an aesthetician. Free introductory lectures for chiropractic, acupuncture, naturopathy, Feldenkrais®, yoga, and meditation are offered and classes are taught in health-related topics as Feldenkrais® somatic/movement education, yoga, Pilates exercise, meditation, infant and couples massage wellness and self-care. Although Wellspace has chosen not to employ any allopathic physicians, the intention is to foster collaborative and adjunctive, rather than adversarial or competitive, relationships with practitioners of the mainstream Western medical model. Inspired by an interdisciplinary perspective, Wellspace hopes, by bringing together a variety of CAM practitioners to provide clients with the benefits of being able to combine different treatment modalities. As a practitioner

employed there since October 1998, I have been a participant–observer in the unfolding of Wellspace's interdisciplinary approach. In the discussion that follows, I offer my perspective along with those of other members of the Wellspace community. I have shared case material from my own clients/students and have also included client feedback from surveys undertaken in Wellspace's interdisciplinary Back and Neck Pain Relief (BNPR) Program.

GENESIS OF WELLSPACE

The opening of Wellspace Fresh Pond was the result of years of planning. Mort Rosenthal, the CEO of Wellspace, and his staff organized focus groups in the fall of 1997 in order to sound out different CAM practitioners and community members as to perceived needs. These were followed by open houses in the spring of 1998 at which Rosenthal and others laid out the Wellspace vision for prospective practitioners. According to its mission statement Wellspace was "to provide knowledge leadership and a careful experience" in meeting client needs and providing a professional working envi-

243

ronment for practitioners. The latter would include an aesthetically pleasing environment with laundry and room cleaning services, as well as medical, dental, retirement benefits, and stock options. Another aspect of the Wellspace vision is to foster collegiality and professionalism among practitioners.

At a time when the public continues to seek out the services of complementary and alternative medical practitioners (Eisenberg, Kessler, Foster, Norlock, Calkins, & Delbanco, 1993, pp. 246–252; Eisenberg, Davis, Ettner, Appel, Wilkey, Van Rompay, Kessler, 1998, pp. 1569–75; Landmark, 1998) Wellspace offers an example of a corporate-based model for the delivery of CAM services that appears to be succeeding. Wellspace welcomed its 10,000th client in February 2001 and has been able to turn a profit within its first two to three years of operation. As a result, this new business venture is beginning to gain nationwide attention. Rosenthal was invited to the White House in December 2000 to report on the Center's "success" at a meeting attended by members of the National Institutes of Health, Office of Alternative Medicine and the Congressional Health Commission. According to Rosenthal, Wellspace was the only for-profit CAM center represented at this meeting, while there was discussion concerning the failure of several other for-profit CAM centers. Serving as a panelist along with Robert Atkins, M.D. (originator of the Atkins diet), among others, Rosenthal explained that "in addition in trying to understand our formula for success, the commission is also interested in our sense of policy considerations" (Rosenthal, email to Wellspace employees, November 29, 2000).

Not surprisingly, the original Wellspace vision has undergone some changes as the result of the realities presented by its economic niche, the individual needs of its employees and clients, and the timing of its opening. While many of the original employees continue at Wellspace, others have moved on to other jobs. Wellspace Fresh Pond remains thus far the only Wellspace Center that has opened, but Wellspace as a "brand" is still a possibility, with a business plan that calls for expanding the Wellspace name and quality of CAM services into other venues.

Wellspace offers a business model that is new to the holistic health community and because it appears to be succeeding as a business venture, it warrants a closer look. How did Wellspace come about? What is the philosophy guiding its operation? How is it currently functioning? Where is it headed? How did its opening affect the local and national holistic health or CAM community?

There were a number of co-existing factors that created an interest regarding the opening of Wellspace within the greater Boston holistic health community: (1) there had been a local effort underway for some years to network across alternative disciplines and to upgrade hands-on professions with a state license; (2) practitioners were generally working as sole proprietors rather than as salaried professionals with benefits paid for by employers; (3) interest in complementary alternative practices was growing among the public; and (4) a large holistic educational center, Interface, where many local as well as national practitioners had offered classes and workshops, had closed its doors in the spring of 1997. At the same time, the arrival of Wellspace on the scene created some ambivalence among members of this community. Some felt threatened and wondered what it would mean to their own businesses. This included many qualified practitioners with full practices, who were not drawn to join Wellspace since they already had viable businesses and did not wish to become employees,[1] as well as owners of CAM-based centers who initially wondered

---

1. Many of us in the local CAM community, in fact, have remarked that the field tends to attract independent, entrepreneurial individuals who have sought out CAM so as not to have to answer to anyone in running their own practice.

if Wellspace would take away business from them. After Wellspace had been in operation for a couple of years, I asked two respected owners of such longstanding holistic CAM centers how they now felt about Wellspace Fresh Pond; interestingly, both replied that they felt that their centers had benefited from the extensive advertising and marketing effort Wellspace Fresh Pond had made in educating the public about CAM services. One remarked that he ". . . was thrilled to see someone putting more resources into the profession, thus elevating it in bringing more awareness to it." In so doing Wellspace had also helped to bring their CAM centers and services even more to the public's attention.

The proliferation of holistic or alternative medicine in the United States, which began in the 1960s and 1970s in conjunction with the growth of the human potential movement and incorporating aspects of cross-cultural transpersonal psychologies and mind/body/spirit integration (Berliner & Salmon, 1980; Hastings, & Gordon, 1980), has continued to grow throughout the 1990s and into the present (Leviton, 2000). Recently, however, the term "alternative medicine" has begun to give way to "complementary and alternative medicine" (CAM), a shift that represents holistic practitioners' growing desire to view their services as adjunctive to those of allopathic medical services, rather than seeking to replace those services; this in turn entails cultivating mutual respect and collaboration between the practitioners of these two different medical models for the good of the public. "Integrative medicine" is another term reflecting this desire for collaboration among practitioners of both allopathic and complementary alternative medical paradigms that has recently come into use. Two examples of this are the recent establishment at Harvard

Medical School of the Division for Research and Education in Complementary and Integrative Medical Therapies by the Bernard Osher Foundation[2] and a collaborative, cross-disciplinary, nonprofit group of conventional and CAM health care providers in and out of hospital settings in the Boston area called the Integrative Medicine Alliance (IMA). Among the very important goals of this collaborative effort is the sharing of information between conventional health care professionals and CAM health care professionals who are working with the same patients/clients, thus reducing the likelihood that they will be inadvertently harmed due to interactive effects of medications and herbal supplements.

HOLISTIC AND SYSTEM'S THEORY PARADIGM SHIFT

These nonallopathic approaches are part of a paradigm shift that began early in the twentieth century. The holistic perspective has found a place in mainstream Western scientific thought in the form of systems theory, a cross-disciplinary perspective that has evolved since the 1930s. Bertalanffy (1950; 1968), the originator of general system theory (GST), believed that this way of thinking constituted, when it was first proposed, a departure amounting to what Kuhn (1970) would later call a "paradigm shift." Defining GST as the "scientific exploration of 'wholes' and 'wholeness' which, not so long ago, were considered to be metaphysical notions transcending the boundaries of science," Bertalanffy (1968, p. xx) noted that GST arose simultaneously within and affected many disciplines, offering "a new scientific paradigm (in contrast to the analytic, mechanistic, one-way causal paradigm of classical

---

2. In 2001, the Bernard Osher Foundation gave $10 million to Harvard Medical School for the study of integrative medicine, leading to the reent establishment of a Division for Research and Education in Complementary and Integrative Medical Therapies and additional plans for the establishment of the Harvard Medical School-Osher Institute for Research and Education in Complementary and Integrative Medical Therapies (*Harvard Gazette* May 10, 2001).

science)" (p. xxi). According to Bertalanffy, "Modern technology and society have become so complex that traditional ways and means are not sufficient anymore but approaches of a holistic or systems, and generalist or interdisciplinary nature became necessary" (p. xx). Moreover, with twentieth-century discoveries such as Einstein's theory of relativity and quantum mechanics, Newtonian views of reality have been challenged.

According to Ferguson (1980), holistic medicine also had its philosophical roots in the concept of "holism," a term that was introduced in 1926 by Jan Christian Smuts, a Boer general, philosopher, and twice prime minister of South Africa, to describe a "powerful organizing principle inherent in nature" (p. 49). With this theory, Smuts sought to explain the rapidly emerging, paradigm-shifting scientific discoveries of his day, such as quantum mechanics and the Heisenberg uncertainty principle, asserting that "if we did not look at wholes, if we failed to see nature's drive toward ever higher organization, we would not be able to make sense out of our accelerating scientific discoveries" (Smuts, cited in Ferguson, 1980, p. 49). Ferguson points out that Smuts also observed that "there is a whole-making principle in mind itself. . . . Just as living matter evolves to higher and higher levels, so does mind, [which is] inherent in matter, Smuts [in *Holism and Evolution* (1926)] was describing a universe becoming ever more conscious" (p. 49). Gordon, a Harvard-trained holistic physician who examined the paradigm of holistic medicine, stated that "to Smuts, holism was an antidote to the analytic reductionism of the prevailing sciences . . . [and] a way of comprehending whole organisms and systems as entities greater than and different from the sum of their parts" (Gordon, cited in Hastings, Fadiman, & Gordon, 1980, p. 3). In other words, holism is a synergistic model (Benedict, 1970).

Systems Model and the Research Study Model

What a holistic or systems perspective offers is a way to deal not only with the many "elements" within a given system (such as Wellspace Fresh Pond), "but [also] their interrelations . . . say, the interplay of enzymes in a cell, of many mental processes conscious and unconscious, the structure and dynamics of social systems and the like" (Bertalanffy, 1968, p. xix). Dealing with the interrelationships between variables also offers a new way to deal with problems or outcomes, one that takes into account synergistic effects where the whole is not merely the sum of the parts. Applying a systems approach to this self-study thus deals with the complexity of a multilevel system like Wellspace. Each member of the Wellspace community is considered not only as a separate individual, but also synergistically in relation to various elements: a given healing environment, the healing energies of particular practitioners' bodies of healing knowledge, other modalities, clients, colleagues, and community.

I have utilized a relational "connected knowing," as contrasted with a "separate knowing," perspective (Belenky, Clinchy, Goldberger, & Tarule, 1986; Goldberger, Tarule, Clinchy, & Belenky, 1996) in my role as participant-observer to delineate my biases and to help me empathize with the differing viewpoints of respondents within the Wellspace system. I also use "connected knowing" in my individual and group work with clients/students. Both "separate" and "connected knowing" are a kind of "procedural knowing." "'Procedural knowers' end their isolation and engage in the procedures that allow them to enter the realm of discourse and evaluate and create knowledge" (Wright, 2000, p. 3). In contrast to "separate knowing . . . reflect[ing] a 'masculine' ethos of the autonomous self: objectivity, impersonal reasoning, doubt, argument, judgment, and control, . . . connected knowing reflects our culture's 'feminine' ethos, involving a self-in-connection and the valuing of personal experience, empathy, trust, understanding, acceptance, and collaboration" (Wright, 2000, pp. 3–4). Connected knowing depends on the knower's being able to empathize with others, which, in turn, implies their being "developmentally ready" (Nesbit, 2000, p. 13). Otherwise, we may remain inside of our subjective knowing rather than testing our knowledge in relation to others' through procedural connected knowing. This involves, in part, learning not only to empathize with others but also to empathize with oneself.

WELLSPACE RELATIONALLY CONNECTED KNOWING GENESIS RESEARCH STUDY

To better understand the Wellspace vision and how it is being actualized, I interviewed members of its corporate and support staffs, practitioners, and clients while continuing to teach and conduct my private Feldenkrais® somatic/movement education, massage, and integrative bodywork practice at Wellspace Fresh Pond. Wellspace Fresh Pond interests me as both practitioner and researcher, as the Center has sought to be–and apparently is currently perceived to be–in the vanguard of providing interdisciplinary CAM holistic health services to the public as an adjunct to conventional allopathic medicine.

Selection of Subject for Study

Respondents for the current study were solicited and/or volunteered to be interviewed. Names of staff and practitioners were used with the respondents' permission, but clients' names have been not been used to protect their confidentiality. In conducting these interviews, I am attempting not only to elucidate Wellspace's strengths, but also to provide feedback from a wide range of par-

ticipants that can help to shape its future. I also hope that this will illustrate the potential for Wellspace to serve as a resource for ongoing study of the delivery of CAM medical services to the community.

At this beginning stage of the research, I wanted particularly to learn about the earliest days of Wellspace, including its development phase and how the original vision had manifested in determining the physical and organizational environment of the Center. I therefore chose to interview the CEO and several other key people both inside and outside of the corporate structure who were influential in bringing this about. I then juxtaposed the comments of several clients, gathered from both interviews and survey results. In so doing, I hoped to see what kind of fit there was between clients' experiences and perceptions and Wellspace's original vision. How did clients describe their experience and what did they consider "success"? How has connected knowing, in addition to subjective knowing and meaning-making, been a part of their experience?

What have they learned, if anything?

Each respondent, with his or her own version of the vision of Wellspace and how it has changed as well as a particular way of articulating it, offered different facets of the greater whole. When each individual's vision is seen as part of this greater whole, one begins to get an idea of the complexity and richness of the "Wellspace vision." For instance, in my interview with Mort Rosenthal, the CEO of Wellspace, he spoke of the Wellspace vision largely from the economic viewpoint, but a fuller picture of Rosenthal emerged as others recounted their relationships with him and the Wellspace idea.

CEO of Wellspace

Rosenthal, who holds an MBA and described himself to me as one who likes to invent and to create new ventures, noted that he had developed an interest in CAM while using the services of many CAM practitioners to help him manage his stressful life as an entrepreneur. In the mid-1990s, having already made a success in software, he "was looking around for new, largely untapped markets and found one where on the one hand, there was a need for a brand, on the other there was a need for professionalism, and there was an unusual circumstance of both undersupply and overdemand," but people often did not know a trusted source of these CAM services.

Continuing, Rosenthal recounted how he had observed the complementary needs of CAM practitioners and the public. On the one hand, he had noted both that many CAM practitioners were having difficulty making a good living and that there was a need to upgrade the CAM professions for more efficient and accessible delivery of service. CAM practitioners were, in his experience, "competent and skilled, but poorly consolidated and not professionalized." On the other hand, he had noted that, although CAM services had captured the interest of the public and were frequently in the news, he doubted that people were able to get very far with the many self-help books on the market without the help of an expert, and "there was no Harvard teaching hospital that you could go to to make sure whom to go to for help." Having thus determined his new market, he began to consider how he could use his entrepreneurial talents to develop it. The idea, hatched in 1996, expanded in 1997 and 1998 by interesting a group of investors in his idea and hiring a corporate staff to bring the idea of Wellspace to fruition. The team he assembled consisted of some people he had known and worked with before, as well as a number of new consultants. Their first goal was to come up with an appropriate business plan and criteria for hiring practitioners.

V-P of Design and Experience

Peter Agoos, Vice President of Design and Experience, found himself interested by Rosenthal's idea for a new business venture in the field of CAM and, when invited, decided to join him. He felt this would be an opportunity to be part of a different vision, one that ensured much more open access to practitioners than the allopathic model offered and that put the needs of the patient, rather than the system, first. According to Agoos, "the vision is to promote widespread acceptance of CAM and to prove that there is an economic way to deliver services that provide excellent care for patients and work for practitioners without many of the hassles and pitfalls of managed care."

In his new position, Agoos worked closely with the architect of Wellspace, Douglas Lemle, to create a facilitating environment both outside and inside its doors. Agoos' job was to bring the perspective of design into these initial conversations about Wellspace– "the look and feel" of the space and how that would affect one's experience. He described how, for an early brainstorming session during which the group was trying "to write the program of the design of Wellspace" as a facilitating environment, he had written three different "stories" describing a typical Wellspace experience to get the ball rolling.

V-P of Therapeutic Practices

Rosemary Drinka, Vice President of Therapeutic Practices, made a point of mentioning one of these stories that had made a particular impression on her. Agoos envisioned a space that "would allow one to disconnect for a while from what was outside its walls" and offer "an enfolding kind of experience where clients would feel well cared for." As he put it, "we were trying to create something that was quite transparent for patients, easy to access and self-directed." During our interview, Agoos underlined how important the issue of choice would be at Wellspace in contrast to managed care facilities and made the point of tying Wellspace's "success" to its different way of treating patients:

Managed care does not allow one to make the choices of one's care. If you are insistent you can get what you need maybe, but only after a lot of work, and experiencing a lot of roadblocks. There are so many steps involved, which only complicate the process and divide the dollars up. To the extent that Wellspace is not like that, we can speak in terms of some "success."

Agoos also spoke about the fact that Wellspace was trying to provide a different way of orienting clients to different modalities than the triage system in allopathic managed care. In listening to him, it was apparent how much his opinion had been formed by frustration with managed care:

It's the difference between someone doing triage as a barrier, versus someone doing it as an entry point to help you get informed to make decisions. If you end up in an ER, you will be investigated and find only the minimum intervention. At Wellspace you will be offered some understanding of all the options that are open to you for your problem and the different paths they will take you down–and make a choice from there. There are different ways to address tough issues, and choices can be very personal depending on how you wish to engage with yourself and your own body so you can make a more informed choice. Allopathic medicine does not do this. It uses a more mechanical model.

After Agoos and others began to join in the early talks, Rosenthal hired Rosemary Drinka, a nationally certified licensed massage therapist, to assist in the development of the therapeutic side of Wellspace; she has since become Vice President of Therapeutic Practices. Drinka had extensive training and experience in teaching massage. Her initial role was to oversee the hiring of qualified practitioners for all practice areas and be responsible for therapeutic quality within the center. This entailed speaking for both the practitioner's and the client's point of view, hiring "coaches" to supervise practitioners, and program development.

In our interview, Drinka stated that the idea of Wellspace was to create "an exceptional, honoring environment for practitioners to do their craft, to raise the bar professionally and to create an interdisciplinary health care practice where practitioners understood, learned from and integrated other practices into their client's treatment plans, where appropriate." Wellspace was to be "a vehicle through which someone could find a higher level of health. On the client side, the vision was to create a safe and healing environment where they are supported as they move along their continuum to better health." She recalled how one of Agoos's proposed scenarios for Wellspace had struck a chord with her. It pictured a scene "where clients' needs were anticipated even before they realized them": "a mother coming with her little daughter, helping herself to a healthy fruit drink for her daughter before receiving a massage or acupuncture treatment and a well-deserved break."

Unlike many CAM practitioners, Drinka was aware of the business end of starting a center. Drinka stated that she now understood how difficult it was for CAM practitioners who lacked the necessary business background to attract investors to back such a venture; it had taken someone of Rosenthal's caliber to accomplish this. With Rosenthal's expertise, reputation, and backing, Drinka remembers appreciating Rosenthal's term "at Wellspace we can be 'high touch' and 'high tech' at the same time."

Drinka described how they each had to learn to think from a business perspective as well–for example, the cost of adding several square feet to each treatment room. She spoke of the challenges she initially encountered in representing the practitioner point of view.

The corporate staff was interested in understanding what practitioner client needs are but we came up against the conflicting needs of different priorities, like controlling build out costs combined with making sure the treatment rooms were comfortable to practice in. How to balance cost with treatment room needs like natural light, ample space, and fresh air. One example of a great collaboration was the resolve around the desire for treatment rooms to have as much natural light as possible. Agoos, and Lemle, designer and architect, utilized an opaque treatment room ceiling material that allowed natural light into the treatment rooms via the skylights within the center.

Practitioner Management Inclusion Group

Drinka also spoke of the difficult period in the first year of operation when it had become clear that downsizing at all levels—corporate staff, support staff, and practitioner—was imperative to maintain the organization's financial viability. After an initial period of awkwardness while all were figuring out the best way to bring in a practitioner voice, the Practitioner Management Inclusion Group (PMIG) was created out of a collaborative effort between practitioners and management. Representatives were chosen among practitioners by practitioners to present their point of view regarding compensation, benefits, and work environment at meetings with management. Since the spring of 2000, this group, comprising of practitioner representatives and members of management, have met once a month to discuss common needs and concerns. Furthermore, with the downsizing of corporate staff, some new opportunities have arisen for practitioners to take over aspects of some of those roles: one has been hired part-time to introduce new practitioners to Wellspace's computerized record-keeping system; another has taken over outreach. Since then, Drinka has also welcomed initiative from practitioners in other ways. For instance, two practitioners have volunteered to organize a formalized exchange system among practitioners, both to help acquaint them with each other's work in order to facilitate the making

of referrals and to prevent burnout. Drinka believes that joint efforts like these on the part of all Wellspace staff have largely been successful. She marvels at how, "There is a flame here."

> It gives me pause . . . it can still takes my breath away . . . what happens on a daily basis in our treatment rooms [how] someone's quality of life can change and improve via the quality of their health. And we are some of the providers for that. It's an incredibly satisfying experience to be part of something that good.

Health Guide

In July 1997, Rosenthal also hired Joyce Singer, an acupuncturist he had known for several years, to help envision the Wellspace business plan, actualize the client/practitioner environment, and build the acupuncture practice. The role of Wellspace "Health Guide" was created in the early talks to help with consultation and referral of the public to the appropriate practitioners and modalities.

Coaches

Elizabeth Valentine, a teacher and practitioner of massage and integrative body work with 20 years' experience, had met Drinka when both were practicing massage and leasing space in the 1980s at Market Street Health in Brighton, MA. Drinka recruited her and she joined Wellspace in February 1998 in a supervisory capacity as the first of four "coaches" who were eventually hired. Initially, she was to be responsible, with Drinka, for envisioning the Wellspace experience for massage practitioners and clients and hiring and helping to supervise 35 to 40 qualified and certified practitioners in bodywork, massage, and somatic/movement education by the following September. She also helped to tailor the language of Wellspace's secure, computerized record-keeping system to fit practitioners' needs. After the hiring phase had been completed, she and three other coaches would act in a supervisory capacity with practitioners. She was also to help build a client base by transferring her well-established practice to Wellspace; once here, these clients were to be treated by other practitioners of her designation.

Valentine was drawn to Wellspace because of her own vision of wanting to be a bridge to the allopathic medical world. "The timing was right for me when, after practicing for 20 years, Wellspace came along with the vision of integrating various hands-on movement reeducation modalities along with Eastern viewpoints in the context of addressing the whole person." In addition, they were open to considering the possibility of thinking in terms of an adjunctive relationship with the mainstream medical world. "I was thrilled they wanted to articulate and create a new term for alternative medicine." With her progressive educational experience and dance background, Valentine was also drawn to "the creative quality of Wellspace" and inspired by the planning team's "imaginative outlook." She found that this group's "extremely thoughtful and artistic background" jibed with her own. Among other things, "They were . . . being creative about the relationship with clients." According to Valentine, the physical environment was another piece of the Wellspace "thoughtfulness": "The environmental piece added dimension for me, and I like the fact that we envisioned Wellspace from the very beginning as a transformational and educational model."

Kate Davies Rivera was hired in June 1998, as the second coach. She already had experience overseeing massage and bodywork practices but would now be working with practitioners of additional modalities and utilizing an interdisciplinary approach. "This truly excited me. I was eager to help create a community of healers working collaboratively and sharing their talents. I also had a strong interest in helping to create a healthy working environment that could

enhance the life of both practitioners and clients!"

In our interview Rivera recounted how, when approached to join the management team at the newly forming Wellspace, she had been an active participant in the CAM field for 25 years, first as a massage therapist and, over time, as teacher, workshop leader, and coach in many settings in both the United States and in Europe where CAM offerings were presented. During these years, she had become increasingly aware of the importance of two aspects of practicing in the CAM field that she believed needed to be developed substantially in order for CAM to reach its full potential as part of the overall health delivery system: the importance of the relational aspect of healing (both the relationship between practitioner and client and the relationship of the client to her or his own body/mind) and the importance of collaboration (both between practitioners of different forms of CAM therapies and between the CAM world and that of allopathic medicine). She understood that the vision offered by the founders of Wellspace supported both of these areas of concern.

Rivera also believed that two other aspects of the Wellspace plan offered great promise for the further professional development of CAM. Wellspace offered its practitioners support in the form of coaching. She was hired originally as one of a team of four coaches whose function it was to help each practitioner reach her or his full professional potential as a therapist and as part of the Wellspace team, while at the same time identifying and sustaining a quality of life that allows for balance and fulfillment. This willingness to take into account the full personhood of each practitioner matched what Rivera had come to believe would optimize the chances of success for both individual therapists and for Wellspace as a viable business. Rivera was also excited by the plans to bring Wellspace into the forefront of the use of communications technology to support the CAM field. All told, Wellspace offered great professional opportunity, and Rivera was excited to become part of it.

Rivera had conducted her massage practice in many environments including the choir loft of a church, a private home-based practice, hospitals, clinics, retreat and fitness centers, and holistic massage centers in the United States and Europe. "I watched massage grow from the time when the inspectors from the Cambridge Health Department had difficulty understanding that massage could possibly be occurring in a church setting (I reminded them that "laying on of hands" was mentioned in the Bible) to today's widespread acceptance." As a seasoned massage practitioner she knew that it was difficult for many practitioners to create and maintain a successful practice on their own and was committed to developing ways in which this important work could be made more widely available, and at the same time provide therapists with a high quality of life.

General Manager Insurance and Managed Care Liaison

Jamie Barber, Vice President and General Manager of Wellspace since January 2001, was originally hired in November 1998, shortly after Wellspace had opened, to work with insurance and managed care. Barber had had experience in the managed care field, both with hospitals and payers, serving as a liaison between senior management and providers. Barber underlined the existing problems vis-a-vis managed care in the delivery of conventional medical services that made him shift his career to further CAM and integrative medicine—where conventional and complementary medicine would work hand in hand. While working in conventional medicine, he nonetheless was pursuing studies to become more knowledgeable regarding CAM services in relation to conventional medicine, having come to feel that the allopathic system for delivery of health care was "broken" with the advent of and dominance of managed care in its cur-

rent iteration. In 1994, he took a class on alternative health care at BU School of Public Health, where initially it "seemed alien to read about homeopathy" and other CAM models, but his interest grew the more he read about results and his own initial skepticism had been affected by becoming acquainted with existing research in CAM. "I find the findings regarding the efficacy of using moxabustion to turn breech babies and in using acupuncture with infertility impressive." He noted that working with different CAM paradigms also necessitated different research designs—such as with acupuncture.

"We view our services in the way that we have been brought up in our Western ways of thinking. Acupuncture has been around thousands of years. But we cast our 'scientific' doubts on everything and classify disease according to the ICD9 codes." Barber began to look around for opportunities in CAM. After seeing an article in the spring of 1998 in the *Boston Globe* concerning new examples of CAM services and mentioning Wellspace as one of a couple of different CAM service-providing models, Barber decided to check Wellspace out. Barber shared with me his "Wellspace 'wow' experiences" when he first walked in the door of the corporate headquarters in nearby Somerville, and then at Fresh Pond. This was the term that he chose to encapsulate the total effect the Wellspace Fresh Pond environment had on him, where earth tones are contrasted with bright calendula and Feng Shui, the Chinese art of placement. "Mort was very clever in having me come to the second meeting at Wellspace Fresh Pond. This 'Wellspace wow experience' played an important part in my decision to accept Mort's offer."

Barber joined Wellspace Fresh Pond largely because he wanted to take CAM services to the next level of professionalization and because he saw a great market opportunity. He also spoke how he had been drawn to Wellspace because of his commitment to bringing about a new vision of medicine, one that would emphasize developing wellness as much as or more than treating illness alone. Along with Rosenthal and Agoos, Barber spoke passionately about his disappointment with the way that conventional medicine was currently practiced. He felt that "managed *care* is a misnomer" and shared his initial pet peeve, "MDeification," where doctors were deferred to whether they deserved it or not leading patients to take little or no responsibility for their own health care. In his opinion, "when you attribute that status to someone, it creates an expectation that one cannot easily live up to." He felt that conventional medicine had suffered and some of the original trust had been eroded between doctor and patient. Barber shared, however, how a more compassionate perspective soon tempered his critical opinion of doctors. By interacting closely with doctors in the hospital as their liaison with insurance companies and HMOs, he came to understand them better and empathize with their plight in a managed care dominated industry.

Barber also raised the issue of "dis-ease" as part of the CAM model and its role in affecting one's health due to the effect mind has on body. He pointed out that a "separation of mind and body have intrinsically been a part of our society in the West [in] that they are two separate things."

> The conventional model is based on a model that doesn't work—"sick" care and treating sick people rather than promoting health—and 99% of doctors are trained to combat disease rather than promoting health. *That* should be the ultimate goal of the healer—to help someone understand what health and disease are. It is not necessarily about a particular disease but the state of dis-ease.

Barber noted that often practitioners in working with skeptical clients "have to overcome that mental dis-ease as well as physical dis-ease. "Thus, how we make meaning of

our symptoms influences how we think they "should" be treated and can affect our health in that, our own unchallenged rigid belief systems can get in the way of our seeking help." In talking about his own and others' initial resistance to accepting that CAM services could work, he recounted that he had first tried acupuncture only after he had an acute injury and all the massage therapists whom he would normally work with were busy. He was amazed at the result. "My pain immediately went away. It was miraculous!" Barber raised the interesting point that clients often feel better after receiving CAM treatment at Wellspace in spite of their skepticism about the effectiveness of these treatments. He emphasized Wellspace's role in educating the public, often in spite of themselves: "You can win over a skeptic just by the service offered [for] the greatest selling point is by definitively showing the efficacy of the service— [that] it works." Clients in Wellspace's Back and Neck Program echo Barber's words. MS, surveyed in May 2001, reports feeling "better" with a 70 percent improvement within two months with chiropractic only. However, he is guarded in attributing his "success" to his chiropractor:

> I remain somewhat skeptical about chiropractic theory and I am tempted to attribute much of my improvement to the physical exercise taught to me by the chiropractor. But the fact remains that he was able to prescribe effective exercises based on a structural analysis of my body, which is something no conventional doctor has been able to do before.

Barber believed that skeptical conventional physicians also would benefit in "be [ing] educated that it [CAM] is not a threat to their practices, and CAM treatment works whether you call it psychosomatic or placebo effect or what," and he believed that CAM's efficacy would be proven also "if we could get more MD's to get the [CAM] services when *they* are suffering. . . ." He reiterated that Wellspace did not want to alienate traditional health care or replace it–it sought to forge a partnership for the benefit of the patient ". . . especially in treating such conditions as chronic pain." Barber expressed surprise that physicians don't recognize Wellspace's usefulness except, he averred, that it might be due to the fact that they are aware that patients must pay out of pocket for Wellspace services–"or because MDs are concerned that CAM is taking part of their market share." Barber also expressed frustration with the fact that managed care too often refuses to cover CAM services–or makes token efforts at best–and underlined how the public's growth in interest in receiving CAM services is important for the continuing success of Wellspace.

Practitioner Management Inclusion Group

Regarding the morale of Wellspace, and the role of practitioners, Barber pointed toward the positive step of establishing the Practitioner Management Inclusion Group (PMIG) in the winter of 2000-01 as a welcome result that grew out of the practitioners' desire to have more of a voice in decisions that affected them. "The PMIG was a creative solution that filled a need that had been identified during a time of much change at Wellspace Fresh Pond." Barber prided Wellspace on its "trying to be different" so as "not [to] get caught in the pitfalls of other systems. We can talk openly about things even when we have heated issues on the table including compensation–and laugh together in the PMIG." Barber felt that "This shows the evolution of Wellspace, which is due to a conscious evolution, not just by chance, and due to a lot of hard work and dedication to forge this and not let it be a place where people do not feel listened to or feel that they have a voice. This has evolved into something that is more successful because of compassionate listening."

Achievement Awards

Barber also expressed being pleased at the way a new idea–instituting an "employee of the month" award–seemed to be gathering momentum. He saw this as one of a number of morale-building processes and observed that "this month [July 2001] I heard from more practitioners than ever about their nominations. Moreover, people wrote the longest reasons as to why people should pick their candidate." Barber saw these descriptions as a way for people to learn more about the talents of their fellow practitioners. He saw this as especially helpful in acquainting new hires with other Wellspace practitioners, thus helping to build community among practitioners–another Wellspace goal.

PERSONAL GENESIS AND JOURNEY TO WELLSPACE

At the time I became aware of Wellspace I was very interested in building community especially among like-minded holistic practitioners. I had been in private practice as a holistic practitioner and psychotherapist for over 20 years. Prior to that, after study abroad and completing a Masters in French, I had been a high school language teacher, and although I found great satisfaction in this work, I realized in the early 1970s that my interests were being drawn elsewhere. A massage session I received as a gift in 1973 turned out to be a life-changing event, leading me to a different way of experiencing my body, my soul, and myself. Massage soon became my healing lifeline, and I decided that I wanted to be able to pass along the benefits of this practice to others. That same year I began to study massage at Ananda in Cambridge and Interface in Newton. Having also decided to obtain the necessary foundation in counseling, I enrolled in a C.A.G.S.

degree program at the Harvard Graduate School of Education. By 1977 I was in private practice as a massage therapist, was licensed in 1980 as a psychotherapist, and became licensed and nationally certified as a massage therapist in 1994. I decided to enhance my practice in both areas by training with Moshe Feldenkrais, D.Sc., becoming certified in 1983 in the Feldenkrais Method® of Somatic/Movement Education, and I received my EdD. in Counseling Psychology from Harvard Graduate School of Education in 1995. This included training in Behavioral Medicine at the Cambridge Hospital in Cambridge, Massachusetts. My private practice and teaching thus derived from my own holistic learning and evolved into ways of teaching and serving the whole person through the use of a variety of different tools.

Prior to Wellspace, interdisciplinary alternative centers had been formed where practitioners of different modalities, including myself, while joining their practices under one roof, continued to conduct their businesses individually. Many of these centers have not only continued to exist, but have been helped by Wellspace's entry to the scene. They are either leased by a group of practitioners or privately owned. Practitioners as independent contractors rent space and are individually responsible for managing their own practices, paying taxes, providing insurance and medical benefits, and saving toward retirement. They may volunteer to attend meetings with landlords to represent their interests, or to help run the centers, or to share approaches and discuss cases. Among the most important benefits of such interdisciplinary centers are the increased opportunities for networking, making and receiving referrals, and arranging for exchanges.

In this spirit, some of us had formed the Massachusetts Coalition for Professional Hands-on Practitioners in 1990 in response to a proposed legislative challenge from massage therapists to require all hands-on practitioners to be licensed in massage ther-

apy. Out of this disagreement, a cross-disciplinary group (of which I was a part) formed, including practitioners of Western massage, somatic/movement educators, body-oriented psychotherapists, Polarity and Shiatsu practitioners, and others practicing Oriental bodywork and massage. Together, we worked to create a licensing bill that would both ensure the quality and scope of practice and protect the public. Although this bill ultimately was not enacted, its "model regulations" for licensing "massage therapy and somatic practice" were adopted by some cities including Cambridge, Massachusetts where Wellspace is licensed as an establishment. The members of the Coalition developed a mutual respect and understanding for each others' differences and practices and learned to work together politically over a period of seven years. Moreover, it was clear that all welcomed a chance to take themselves and alternative practices to the next level professionally.

This next level involved a shift to seeing holistic practices as complementary and adjunctive in relation to the allopathic medical model, and a new term–"Complementary and Alternative Medicine" (CAM)– began to be used. Although the word "alternative" is still part of the term, it was becoming more an acknowledgment of the fact that differences do indeed exist between the two models than a declaration that one should replace the other. The goals of Wellspace as stated by Rosenthal, its CEO, reflected this change in emphasis. Thus, when I was approached in the spring of 1998 by Drinka, to join the Wellspace Advisory Board as the only hands-on practitioner among a mixture of business, medical (including both the CAM and conventional medical fields), and lay people, I accepted willingly because it seemed to provide an opportunity for practitioners to have a voice in shaping the Wellspace model. Then, encouraged by the fact that colleagues I knew and respected had already joined Wellspace Fresh Pond, I, too, decided to attend an Open House that same spring to see what it might offer to me as a practitioner.

At the Open House, I introduced myself by saying jokingly that I had been acting for several years as "my own holistic health center in one" in that I would often use different approaches with the same client at different times in order to address their body, mind, and spirit. Some clients I would refer out, when it was inappropriate for me to be doing more than one thing with them–especially when working with clients who were survivors of sexual abuse where maintaining clear boundaries was particularly important. I networked as much as my schedule allowed with other alternative practitioners, traditional psychotherapists, and allopathic health care providers in working with clients, but managing all the details of my own increasingly busy interdisciplinary practice was very time-consuming and left me with less and less time to network. Although I loved the freedom and creativity of maintaining my own practice, I was finding it increasingly expensive and time-consuming to be a sole proprietor in private practice. In addition to maintaining a bodywork practice as a Feldenkrais somatic educator, I was teaching several weekly classes in different locations and leading workshops for the public and health professionals. After joining the faculty of the Mind/Body Department at the Longy School of Music in Cambridge, Massachusetts, in 1997, I nonetheless still had to pay for my family's medical insurance as an individual and make provisions for retirement on my own.

At the Open House I attended, Rosenthal described his vision of a healing environment, part of which entailed utilizing current technologies in the service of both client and practitioner. As I listened, I saw a possible solution to the problem of communicating with other caregivers sharing the care of a client. Even if one were fully booked, we could correspond about our clients through email and through sharing client records with the secure computerized system that

was being set up. Moreover, Wellspace would potentially provide a site to do research into CAM services, which might allow me to build on my doctoral research. We could easily collect data as to what services clients were using for what conditions, track different combinations of modalities for different conditions, and develop greater clarity about our interdisciplinary approach. This would allow us potentially to further the field of CAM beyond anecdotal evidence and provide better service to the community.

Perhaps most important, however, I joined Wellspace because of valued connections–previous respected relationships with CAM colleagues. As these respected colleagues in various CAM disciplines with whom I wished to collaborate more formally had already decided to join Wellspace, I decided to follow them there in that the Center offered the possibilities of furthering collegiality, and the professionalization of CAM services while promoting a collaborative relationship with allopathic physicians. Furthermore, I could move my Feldenkrais classes to the group facility at Wellspace Fresh Pond, and I welcomed the opportunity to receive medical, dental, liability, disability insurances, paid time off, retirement benefits, and stock options. For all of these reasons, I decided to move my private practice and teaching to Wellspace Fresh Pond beginning in October 1998, shortly after it had opened.

WELLSPACE FRESH POND TODAY

Wellspace seeks to educate the public about self-care including home care/self-care. In addition to private appointments, the Center offers free introductory lectures in chiropractic, naturopathy, acupuncture, Feldenkrais, yoga, etc. as well as a series of classes, and workshops in health-related subjects such as, yoga, t'ai chi, Feldenkrais, meditation, nutrition, and the like as a cost-effective way to learn about self-care. Family members or friends who accompany clients can also sit comfortably in the large waiting area, or browse in the retail area where supplements, health aids, and books on health-related subjects are for sale. Wellspace offers several cost-reducing discount programs as well in an effort to make its services affordable to a greater number of people. Clients/students may also participate in any of the Wellspace interdisciplinary programs, such as the BNPR Program described below, to address their health needs. Most Wellspace clients pay for services out of pocket as their insurance most often does not cover CAM services. Recently, however, some chiropractic services have begun to be covered by insurance.

Wellspace Fresh Pond first opened its doors in Cambridge, Massachusetts, in July 1998, offering treatment in Complementary and Alternative Medical (CAM) services. It is housed inside a renovated warehouse (that looked a little like the Musee de Pompidou in Paris!) with bright colors and external pipes. However, renovations by the architect, Douglas Lemle, with the assistance of design consultant and Wellspace Vice President, Agoos, have created an ingenious illusion: when one walks up to the second floor and looks down, the roofs of the individual treatment rooms are visible, reminding one of huts in a tribal village. Initially there were 40 practitioners sharing 27 treatment rooms, offering a variety of approaches based on Eastern and Western holistic healing paradigms, including massage, bodywork, movement/somatic education, naturopathy, and acupuncture. Chiropractic services were added in January 2000. During the first couple of years, the number of practitioners has fluctuated. As we go to press, however there are once again 40 practitioners including Singer and three chiropractors, four acupuncturists, one naturopath, 28 practitioners under the category of massage therapy, bodywork, somatic/movement education—including two Feldenkrais somatic/movement educators, two registered dieticians, and one aesthetician.[3] In addition, there is one large group room where classes are offered and a sauna located between the men's and women's facilities. In between sessions or classes, clients are invited to use the sauna and/or the group room, if vacant. Use of the sauna is included with any visit to Wellspace.

Wellspace Fresh Pond is convenient to community life by being located at the back of a mall; a movie theatre is adjacent to it, and a whole foods supermarket is located at the other end of the mall. Painted in bright cream and yellow, Wellspace stands out from its surroundings due to its bright colors and landscaping with a variety of trees, shrubs, and flowers. Inside, the predominating colors are yielded by cedar floors, and a sunny bright calendula orange-yellow as a backdrop to earth tones. Cushioned benches in the spacious waiting area face a large fireplace and a water cooler, and self-help books and useful health aids are for sale in a retail area near the reception desk as one enters the building. In addition to the fireplace and water cooler, there is a waterfall wall in one of the windows in the waiting area, natural objects from the earth, such as birch bark, cedar, and stones, plenty of open space in the waiting and retail area, and a high ceiling that stretches up above the second floor. Barber spoke of his own "Wow experience" when he first walked in, and Drinka recalled that a lot of attention was paid to creating an esthetic facilitating environment. This included utilizing the principles of Feng Shui,

---

3. Rosenthal and Agoos readily admit that they and other original planners of Wellspace overestimated the growth of the CAM market, and it was with regret that it was found necessary to let go a few practitioners within the first year. In fact, it has taken three years to find the right balance so that Wellspace Fresh Pond can now operate at a profit.

the Chinese art of placement, and included symbols of the five Chinese **elements**– earth, air, fire, water, and wood. Wellspace has silk wall hangings and a majestic bronze peacock that oversees all activity from its location on the second floor landing. Wellspace also makes a point of exhibiting the work of local artists throughout, including the artwork of some of its practitioners. Art exhibits are continually changing and carefully chosen to fit in with the facilitating environment of Wellspace. As one of my clients described it, "The atmosphere and physical space of Wellspace is calming and restful. It's very powerful when you walk in the door."

WELLSPACE INTAKE PROCEDURE

All Wellspace clients schedule with practitioners through the front desk and check in at the front desk whenever they have an appointment. Those who are new to Wellspace receive a brochure and an intake form regarding health history to fill out, which is then handed to the Wellspace Health Guide or to the practitioner giving the session. Clients who are new to Complementary Alternative Medicine services and need help deciding who is the appropriate practitioner can schedule a free fifteen-minute appointment with the Wellspace Fresh Pond Health Guide. After meeting with the client, the guide makes a referral and the client returns to the front desk to schedule an appointment. The guide also oversees three interdisciplinary programs, the Back and Neck Pain Relief (BNPR) Program, begun in spring 2000, the Menopause Wellness Program, begun in fall 2000, and the Headache Relief Program, begun in spring 2001 where a client might ostensibly book appointments with more than one practitioner, upon her recommendation.

Not all Wellspace clients feel the need to

schedule an initial appointment with the Health Guide. Many set up their initial appointment with a particular practitioner or for a particular type of treatment because of a friend's recommendation, or because they have been referred by another CAM or conventional medical professional. The practitioner, paged at the time the client checks in with the desk, greets the client and introduces him or her to the facilities before escorting the client to the treatment room to discuss the presenting problem and to begin a session. If they wish, clients may help themselves to robes provided in the changing facilities or the treatment rooms. During a session, practitioner and client come up with a treatment plan for conditions requiring a formal treatment plan. Afterwards, practitioners enter SOAP notes into the computer, entering data under the standard categories used in medical notes: *S*ubjective, *O*bjective, *A*ssessment, *P*lan for each session in the secure Wellspace computerized record-keeping system. Both CAM and conventional terms are included in the system so as to make the Wellspace record-keeping system compatible with conventional medical record-keeping to facilitate sharing of information when patients/clients are seen by both allopathic and CAM health care providers.

THE BACK AND NECK PAIN RELIEF INTER-DISCIPLINARY PROGRAM

Wellspace's Back and Neck Pain Relief (BNPR) Program began in spring of 2000 and has thus far welcomed 129 participants. According to Singer, it has not been possible to keep track of everyone in the program because respondents do not always return phone calls, or emails. She has been able to be in touch with the 60 active participants and survey 69 inactive participants in the program to find out how their participation in the BNPR affected them. The client feedback we received helps to flesh out their experience at Wellspace Fresh Pond in relation to the vision laid out by those who co-created Wellspace.

As Guide, Singer receives referrals for health consultations from practitioners, from the Front Desk receptionists, or directly from answering intake calls. Wellspace offers to new clients who are undecided a free fifteen-minute consultation with Singer about who is/are the best practitioner(s) to see regarding their presenting problem; clients also have the option of coming for free fifteen-minute consultations more than once or of paying for a longer, more in-depth health consultation. For participants in the BNPR program, Singer offers a free thirty-minute session (which can be repeated). Singer keeps in touch with practitioners and clients to facilitate ongoing treatment. Other responsibilities include chairing case discussions and welcoming and introducing new participants to Wellspace classes and to the facilities, as well as gathering survey data.

Wellspace's Back and Neck Pain Relief (BNPR) Program illustrates how clients presenting with similar pain may combine different modalities in treatment for optimum results. Singer remarked on the effectiveness of the BNPR Program in offering treatment that truly helps people: "It never ceases to amaze me how I see people who can barely walk come in here and receive true help so they can walk out of here looking like a completely different person a couple of hours later." Singer, as Health Guide, emphatically stated that she views her role as "primarily educational." This is especially true with the BNPR Program clients. She explained that:

> The BNPR Program was designed for several reasons–the first being to use our skills to help people feel better and get to a new level of comfort in their bodies. It was also designed to build team work, collect data regarding the synergistic effect of using more than one modality to heal and allow clients to make an informed choice about their treatments. It seemed important to

educate existing clients and people new to Wellspace that to achieve lasting results, one must commit to 2-3 treatments per week for at least a month to six weeks. Then one can reduce the number of appointments to maintenance only.

She explained that some of the participants in the BNPR Program are already Wellspace clients who, in the past, would occasionally schedule a relaxation massage or a deep tissue problem-specific session to "fix" an acute problem. Singer explained how such clients would then stay away from treatment until pain or discomfort forced them to come in for another appointment. No learning concerning how to change the pattern was taking place, however, and their back pain would recur. Other clients who have been helped by the BNPR have more chronic problems. Participants in the BNPR Program receive individualized treatment plans suggested by each practitioner they are seeing for treatment. Clients learn about self-care and continue to check in regularly with their practitioners and with Singer. They are able to learn new ways of moving and being that reduces their pain and discomfort. Laura whose case follows reports feeling a sense of "success" after continuing to participate in the program for one year.

ROLE OF THERAPIST

In my opinion, Wellspace wishes to foster empathic connected knowing in the way that practitioners seek to educate clients about their presenting complaints. CAM practitioners use procedural connected knowing in examining the whole picture of the client/student's health situation: for example, in understanding the connection between primary and secondary complaints–i.e., between neck and back pain due to nerve pathways and/or body mechanics, or noting how stress and the consumption of caffeinated products affects muscle tension. Practitioners attempt not only to develop their own capacity for connected knowing, but also to co-create conditions for clients to learn to apply informed connected knowing to their health concerns. Empathic somatically-based connected knowing or "somatic empathy" (Cheever, 1995, Cheever, 2000; Cheever & Cohen, in press) includes aspects of emotional intelligence such as self-awareness and empathy (Goleman, 1995), and includes also kinesthetic intelligence, and spatial intelligence (Gardner, 1999) and the care of the soul (Moore, 1992). Empathy entails "movement-in-relationship" (Jordan, 1991). Somatic empathy entails moving as one whole embodied self in relation to another whole embodied self. This involves teaching clients/students how to empathize with, or feel into, what they are sensing physically and somatically, as well as emotionally and spiritually (Cheever, 1995, 2000), and to understand it in relation to what is known scientifically about their problem. If the client is capable of participating in this type of knowing with a practitioner, it enables him or her to move beyond subjective knowing (Belenky et al., 1986) and respond more fully to what the practitioner knows about treating the client's condition and/or educating the client. In so doing, practitioners attempt to facilitate the clients' healing not only through specific techniques and technologies, but also through the quality of their relationships with clients.

A facilitating relationship that practitioners attempt to build with their clients should provide a safe place for each to look at the meaning for the client of what has led him or her to seek treatment and to continue to seek help. For, the holistic CAM paradigm recognizes that healing for the whole person involves, in part, understanding how the client is making meaning of both the experience of illness, or "dis-ease," and the experience of healing (Benson, 1996; Borysenko, 1987; Dossey, 1991; Gordon, 1996; Kabat-Zinn, 1990; Pert, 1993).

Within the context of a facilitating rela-

tionship, the client/student can be guided into learning how to experience and cultivate pleasant feelings, or a sense of well-being, as an important part of CAM wellness. A CAM practitioner can help the client/student to focus in on his or her somatic experience by guiding the latter into a body scan. For example, when the client says, "I feel good" or "I feel better" after a massage, movement education, or acupuncture session, etc., the practitioner can help the client to sense what his or her experience of embodied well-being feels like in contrast to his or her state of dis-ease. These clients are then better able to recognize feeling better and to be able to return to this state of ease in the future.

When the facilitating relationship works, both the practitioner and the client feel "happy," "good," "well," or "energized." Feldenkrais (1981, p. 8) gave an example of this in describing his form of somatic education. When one connects with a client through the hands-on component of the Feldenkrais Method through it the use of touch to guide the client's movement, is like dancing with someone one wants to dance with and feels good dancing with. In this metaphor, Feldenkrais was also emphasizing the importance of continually learning how to move toward pleasant sensation, through decreasing effort (1980, p. 5) rather than merely being preoccupied with moving out of pain. The following case exemplifies this process.

CLINICAL CASES

Regina

Regina (a pseudonym) provides an example of a student of mine at Wellspace who through the Feldenkrais Method® is learning to use connected knowing to regain functioning by decreasing pain and by moving toward greater ease. Regina, a 37-year-old single instrumentalist, relates the presenting symptom of chronic myofascial pain of unknown origin since 1995. A professional string player, she at one point had to completely desist from playing for five months due to the extent of her pain (which, in her words, was often at a level of "9.9999 on a scale of 10"). After she was referred to me for Feldenkrais by her psychiatrist, I referred her to a rheumatologist, who ruled out fibromyalgia. Regina shared with me that she had been orally raped when she was five years old. After six years of psychotherapy and one-and-a-half years of participation in a group for survivors of sexual abuse, she was still in chronic pain and despairing of ever being pain-free. Nonetheless, by means of Feldenkrais® lessons where I guided her movement, Regina learned to listen to and experience her embodied self with less or no pain within eight months of coming for lessons once or twice a week. Her health plan was also supplemented by attending my weekly Feldenkrais Awareness Through Movement® (ATM) class; this, in turn, had led her to feel empowered. The Feldenkrais Method® is an educational rather than a treatment model that teaches "students" how to reduce extraneous effort as they move; a certified Feldenkrais® practitioner conveys a sense of easy, comfortable movement kinesthetically to the student through guided movement, and in so doing co-creates the conditions for the student to learn new movement options.

As we worked together it became apparent that her pain related to the areas where she had memories of being held down by her perpetrator. Feldenkrais touch conveys a kind of listening that goes beyond verbal conversation, a process that Feldenkrais practitioners refer to as "conversing with" someone's nervous system. As Regina put it,

I just had the sense that you understood me from the inside out. . . . You listen between the lines. . . . You listen to my body language and everything. So I think I started to value my thoughts a little more because I felt

heard. . . . And that gave me the sense that maybe I should do that for myself. I should really listen to my voice and what I'm really saying. . . . And so I felt that all the cells in my body felt heard. I think for trauma and abuse and maybe life, everyone wants to be known and heard for who they really are. . . . Lots of therapists don't know how to listen and don't have a clue. . . . I started to take that on and started to listen to myself more. (Personal Communication, April 2001)

As I guided this student into new movement patterns in the context of a facilitating relationship, she was learning the difference between moving out of pain and moving toward pleasant sensation. In so doing, she was learning how to empathize with herself and to experience her body or "soma" (Hanna, 1985, 1988) as a safe place, thus engaging in "somatic empathy." This shift in perspective, which other Feldenkrais students have reported as well (Cheever, 2000, pp. 20–22), represents an important part of healing from the trauma of sexual abuse. She was moving beyond her own subjective knowing, which included extremely negative self-criticism and self-talk, and learning how to witness without judgment how she was moving. Subsequently, she has been able to develop a more neutral, less self-punishing attitude toward her playing, and, as she has been able to reduce and manage her pain, she has resumed her career as a professional musician.

Recently, when she had a flare-up, rather than panicking, she engaged in Feldenkrais Awareness through Movement® (ATM) movements:

In the ATM class, I started to really notice that my shoulder blades move and my neck moves a little when I am moving my legs. That has been really helpful to realize that these things are moving even when my shoulders are in tons of pain. Just to know that my shoulders are moving a little when I move my legs is actually a comforting feeling. So I've been able to reverse some of the pain by doing those ATMs. (Personal Communication, July 2001)

Laura

Laura is a 40-year-old married business consultant who sought help for acute back spasm at Wellspace in the spring of 2000 and was referred by Singer to me for massage therapy and to Dr. Kevin Gregg for chiropractic. When I interviewed her in spring 2001 about her experience in the BNPR, she described a process whereby she had learned to move beyond her own subjective knowing stance–e.g., an initial attitude where: "my back pain [which she had experienced since her teens] is inevitable because I am like my father who suffered from back pain all his life, etc. etc." to a connected knowing stance–e.g., "I'm trying to pay attention. I can feel it when the 'big one' is coming and I take it as a warning and take preventive steps." Laura has developed connected knowing and somatic empathy–in developing awareness and learning to sense what she is feeling somatically in conjunction with what she is receiving and learning from practitioners of two modalities. This has helped her to make some life-style changes and to focus on preventing the recurrence of back spasms. Laura's case also provides an example of the need to work from a holistic mindbody approach to alleviate her back pain. For, in order for her to prevent continued reinjury to her back, she had to get in touch with her lack of awareness about her fatalistic attitude that she had no choice but to do as her father had done and give in to her back pain. She came to realize that she had a belief that the problem would continue to recur for the rest of her life and "I would just have to grin and bear it."

In our interview, Laura recounted how she, had driven by Wellspace many times on her way to various consulting jobs and always wondered about it, but that she waited until she ". . . was pretty desperate when

I decided to check it [Wellspace] out–in the middle of a really bad episode with my back which was not going away after two weeks." Laura began her investigation with a free consultation with Singer and then decided to pay for a more extensive evaluation. After going over Laura's history together, Singer referred Laura to the Wellspace Fresh Pond Back and Neck Pain Relief Program, with a specific recommendation to see me for massage or Feldenkrais and Gregg for chiropractic. Laura explained to me that she would "ignore it until the pain was so bad that I could not stand it anymore. Then I'd go to my brother's chiropractor for one adjustment. There was nothing offered there about prevention or how to practice self-care." In contrast, after receiving one massage from me and one chiropractic appointment from Dr. Gregg, she immediately felt relief: "I was amazed at how quickly I felt a difference after seeing you for massage and then Dr. Gregg for chiropractic."

Laura also learned, however, that she would not be able to effect lasting change regarding her symptoms unless she made a longer-term commitment to meet her needs with regularly scheduled sessions. After coming several times for massage with myself and chiropractic, Laura at first found herself going right back to her stressful life-style, as was her habit. Within days, she found herself back at Wellspace and in a chiropractic session with Gregg. "I broke down in tears. . . . After that I really began to listen to my body and scheduled regular sessions with both of you." As she was experiencing and learning new options in the way she moved relative to her back, she was practicing on her own at home the exercises given to her by Dr. Gregg and the Feldenkrais Awareness Through Movement® (ATM) sequences she had learned when she attended one of my classes. Informed by her connected knowing, she had subsequently continued to make some life-style changes, including joining a health club taking up walking for exercise, and going back on a diet.

She reported, since beginning treatment a year ago, "I have not suffered another such pain episode in one year. I'm much, much better, I'm not in that kind of pain anymore, there's been no recurrence, and I do things preventatively, (which is new for me!). I have taken up walking, which helps a great deal."

Besides showing the usefulness in learning to move from subjective to connected knowing, Laura's case also illustrates how working with more than one modality appears to have synergistic effects, since using only one modality in the past–chiropractic–did not shift her pain pattern. In her words:

> This was a real learning experience–and I'm taking better care of myself as a result. The key was moving from just pain management to ongoing maintenance of my back. It's made the difference–also the combination of the two modalities–massage and chiropractic–seemed to have a much longer lasting effect, and ultimately has contributed to being pretty pain free most of the time now. Occasionally I have a tough day, but seem to snap back from it quicker.

In working as an interdisciplinary team, some of the logistics still have to be worked out. It has been difficult to schedule a face-to-face meeting between the two practitioners, and/or with the two practitioners with the client. Laura, in her feedback concerning the BNPR Program, expressed the importance of knowing that both practitioners working with her were also in touch with each other and felt that she would have liked more evidence of this. Based on this feedback, I have suggested to her and to Dr. Gregg that we stay in touch with each other via email regarding her process, questions, etc. so as to keep each other in the loop and truly integrate our sharing of information. All three of us have agreed to try this approach. We will also keep Joyce Singer, as the Guide, in the loop.

CAM RESEARCH POTENTIAL AT WELLSPACE

Wellspace is conveniently located near several colleges, universities, medical schools, hospitals, acupuncture and massage schools in the Boston area who are enrolling students interested in some aspect of CAM health care and/or health education. For example, in Cambridge, CAM massage students at the Muscular therapy Institute, and graduate students enrolled in the Holistic Health Studies Certificate Program at Lesley University can observe Wellspace among other models in the area for CAM delivery of services.

Wellspace provides such an opportunity to have its practitioners participate in studies of the effects of different modalities. Wellspace could be a useful site in responding to the call for building CAM research skills into massage and somatic educational training programs. Unlike some other CAM centers, Wellspace has a computerized record-keeping system to organize the data. As an interdisciplinary center, Wellspace could offer researchers of Eastern and Western modalities an opportunity to conduct studies using different paradigms. For example, if a client/student were combining acupuncture and massage, it would be possible to observe the effects on him or her from the perspective of both paradigms.

For Wellspace practitioners to participate in internally and externally-initiated studies will require some coordination in scheduling. Nonetheless, with careful planning, and using appropriate research methodologies to "measure" what happens in sessions, Wellspace can serve as a potential interdisciplinary "laboratory" and as a training ground for CAM and other researchers. One of the challenging questions that faces any researcher in and out of CAM programs, however, is that when dealing with different paradigms in trying to set up "scientific studies"–it is necessary to use the appropriate methodology and outcomes that are appropriate for the modality one is researching. Moreover, qualitatively-based findings provide a different, but I maintain, equally important database as quantitative.

If medicine in the twenty-first century is to be truly integrative allowing patients/clients/students to reap the benefits of combining both conventional and CAM approaches, then the research models used to collect the data must also be integrative—taken from Eastern and Western perspectives and based on different paradigms. Building a research base beyond anecdotal evidence is necessary for CAM to gain validity and become accepted in mainstream medical circles. Appropriate outcome studies need to be undertaken. But as Barber points out not all aspects of CAM can be researched according to the Western scientific method—nor should they be. Furthermore, any research must take into account the well-being and privacy of the client and follow protective research guidelines, and not interfere with serving the client.

SUMMARY

In the first part of this chapter some of the planners of Wellspace explored their intentions were explored as they envisioned Wellspace. Certain of these intentions are included in the Wellspace mission statement "to do remarkable things in health care" and in its core values: (1) "to provide knowledge leadership" in CAM in conjunction with conventional medicine; (2) "to provide *careful* experiences for clients" while providing a facilitating environment for clients/students from knowledgeable, licensed practitioners, which would leave clients feeling empowered and cared for. Another intention, voiced by many quoted in this chapter, was (3) to help practitioners make a better living, in professional surroundings and have a balanced life while (4) finding appropriate ways for practitioners to have a voice in shaping policies which affect them. (5) Finally,

Wellspace as a model hoped to take CAM to the next level of professionalism.

Regarding Wellspace's goal to "provide a care-ful experience" in a facilitating environment for both client and practitioner, I have presented two cases to illustrate a couple of clients' experiences as an example of learning that may take place in the interaction between client/student and practitioner. This process is helping the client to move from subjective knowing to empathic, informed, embodied connected knowing in relation to their health. We have heard from both clients that they feel a connection that they are learning to change habitual behaviors and learning new options. One client is a Feldenkrais student, the other a massage client. Other clients are appreciative of the service they received but were limited in not having insurance coverage.

Regarding Wellspace's intention to better the lot of the CAM health care provider, in my opinion, Wellspace provides a very real step up for practitioners in offering a benefits package to full-time employees (including a reduced benefits package for part-time practitioners). This includes medical, dental, disability, and liability insurances, paid time off, family and medical leave (FMLA), and stock options. It is thus perhaps not surprising to note that since its opening, several Wellspace employees have taken advantage of FMLA leave.

I asked Joelle Hochman, a massage practitioner and teacher who joined Wellspace in September 1998, having trained in massage at Kripalu in Lenox, MA, as to whether becoming a practitioner at Wellspace had helped her make a better living. She joined Wellspace, in part, because a friend of hers was joining. Similar to myself, she was tired of the time-consuming tasks in running her own business. After eight years in practice, renting space in a small office with other practitioners, she still felt that she "could have used a fuller practice and had never quite been able to make a living with massage," so she "always needed to take a second job." Hochman, herself, is at this writing, now pregnant and about to go on maternity leave. Prior to her coming to Wellspace, although she and her husband had thought of having a child, they had not felt ready to take on the financial responsibility. Now, however, with the benefit package including FMLA leave offered by Wellspace, they have felt ready to start a family.

Regarding the effort to upgrade the CAM profession in giving practitioners more of a voice in determining policies which affect them: it would seem that with the formation of the PMIG, practitioners are being heard through the PMIG monthly meetings. Practitioners can funnel any concerns regarding compensation, benefits, and the working environment to the PMIG.

Barber and Drinka, especially, made a point of mentioning their support for the effectiveness of the PMIG and supporting this practitioner initiative, among others. Another practitioner initiative, a formalized exchange system, promises to be helpful. Among different groups of practitioners, peers exchange help with each taking turn in helping the other. Exchange sessions are scheduled when practitioners are off the schedule so it does not interfere with their availability to clients during their shifts. Through sharing in this way, information about the work of each practitioner is circulated through the Wellspace system, the better to make referrals, through having experienced each practitioner's way of being vis-a-vis his or her modality. This also helps prevent burnout. Wellspace also tries to do its part in preventing burnout through a special health benefit where full-time employees receive discounted CAM services at the Center up to $550 and part-time employees receive up to $250 per annum, at a $20,000 cost per annum to Wellspace.

Relationship with Allopathic Medicine and Managed Care

Regarding Wellspace's wish to be of ser-

vice to the allopathic community and to be able to work in partnership with them: Barber, like Agoos, expressed regret that Wellspace had not yet been able to forge the alliance with conventional medicine that it wanted to, although certain referrals are happening in that an OB-Gyn Service nearby refers patients to Wellspace for pregnancy massage. Thus, Wellspace has begun to make some inroads in receiving referrals from conventional medical health care providers. Wellspace hopes to continue to expand its role in offering complementary service to allopathic health care professionals, in addition to making appropriate referrals, and working with clients'/students' primary care physicians.

Barber felt that Wellspace's acceptance is, in part, tied to the larger issue that CAM approaches have not been accepted due to the need to accept the validity of other paradigms requiring different methodologies when determining outcomes. As Barber pointed out, the two systems with different paradigms working hand-in-hand could ostensibly provide the patient with more than either one alone: "We don't want to replace conventional medicine. We can work best as a complement and also to be here for patients who are tired of the other system or who want to take more ownership for their health choices." Likewise he pointed out that: "We don't want someone who has cancer to abandon treatment to come here." As an adjunct, "what we can offer is comfort, and additional healing through herbs or body treatment which can add to conventional medicine–especially with chronic pain."

Some of the voices in this chapter seem to agree with Barber's words that Wellspace can be and has been a helpful adjunct in offering CAM in a healing environment; others speak of connection; many also speak of learning. It would seem that the essence missing in managed care is where Wellspace begins–in connection and caring. As cited above, clients/students mention as one of the strengths of Wellspace that they feel that they are cared for and paid attention to in ways that they have not been before with their HMO. As one client said, "With my HMO, I got tired of feeling as if I was on an assembly line. I had to continually advocate for my own treatment. It was exhausting and frustrating." In contrast, Wellspace Fresh Pond seeks to create conditions ensuring caring and connection between client and practitioner, or "care-ful experience," as stated in the Wellspace business plan.

Many allopathically-trained physicians are also calling for a change in the way that health care professionals relate to the patient/client/student (Benson, 1996; Hallowell, 1999; Gordon, 1996; Weil, 1995). In our interview, Rosenthal remarked that a doctor he knows who is on the staff of a Harvard teaching hospital and for whom he had "a great deal of respect," was "increasingly frustrated with the managed care system and was thinking of leaving medicine altogether."

Restoring the importance of the relationship with patients/clients/students to its rightful place is perhaps another way that Wellspace and allopathic physicians can find common ground. Historically, this relational value is not new to allopathic conventional medicine. The importance of relating compassionately was the one of the most important core values of conventional allopathic medicine at Harvard Medical School as voiced by one of its most honored physicians and faculty members in 1925. Francis W. Peabody, a graduate of Harvard College and of Harvard Medical School in 1903, was highly influential to medical students of his day through his teaching, both in word and by example, concerning the importance of relational factors in the healing process. His original lecture, "The Care of the Patient," made such a strong impression when it was first delivered at Harvard Medical School in 1925 that it was published in the *Journal of the American Medical Association* in 1927, thus reaching a far wider audience. Subsequently,

this lecture and article have been frequently used in the teaching of medical students, and, indeed, it was reprinted as recently as 1984 as a "Landmark Article" in the same journal (Paul, 1991*, p. 120). What is primary to the practice of medicine, in Peabody's opinion, is the doctor-patient relationship: "the practice of medicine in its broadest sense includes the whole relationship of the physician with his patient" (Peabody, 1923, cited in Paul, 1991, p. 156). He began his 1925 lecture by saying that:

> The most common criticism made at present by older practitioners is that young graduates have been taught a great deal about the mechanism of disease, but very little about the practice of medicine–or, to put it more bluntly, they are too "scientific" and do not know how to take care of patients. (Peabody, 1923, cited in Paul, 1991, p. 155)

While Peabody recognized the importance of "an understanding of the sciences which contribute to the structure of modern medicine," he nonetheless felt that "it is obvious that sound professional training should include a much broader equipment" (Peabody, 1923, cited in Paul, 1991, p. 157). His understanding of this situation led to an interest in whether this larger perspective might be addressed from the standpoint of the medical curriculum of his day, including a broadening of medicine's province beyond a focus on any one people or nation. Thus he queried:

> Can the practitioner's art be grafted on the main trunk of the fundamental sciences in such a way that there shall arise a symmetrical growth, like an expanding tree, the leaves of which may be for the 'healing of the nations'? (Peabody, 1923, cited in Paul, 1991, p. 157)

This tension in medicine in Peabody's day arose between the necessity to maintain, on the one hand, a caring relationship with patients–Peabody's "art" of medicine–and the necessity to master a large body of scientific knowledge, on the other–Peabody's "science" in medicine. Currently with managed care, allopathically trained physicians must shorten the amount of time spent with patients. They must conduct an examination in a shorter and shorter amount of time allotted for appointments and, at the same time, maintain a caring, empathic connection with patients. They, too, along with CAM health care professionals are calling for a change due to "medicine's spiritual crisis" (Benson, 1996, pp. 105–107). Perhaps both CAM and conventional medicine are all looking for the same thing–to restore the art to the science of healing–no matter which approach–that which Peabody called "the care of the patient."

CONCLUSION

In the three years since its opening, Wellspace Fresh Pond has become a nexus of educational as well as health services for the community. This chapter has only begun to look at one small part of the Wellspace system–how its original vision–as voiced by some of those who had a hand in shaping it– has played itself out in relation to preliminary client feedback.

Financial Limitations

As a business, notwithstanding the fact that Wellspace Fresh Pond has undergone growing pains, and in so doing has had to amend its original business plan which involved the opening of several Wellspace Centers nationally within the first two years, Wellspace Fresh Pond as a freestanding center seems to be a "success." Rosenthal and Agoos readily admit that they and other original planners of Wellspace overestimated the growth of the CAM market. The original business plan in envisioning several Wellspaces opening up in different geographical areas meant that the monies would be dis-

tributed to several Wellspace Centers. Agoos spoke wistfully about a feeling he had of "still trying but not quite succeeding to reach the brass ring." Thus, it was with regret that after overhiring especially in regards to bodyworkers, and supervisory coaches, a few practitioners and corporate staff had to be let go within the first year.

It has thus taken three years to find the right balance between the different elements so that Wellspace Fresh Pond can now operate at a profit. However, according to Rosenthal, its capacity for further growth is limited. He pointed out to me that "Wellspace Fresh Pond is probably pretty near optimum capacity" with 40 practitioners divided between part-time and full-time. Thus, Wellspace Fresh Pond does have a cap as to the amount that it can bring in financially. He explained that unlike with lawyers, where the public is willing to pay a high price for the expertise of a senior partner in a law firm, a CAM health care practitioner cannot bill out at two to three times the cost for his or her consultation. In providing CAM health care, one bills out at only slightly higher so that the margin for profit is very slim. Unlike with conventional medicine most CAM services are not reimbursed by insurance companies, so the public ends up having to pay out of pocket for CAM services. Rosenthal pointed out that although this might not seem fair when one considers the case of a qualified acupuncturist with as much as 30-40 years' experience in a field that has been existing for thousands of years, and the best education in the field, one nonetheless can only charge as much as the market will bear. Thus, he and his team still wish to expand the Wellspace name into other venues. He is looking to find more cost-effective ways to expand in addition to freestanding centers such as Wellspace Fresh Pond.

It would seem, however, that Wellspace is moving in the direction of fulfilling its goals to: "provide knowledge leadership"; "do remarkable things in health care"–in contrast to the erosion of medical services with managed care; and "provide a care-ful experience," in order to take CAM health care to the next level of professionalism. But what about those voices we have not yet heard from–those who do not have access to CAM services as yet? For the most part, Wellspace still remains accessible only to those who can afford its services. CAM/holistic health services are not often covered by insurance and even those who are insured often cannot afford to pay out of pocket for these CAM services. The uninsured remain shut out of both systems. We at Wellspace share the widespread frustration with the unwillingness of the managed care system to cover CAM services and hope that changes will soon be made. In the meantime, we need to continue to find ways to make our services accessible to all. To help reduce the cost, Wellspace offers discounted series, or discounted introductory sessions. Practitioners also have the option to offer discounted vouchers to clients and share with Wellspace the cost of the discount, but these certainly do not provide the degree of accessibility that most of us envision.

In traditional societies, healing is available to all and does not depend on ability to pay. Healers do not receive money for their services; instead, the tribe looks after their needs. To collect money for healing, in fact, is considered to be an abuse of the healing power. Money of course, drives capitalistic economies, but within this context, Wellspace provides a for-profit model of a corporation attempting to use its financial resources to expand the resource of healing to the community by such means as free lectures, discounts, special introductory offers, and a make-up policy between classes.

The Synergy Phenomenon

Nonetheless, as Barber put it, perhaps the most surprising thing about Wellspace is the way that it has flourished in unexpected ways. Barber attributes it to synergy. In gen-eral terms, synergy describes a pattern by which phenomena relate to each other in a mutually enhancing way: "A synergistic pattern brings phenomena together, interrelating them, creating an often unexpected, new and greater whole from the disparate, seemingly conflicting parts. In that pattern, phenomena exist in harmony with each other, maximizing each others' potential" (Katz, 1983/84, p. 202). Such "phenomena" include human interactions, which have been studied for their synergistic elements by various theorists (Benedict, 1970; Fuller, 1963; Katz, 1982; Maslow, 1971, cited in Katz, 1983/84).

As Barber put it, at Wellspace Fresh Pond, there is no logical reason that such disparate elements "such as a corporate business model and a group of healers who are artists in their own right" when taken separately should co-exist with one another as well as they do at Wellspace. It *must* be due to synergy: "Thus, the fact that it is working must mean that synergy is operating here because the whole must *really* be greater than the sum of the parts in order for that to happen."

It's important to focus on the fact that we are in this as a for-profit business and that we are doing a surprisingly good job at operating as a for-profit business while not losing sight of our mission: to do remarkable things in health care. Practitioners at Wellspace, despite working for a for-profit business, are encouraged to be the individual artists they are while making a better living than most of them would be making on their own–all while participating as part of a true community. Through synergy these disparate parts come together, and I think that is perhaps the most pleasantly surprising result of Wellspace Fresh Pond: the whole *is* truly greater than the sum of the parts.

REFERENCES

Benedict, R. (1970). *Patterns of culture.* Boston: Houghton Mifflin.
Benson, H. with Starg, M. (1996). *Timeless*

Healing: The power and biology of belief. New York: Scribner.

Berliner, H. S., & Salmon, J.W. (1980).The holistic alternative to scientific medicine: History and analysis. *International Journal of Health Services.* 10(1).

Bertalanffy, L. von. (1950). An outline of general system theory. *British Journal of Philosophical Science, 1*, 139–164.

Bertalanffy, L. von. (1968). *General system theory: Foundations, development, applications* (rev. ed.). New York: George Braziller.

Borysenko, J. (1987). *Minding the body, mending the mind.* Reading, MA: Addison Wesley Press.

Cheever, O. (2000). Connected knowing and "somatic empathy" among somatic educators and students of somatic education. In *ReVision*, Spring 2000, Volume 22, Number 4, pp. 2–5.

Cheever, O. (1995). Education as transformation in American psychiatry: From voices of control to voices of connection. EdD diss., Harvard Graduate School of Education. UMI.

Dossey, L. (1991). *Meaning and medicine: Lessons from a doctor's tales of breakthrough and healing.* New York: Bantam Books.

Eisenberg, D. M., Kessler, R. C., Foster, C., Norlock, F. E., Calkins, D. R., & Delbanco, T. L. (1993). Unconventional medicine in the United States. *New England Journal of Medicine, 328*(4), 246–252.

Eisenberg, D.M., Davis, R.B., Ettner, S.L., Appel, S., Wilkey, S., Van Rompay, M., Kessler, R.C. (1998). Trends in alternative medicine use in the United States, 1990-1997. Results of a follow-up national survey. *Journal of the American Medical Association*, November 11; *280*(18); 1569–75.

Feldenkrais, M. (1949). *Body and Mature Behavior: A study of anxiety, sex, gravitation & learning.* (1949/1977). New York: International Universities Press.

Ferguson, M. (1980). *The Aquarian conspiracy: Personal and social transformation in the 1980s.* Los Angeles: J. P. Tarcher.

Gardner, H. (1999). *Intelligence reframed: Multiple intelligences for the 21st century.* New York: Basic Books.

Goleman, D. (1995). *Emotional intelligence.* New York: Bantam Books,

Gordon, J. (1996). *Manifesto for a New Medicine:*
Your Guide to Healing Partnerships and the Wise Use of Alternative Therapies.

Hallowell, E. (1999). *Connect.* New York: Pantheon Books.

Hanna, T. (1985). *Bodies in revolt: A primer in somatic thinking.* Novato, CA: Freeperson Press.

Hanna, T. (1988). *Somatics: Reawakening the mind's control of movement, flexibility, and health.* Cambridge, MA: Perseus Books.

Hastings, A.C., Fadiman. J., & Gordon, J.S. (Eds.). (1980). *Health for the whole person.* Boulder, CO: Westview Press.

Jordan, J. V. (1991). Empathy and self boundaries. In J. V. Jordan, A. G. Kaplan, J. B. Miller, I. P. Stiver, & J. L. Surrey, *Women's growth in connection* (pp. 67–80). New York: Guilford.

Kabat-Zinn, J. (1990). *Full catastrophe living: Using the wisdom of your body and mind to face stress, pain, illness.* New York: Bantam, Doubleday, Dell Publishing Company.

Kahn, J. (2001). Research matters. *Massage Magazine* July/August (92), 65–69.

Katz, R. (1981). *Boiling energy, community healing among the Kalahari !Kung.* Cambridge, MA: Harvard University Press.

Katz, R. (1982a). Accepting "boiling energy": The experience of !kia-healing among the !Kung. *Ethos, 10*(4), 344–368.

Katz, R. (1983/84). Empowerment and synergy: Expanding the community's healing resources. *Prevention in Human Services, 3*(2/3), 201–226.

Kuhn, T. S. (1970). *The structure of scientific revolutions* (2nd ed.). Chicago: University of Chicago Press.

Leviton, R. (2000). *Physician: Medicine and the unsuspected battle for human freedom.* Charlottsville, VA: Hampton Roads Publishing Company.

Moore, T. (1992). *Care of the soul: A guide for cultivating depth and sacredness I in everyday life.* New York: Harper Collins.

Moyers, B. (1993). *Healing and the mind.* New York: Doubleday.

Nesbit, M. (2000). Connected Knowing and Developmental Theory. In *ReVision*, Spring 2000, Volume 22, Number 4, pp. 6–14.

Paul, O. (1991). *The caring physician: The life of Dr. Francis W. Peabody.* Cambridge, MA: Harvard University Press.

Pert, C. (1997). *Molecules of Emotion.* New York:

Simon & Schuster.

The Landmark Report on Public Perceptions of Alternative Care, (1998). Landmark Healthcare, Sacramento, CA.

Weil, A. (1995). *Spontaneous Healing.* New York: Alfred J. Knopf.

Weil, A. (1972). *Natural Mind.* New York: Houghton Mifflin.

Weil, A. (2000). *Eating well for optimum health.* New York: Alfred A. Knopf.

Wright, P. (2000). Connected Knowing: Exploring Self, Soma, Empathy, and Intuition. In *ReVision,* Spring, Volume 22, Number 4, pp. 2–5.

For more information contact:

Wellspace Fresh Pond
1 New Street
Cambridge, MA 02138
(617) 876-4554 x2125
ocheever@wellspace.com

Section III

INTEGRATIVE HOLISTIC
HEALTH PRACTICES

INTRODUCTION

The following three chapters are examples of holistic health practitioners and/or therapists who employ an integrative mindbody, Einsteinian, and combined Era II, III and Einsteinian approaches respectively to working holistically with individuals. These approaches are meant as examples of how three individuals work. They are, by no means, meant to represent the totality of the work extant in complimentary and alternative medicine, but rather to stimulate the reader to formulate his or her own integrative philosophy.

Chapter 16

THE MOVING CYCLE: A MODEL FOR HEALING

CHRISTINE CALDWELL

INTRODUCTION

IN THE LATE SEVENTIES, after two years as a dance therapist in the trenches of a state mental hospital in Maryland, I had begun to question my training and my orientation as a clinician. Though I wanted to be of help, to be a healer, I felt plagued by a feeling that I was showing up each morning to do my groups in ways that did not deeply see or understand the people I was working with. Though I harbored no doubt that my clients were suffering and ill, and I trusted the good intentions of all the staff around me, I couldn't shake the feeling that my whole approach to healing and therapy was at least a bit off. I had assumed in these first two years that it was just a product of my inexperience as a clinician, but as I gained skills this feeling got even worse.

Modern Western psychotherapy models itself from the views of modern Western medicine, which in turn has taken its inspiration from Western scientific thought. Science, as we in the West have shaped it, inclines itself towards reductionism, liking to take things apart and study them as parts. It values critical thinking, an essential tool in any method of inquiry. It also likes to ask what is wrong, or, why do things fail to work? The word therapy itself betrays this

bias. Therapy assumes something has gone wrong, and needs to be fixed. This can be and has been a tremendously useful viewpoint, and it also determines what we observe.

In a "why do things fail?" system of thought, four answers tend to arise. First, that which fails can be inherently defective. In psychotherapy we call this genetics. We somehow inherit a defect. Second, the part wears out from use. In biology this is called senescence. In medicine and psychology we might call this stress or senility. The third cause is being treated badly, and in psychotherapy we favor this answer frequently, calling it abuse or neglect. Lastly, we see an accident as a potential cause, which we usually translate as trauma. Answering the question "How does something go wrong?" has bred many great advances in health and healing, and will continue to do so. In my case, since I harbor a rather contrary nature, I decided those many years ago to look at something different. Along with others, I have been interested in the question "What is occurring as things go right?" Another way to put it is "What does health look like? How does it operate?" As soon as I began to ask myself these questions, a great sense of relief came over me, as well as an unsettled feeling of cluelessness.

273

When I began contemplating this question, I determined that as a somatic psychotherapist I had to look at the process of healing as it occurs naturally in the body, without any external help. Research tells me that overall, many illnesses tend to resolve whether the clinician "therapizes" them or not. What is occurring in these situations? Clearly, everyone possesses self-regulating mechanisms. In fact, the ability to self-regulate stands out as the single greatest hallmark of health. It struck me that the process may be akin to watching a cut on my finger heal. I'm not consciously directing this healing, yet an ordered process occurs, time and again. If this elegant natural process can be studied and named, could therapists then get in alignment with it and model their therapies after it, especially in more complex and severe situations in which self-regulation proves inadequate? Why not model therapy on the ways that the body heals itself? It struck me then that the dance therapy and the psychotherapy I had learned, for all their body-centered practices, were head-driven models, and that I had only to study the physical body to come into a more perfect union with healing.

In the early 1970s, I received my BA at UCLA in Psychological Anthropology, studying cross-cultural healing systems. It occurred to me that many indigenous cultures used this same body-centered, self-regulatory view. Their cures focused, in many cases, on restoring an alignment with natural order. And that recovery process more often than not involved movement and movement ritual. The central theme that kept returning and returning was movement. Something about movement was healing, and a disturbance of movement heralded illness. In my fascination with anatomy and physiology, this movement theme revealed itself on the cellular, tissue and systems level as well. It sounds strange to come back to this very basic view, but in a sense I had to suspend my belief in externally imposed systems of thought in order to find home again, and to build a new house on that foundation. That suspension process conceived the Moving Cycle work, though I had no inkling of it at the time.

Then began a four-year observation project that accelerated tremendously when I moved to Boulder, Colorado (1980) and began teaching at Naropa University, a Buddhist-inspired college that invited me to begin a Dance/Movement Therapy Department for them.[1] By serendipitously landing at an institution that valued and taught meditative and contemplative practices, I began to develop witnessing skills that tapped into wisdom traditions thousands of years old. It was in this womb that the Moving Cycle gestated.

As I observed my students and clients over and over, I came to see that the natural processes I was witnessing were not confined to healing, but were also the same events that generated growth, creativity, evolution, and transformation. Nature does not seem to separate healing from growth and creativity, but puts them on a continuum. I developed the Moving Cycle work as a way to describe and then teach what I was learning from watching natural healing and organic movement. My students helped me to refine it, and continue to do so to this day. The Moving Cycle remains one of the central teaching paradigms of the Somatic Psychology Department at the Naropa University.

---

1. I founded the BA program in Dance/Movement Therapy at Naropa in 1982, and the MA program in 1984. In 1990, we split the department into two majors, body psychology and dance/movement therapy. It thrives to this day, and we are now contemplating a Ph.D. program.

THE THEORY BEHIND THE MOVING CYCLE

"The first responsibility in information, is truth" Adlai Stevenson.

Life is defined by movements, movements such as the beating of the heart, the expansion and release of the lungs with breath, and the electrical pulsations of brain waves. In the physical body, many complex physiological systems move in concert, like instruments in an orchestra, to create a functioning human being. When one or more of these systems cease to move, we die. The physical realities of movement as life can be extrapolated to other physical human processes as well. We also are an emotional body, which manifests as gross vibrational charge/discharge throughout the physical body (e-motion). Thus, the emotion "anger" is an energetic effort to regulate our power; we often become angry as a direct result of disempowering ourselves, and the emotion is a move to get our power back. We also exist as a cognitive body, which manifests as fine energetic flow in the physical body (brain waves), and a transpersonal body, which manifests as space in the physical body. Given this model, we can see ourselves as a series of bodies that progress from the material world through the energetic world to the world of space. All of these bodies require movement to live. And all of these bodies live through interdependent movement interactions with each other. Instead of trying to integrate body and mind into some amalgamated bodymind, we can conceive ourselves as a unified body that exists on a continuum from matter to pure energy to unlimited space.

The Moving Cycle models itself on the way the physical body appears to operate, which manifests as these levels of motion. The Moving Cycle operates on premises that arose from my observations of the movement processes involved in natural healing:

1. Life exists as a body, a body that strives for wholeness.

2. Wholeness occurs through actions that maintain and extend bodily integrity.
3. Integrity operates as a constant oscillation between the organisms existing behavior patterns (organizers) and novel experiments (disorganizers).
4. Illness arises when an organism overorganizes or overdisorganizes or a combination of both, resulting in a loss of the adaptability needed to maintain wholeness.
5. Adaptability is a product of movement, of a body moving cooperatively within itself, and moving in cooperation other bodies and with external forces and relationships.

On a nuts and bolts level, how is lost integrity and lessened adaptability recovered? How is movement used to step forward into a more responsive and responsible life? I could see right off that, though most movement produced positive effects in the bodies, some movements did nothing to reestablish health, and some even contributed to greater fragmentation. I began to tackle these questions by taking a deeper look at different kinds of movement processes in the body.

PHYSICAL MOVEMENT

Biological Movement

Physical body movement comes in three forms and two principles. The first form of movement is biological, the thrummings of the body itself, shaping and creating itself through its various interior metabolic vibrations and pulsations. Biologic movement is our bottom line definition of life. The heart must beat; the lungs must fill and empty. Individuals are required to neurotransmit, to peristalt, to secrete. It is these movements that basically create unique body patterns, the recurring structure over time. Biological movement is shared by all life–nature repeats what works–the dance is much the same. At the same time it stamps everyone with an individual fingerprint. And scientists are only beginning to understand the synchronicity, the entertainment that splendidly occurs across the seemingly vast distances between two live bodies. Humans all sizzle and thrum inside, and when they get in close proximity to each other, they can to do it to a mutual beat.

Most biological movement is by its nature autonomic—it goes on in cells, tissues and systems, responding to various self-regulatory controls, while being blithely uninvolved in human's conscious state. Some biologic movement is under some volitional control, an example being breathing and heart rate, but it can and does occur without a thought, a will, a conscious "Yes, do that now." The first movement principle, therefore, arises from genetic pattern, and biological movement is almost wholly patterned. The constancy of patterned, recurring movement is needed. Humans could never juggle all of their metabolic balls at once consciously, so imprinted movement pattern is depended upon to take care of basic aliveness. Pattern invokes the law of the conservation of energy—patterns are created because they use less energy than novel actions. In a sense, it can be said that biologic movement is human's physical unconscious.

Locomotor Movement

The second form of movement is locomotion. Moving the body through space is required for the networking of life in a larger scale. Locomotion combines reflexes with conscious actions, and comprises the method of relationship to the world. From a sunflower turning its face to the sun to a curious child reaching for a rock, locomotion is movement organized towards contact, contact being an ongoing life need. Locomotion is also highly adaptive. It allows us an almost instantaneous ability to change an individual's relationship to the world, to first make

it more safe, then more nourishing, then more penetratingly conscious. Much like Maslow's *Hierarchy of Needs* (1971), locomotion gets more sophisticated, more blissfully intricate as individuals go up the developmental and phylogenetic scales. All these motions create and affirm current status in the environment, and can span functions from safety, survival, and reproduction, to emotional expression, curiosity, and fun.

The advent of culture in humans (and other species) creates a unique parameter to locomotion. Posture, stance, spacing and gesture all locomote culture. They show movement as communication, nonverbal locomotion. Basic forms of play and creativity can be seen in this movement form. Locomotion is semi-patterned movement in that it is only somewhat hard-wired at birth. A human newborn only knows how to suckle and root and turn its head in an organized way. The more complex the organism, the more locomotive movement must be learned through experience and practice. Culture sculpts many patterns of locomotor movement in many species.

Locomotion can contain within it repeated movement patterns that create an ongoing sense of identity: "I know who I am through my recurring gestures, stances, positions. I am the one who always puts my hand to my mouth when I listen, or I am the one who puffs up and clenches my fists when I get angry." Locomotion also has another special capability, in that it can be either patterned or impulsive. Impulse is the second movement principle. Impulsive movement arises spontaneously, and serves no obvious ongoing need. It moves us for moving's sake. Who knows why Martha Graham raised her hand in front of her face, extending it like a beacon above her head, captivating audiences all over the world? That expressive gesture was born of impulse movement, and it and millions like it are the ingredients of art, human creativity as a species.

Expressive Movement

The third form of movement is almost purely in the realm of the impulse principle. I call it expressive movement. It is movement that is required to be immediately superfluous. It is designed to *de-automatize* a previous movement pattern, to unravel it, to disorganize it. All individuals need pattern to exist, and they also need impulse. Expressive movement generates and nourishes impulse, as impulse is a necessary balance to pattern. Expressive movement may express life's need to de-pattern, to be nourished by randomness, to experiment again with a different and possibly more perfect union. Entropy occurs when individuals express themselves. Expression predicts the death of an event that has moved individuals, moved through them. In this way, expression creates the conditions for future conception, and forms one of the essential features of healing.

Through expressive movement individual, group and species evolution is made possible in a single lifetime. Biologic change often takes generations to alter itself, and all humans need this rooted stability. But they also need rapid change, and expressive movement holds this capacity. Brian Swimme and Thomas Berry (1992) spoke eloquently of this idea in their book *The Universe Story*. In it they examined the second law of thermodynamics, which explains entropy. They introduced the concept of cosmogenesis as a companion to entropy, a balance to the fact that everything disorganizes. Cosmogenesis is the universe's constant of forming, of shaping of creating itself. Cosmogenesis explains a star's formation; entropy explains its eventual collapse. Because of collapse, the raw material for cosmogenesis is made available. Impulse-based expressive movement begets cosmogenesis through its capability to flummox established patterns. Pattern movement celebrates organization and form; impulse movement instigates the raw material necessary for cosmogenesis. The structure of movement can be viewed like this:

Type of Movement	Movement Principle
Biologic	Pattern
Locomotive	Pattern/Impulse
Expressive	Impulse

Expressive movement is perhaps best manifested in the flowings of improvisational dance, as well as music, painting, sculpture, etc. It can also be seen in the movement of free-associational thinking that great scientists and philosophers do. Rollo May (1975) and others have observed that creativity of all kinds requires just such a suspension of the way it is usually done, a disordering of old forms, coupled with dedication and a driving urge to "express" whatever emerges from the rubble.

Expressive movement reaches its pinnacle in free play, and may be the basis of such dance therapy forms as Authentic Movement. I define free play as activity that has no immediate organized function, no enduring rules, and no projected outcome. It is observed in many birds, mammals and all humans, and is often done individually. It can consist of the spontaneous leaps and gambols we see in sheep, horses, and wolves. It is seen in humans as free-associative movement—movement that unfolds not through any external dictates, but motion that arises from a deep immersion in direct experience, following the moment-to-moment stimuli of the senses, of feelings, of images.

THE RECOVERY OF HEALTH

Recovering expressive movement in the physical, emotional, cognitive and transpersonal body may be one of the most important factors in the recovery of health. Expressive movement decreases when our wholeness is threatened. Due to the conservation of energy, our movement becomes more primitive and stereotyped when we are taken up with unfinished trauma and what Candace Pert (1997) calls undigested feelings. The Moving Cycle, like many forms of dance therapy, seeks to not only resolve these movement wounds but to restore expressive (creative) movement capability. Remediation takes the form of restoring a natural oscillation along a bell curve of patterned and impulse movement, and a pyramid of biologic, locomotor and expressive motion. Biologic movement can always be drawn upon to reinforce pattern movement. Indeed, many meditative practices focus on contemplation of biologic movement such as breathing to help the meditator feel more clear, stable, and whole. But large amounts of free play (expressive movement) are equally needed to sustain the healing and transformational properties of impulse. Lots of locomotor movement, which immediately blends pattern and impulse, is also needed. As Mary Whitehouse put it, individuals need to both move and be moved (In Lewis, 1984). Wholeness is operationalized in the laboratory of locomotion. But it is conceived, gestated and born in impulse movement.

Free play is, by its nature, recreational. It recreates. This points to the need that all humans have to engage in nonproductive activities. The contemporary culture has trouble with this concept. The idea that individuals need to do things that are not immediately useful or productive is usually equated with laziness or sloth. And in turn, in many subcultures, recreation has increasingly been associated with drugs (often called recreational drugs), passive entertainment, and mindless consumption. Impulse then perverts into oblivious actions (people often chide themselves for being impulsive, which they equate with mindless disregard). This perversion of impulse may be the origin of addictions and much of the violent behavior in our society.

EMOTIONAL OR ENERGETIC MOVEMENT

The previous paragraphs described physical movement. The next principle behind the Moving Cycle comes from an understanding of emotional or energetic movement. One of the primary ways in which waves of emotional excitation are generated is when a new experience hits a person's organized sense of self and this established form has no reference points with which to process the experience. An experience pressures a person to disorganize, and some kind of shift or change is needed to resolve the dissonance. An example of this is someone telling a person that she is beautiful. This may conflict with her structurally held belief that "I am 'homely,'" and this dissonance gives rise to a feeling of heat in the face, sweatiness, and rapid breathing. These excitatory feelings are an attempt to bridge her old self-concept with new input. They excite her, vibrating her physical body, changing sensation and perception in order to create the option of change. She has an opportunity to modify old imprints, to create new and more satisfying concepts, concepts that match current experience.

If she resists this option and decides to keep her old form as it is, she must get harder and denser so that the vibrations don't travel through her and change things. She will experience these resistive actions as painful and negative. The resistance, which is an effort to stop the excitation, hurts. She might learn from this hurt feeling to fear change and excitation, even though it is her resistance that causes the pain. She then feels justified in continuing to resist further excitation, because she has linked it with negative experiences. If she participates with the excitatory experience by inviting it to flow in an unimpeded manner, she achieves a new and more balanced state of being. In this sense, all emotions have the capacity for satisfying resolution. They all attempt to restore our wholeness.

In individuals' energetic bodies a more relative world exists. Energy molecularly vibrates mass, and in so doing can change its structure and properties (Keleman, 1975). Each happening can be an opportunity to align my form with the external world so that I maximize my contact with it. Events become relative to the energy we put into experiencing them directly.

The movement patterns and impulses of thought come next. We are also a cognitive body. In this body we experience the ability to transcend regular space and time through thought. This particular body's vibration manifests as cognitions, as waves of massless energy. Humans can remember the past, imagine the future, and create whole worlds that exist only in fantasy. The life of this body can be quite limitless. This can be tremendously freeing, and also very tricky. If this body is invested with too much attention in a world further and further removed from the nourishment that is needed from physical, consensual reality, this investment can be seen as insanity.

Other bodies may also exist as well, all of which live through our material body. The next body would be the transpersonal. It deals with space and the creative void. It is revealed in the gap between our thoughts when individuals meditate, and in the spontaneous creative act. The movement of this body exists in the experience of communion with that which is typically experienced as outside of individuals' separate selves. It is a resonant pulsation, and can result in a sense of connection and vaster identity. If this movement is disturbed it can result in a feeling of threatening boundary loss. The spiritual body is perhaps the part of individuals that can transcend any form and completely occupy limitless space. It is at one with all that is because it *is* all that is. There is no separation from anything in this body.

Movement initiated in one body ripples through the others, setting them in synchronous motion, so that thoughts create physical responses, emotions trigger thoughts, etc. This co-operative movement is experienced between bodies as pleasure. It is when the bodies fail to move in harmony that pain is experienced. True pleasure involves the harmonious motion of all bodies, much like the singing of a choir. This bodysong is everyone's birthright and the mechanism of humanity's continuing evolution.

THE MOVING CYCLE DESCRIBED

The above elements formed the basis for my understanding of the "moving" part of the Moving Cycle. I then began to examine successful therapy sessions to see if I could discern any kind of pattern or sequence of events in them. Does healing follow a predictable course across time? I did indeed observe a pattern, and out of this observation came the "cycle" portion of the Moving Cycle. The pattern in time seemed to predict not the content of what a client would experience, but the process of opening, deepening, committing, completing, and integrating. I believe now that when individuals are engaged in healing and are allowed to do so from the dictates of their essential nature, they unravel illness in a sequenced fashion, undoing their injuries and recovering their movement in an individualized yet predictable way. As the name implies, the process of healing involves a cycle or spiral of events. The spirilic nature of healing allows one to orient towards movement as a process, and reinforces the concept that there is no end point, no "arriving," but only increasingly satisfying and nurturing movement.

Healing, growth, and transformation seem to occur in four phases. Each phase must be successfully resolved in order for the next one to occur. Often clients will move into the next phase momentarily, then fall back in order to really complete with the last one. These phases can be seen in physical healing, emotional healing, cognitive healing, and transpersonal/spiritual healing. The phases are the same.

1. Awareness

Awareness is the first step onto the Moving Cycle. It commences as therapy begins, and it begins each session. It moves people to come to therapy, as they tell themselves "Hey, something is going on that I want to take a look at." Often, pain of some sort is what's going on, but luckily not always. Individuals live both in the dark and the light, in the deep cave of the unconscious and the pattern, and in the light of consciousness. They draw towards healing when something that was stored in the dark needs to be exposed to the light. This first phase involves focusing attention on sensations, feelings and thoughts that were not previously acknowledged. Awareness is a light, and attention occurs when a beam of that light is created and shone on some part of a person's existence. All humans share a birthright of the ability to pay unconditional attention to the original details of life. Often individuals' family or culture trains them away from this ability as a way to perpetuate entrenched patterns. Patterns limit attention to conserve energy. If they are trained to stop attending to the raw data of reality then they are unable to participate fully in self-regulation. If they begin their work with the practice of paying attention to their physical, emotional, cognitive, and other bodies, they create a rich experience of consciousness. Consciousness in and of itself is one of the primary components of healing and transformation, the first source of fuel that is needed for the healing journey. Bodies love the light. Another way to put it is that everyone shares a common developmental task–

to live a revealed life.

Focusing attention also involves the development of an observing or "witness" self, because individuals acknowledge that a part of them is "attending" to another part of them that is "experiencing." Witnessing generates healing in and of itself, as it allows clients to acknowledge and go through what they are feeling without fixating upon it as part of their identity. It allows the statement "I am *having* this feeling (it will come and it will go), and I am *not* this feeling (it is not a permanent part of who I am)." This ability to witness allows people to disentangle their pain, which is in the moment and will come and go, from their suffering, which is a fusion of present pain with unresolved past experience (dysfunctional patterns). Suffering results from having views and positions that interfere with their ability to directly and accurately experience it.

Einstein once posited that what individuals decide to look at determines what they see. He also noted that they cannot solve a problem in the same state of consciousness that the problem arose in. The Zen master Thich Nhat Hanh once said that all views are wrong views, but since it is in our nature to have views, we might as well relax and get them as accurate as possible. The Awareness Phase is about just such a relaxing, a surrender to whatever arises in our attentional field, coupled with a willingness to change vantage points so that the view is different, and an understanding that any view is not ultimate truth, but a transient facet of it.

Charles Darwin (1998), when he wrote about emotions, stated that attention or conscious concentration on almost any part of the body produces some direct physical effect on it.[2] A felt shift (Gendlin, 1976) occurs in the Awareness phase, when we let our attention drift over or focus on the less arguable, more concrete qualities of move-

2. One of my favorite quotes from Darwin: "I have no great quickness of apprehension or wit . . . my power to follow a long and purely abstract train of thought is very limitied . . . (but) I am superior to the common run of men in noticing things which easily escape attention, and in observing them carefully."

ment made visible by sensation. For what is attended to is the movement. Sensation is merely information that informs persons that they are moving. And this attention and its concomitant shift in the body moves the client to the second phase of the Moving Cycle.

2. *Owning What Arises*

Owning what arises comes next. Awareness is about a stranger coming to the door. Owning is about opening that door and greeting and welcoming the stranger. The stranger is invited inside; she is given a meal, and asked to tell who she is. On a physical body level, clients deepen their focus on sensation, on movement for its own sake. They commit to an emerging movement sequence, to seeing it through to the end, even if it gets rough, even if it behaves badly. The stranger is sent from their unconscious, still cloaked in imagery and mystery. To make matters worse, she rarely speaks English (or whatever ones language). She uses impulse energy, through the medium of expressive movement, to get acquainted and to pass on information about our healing. The Owning Phase follows Einstein's idea that everyone must change their consciousness in order to solve problems. Numerous therapists, most notably Stan Grof (1985), believe, as many indigenous cultures do, that all healing takes place in an altered state of consciousness. In the Owning Phase, clients descend or ascend out of the pattern of movement they are used to, and this alters their consciousness until new solutions emerge.

Jungian therapists might rightly point out here that the Owning Phase is a dangerous enterprise. A good Jungian will talk about perilous journeys into the wilderness, into the dark, into the dark night of the soul. Humans do tend to resist Owning, for it can be uncomfortable and frightening. It is usually only attempted in safe holding environments such as therapy or with a trusted friend. But safety is not required, and Owning can take place in a prison cell, a concentration camp, and a war zone. That level of owning produces people that can only be known as heroes, as healers of the collective.

In the act of Owning, clients take deep personal responsibility for themselves and their movement. For it is within this ability to respond that the shift from being not owned and unrecognized to being empowered is made. After some time, the stranger is recognized as me. Anne Morrow Lindberg once said that the most exhausting thing in life is being insincere. Owning gives the energy, the next source of fuel, to move sincerely. It generates self-efficacy, and what is called an internal locus of control. In this realm the deepest truths can be told about experience. Interpretation is avoided and rests into the primal nourishment of description. For in description the client and healer can get as close as it gets to what is real and true.

Owning is resisted through classical means such as projection, denial, dissociation, depression, and distraction. The Owning Phase calls up introjected critical voices who will urge humans to go back, or to shut the door on the stranger. The task of this phase is to make the movement sequence more important than any of these voices or urges. The Awareness phase is about a change of attention. The Owning Phase is about a shift in intention. We make a commitment to the emergent expressive movement, and make it more important than the old pattern. What gets stimulated in the moment of intention is the fear of death. Clients are identified with their patterns, and rightly fear their death as personal death. A good Owning Phase will kill the client. It will dissolve the pattern the clients calls "me" in some way, and in its place put new movement that may feel truer, but may also feel more tender, vulnerable, and unfamiliar.

In Owning, the client recovers what architects call structural integrity. If the client's structure, which is a pattern of movement, has deviated from a wholesome relationship to itself and to the world, its structural integrity will be compromised and it is in danger of falling down. When an emergent expressive movement sequence is committed to and not placated or perverted, the client regains original integrity. Perhaps some would say this original integrity is the soul, the person's essence. The Bible has said that the truth will set us free. It certainly forms the core experience of personal and social liberation.

3. Appreciation Phase

When a movement sequence completes, the body relaxes, and satisfaction, if not pleasure, occurs. Clients have returned to a state of increased wholeness. The third phase begins as we learn to tolerate and move with this satisfaction. Marianne Williamson would call it a return to love (1992). I call it the Appreciation Phase, for this moment requires that clients appreciate, welcome, hold, and caress their new-found movement as if it were their own child they had just birthed, one they had known before only as someone buried deep within them and growing. After the labors of Owning, they bond with themselves, they spend time holding and loving themselves.

Many modern therapies ignore this crucial phase, not realizing that most clients need help tolerating and basking in feelings of satisfaction and love. Most individuals have been enculturated by family, society, or religion to limit their positive feelings (Hendricks, 1990). Even when the Owning Phase has uncovered feelings of rage or grief, their moving with those feelings and taking responsibility for them gestates new movement that feels whole, true, and relieving. Appreciation involves spending some time with this movement, and bonding to it. The Appreciation Phase brings us back to a shift of attention. Thich Nhat Hanh has written that attention is like sunlight and water for a plant. What we pay attention to will

grow. If clients want to grow a more whole, satisfied self, they take this time to allow the movement that supports that self to have its way with them.

The Appreciation phase is about basking in whatever experience arises, and forms the essential building block of a bonded relationship. If clients can unconditionally ride whatever experience they are having, then they don't have to protect or control their relationships to others. When they stay in dialogue with themselves, they are capable of intimate dialogue with others. In the body, this stage often involves deep emotional (but not necessarily cathartic) release. Bodies move in a more integrated fashion, because they are not recruiting musculature to defend themselves against unwanted experience or against threatening contact.

4. Action Phase

The fourth stage is Action, and it aligns clients with the very real truth that they have to leave the room now and go back out into their daily lives. When the Appreciation stage is completed, they feel inner healing. In order for this healing to be permanent it must find a place in the outside environment. This means literally using their thoughts, feelings, and body differently, and committing this difference to patterned movement. Only then can clients truly change, and contribute this change to the benefit of the external environment. Contributing to the world may be one of humans' prime directives, and the Action Phase honors this directive. Personal healing has no reference point, no point at all, if it does not extend into the community. It is from personal healing that planetary healing becomes possible.

The Action phase is about transitioning into the outer world, and an intention to manifest self differently within it. Perhaps a client will walk in a more relaxed manner. Perhaps reluctance to self-reveal has melted a bit. This change needs to be practiced and committed to the patterned movement repetoire, or else it will dissolve, as all dreams and impulses do.

The Moving Cycle, though an ordered sequence, is individual to each person in each situation. All are on many Moving Cycles in one lifetime, some which take moments to complete and still others that will complete as individuals lie on their deathbed. Each phase liberates a portion of our energy and applies it to personal healing, growth, and creativity. Tendencies or patterns of obstructing Moving Cycles at characteristic places tend, for example, to have difficulty with the Appreciation phase no matter what the content of the specific situation is. But this ability to focus on the process of wounding and healing, rather than getting bogged down and led astray by the content of the wound, allows clients to heal more efficiently and completely. They are accessing their core nature more than the less-than-accurate reconstruction of their personal history. They are addressing habitual withdrawals from experience which starve their core being, more than chasing down the specifics of each withdrawal.

DIAGNOSIS IN THE MOVING CYCLE

In the Moving Cycle diagnosis centers around the forms and principles of movement. It rests in description, and relies on the postponement of interpretation. Interpretation is nothing more than the repetition of an old thought pattern unless it is postponed until the Action Phase of the Cycle. Meaning does not reveal itself until the completion of an experience, until the stranger has fully revealed herself.

Diagnostic training consists of becoming as clear of a vessel of movement description as possible, combined with an understanding of the movement elements described above. Most dance therapy uses Laban Movement Analysis or the Kestenberg Movement Profile, which also tend to rest into description. In this way we can see dance therapy as profoundly behavioral in its diagnostic work. It luxuriates in the description of observable behavior.

It was important for me, as I developed this work, not to fall into an imposed and projective interpretation of others. Interpretation is the inalienable right of each individual with regard to themselves as they complete an experience, and becomes a projective disempowerment when applied to others experience. Diagnosis then perverts into a method of social control.

Clients are largely assessed in terms of the bell curve of pattern to impulse movement, and on the pyramid of pattern to locomotor to impulse movement. This movement is assessed in all the bodies, and may be integrated with the clients' report of their symptoms and their healing goals. The treatment plan is to use conscious attention and intention to oscillate between entering and relieving the movements we want to study.

TREATMENT IN THE MOVING CYCLE

Therapists may be equivalent to midwives, coaching the birth of the whole client. In this respect, treatment looks a lot like the stages of labor and delivery. In Moving Cycle psychotherapy, treatment is based on working with all the client's bodies to promote movement and to restore orgasmic interdependence. Places of decreased aliveness in these bodies are infused with four successive phases of treatment, phases that correspond to the birth process. The Awareness phase corresponds to the onset of labor. The clients' being is telling them that something needs to happen, to shift, much like contractions awaken us to imminent birth. In the physical body, awareness occurs along the sensory-motor nerves. Desensitization is often a physical choice people make in order to minimize pain or prevent overwhelming or unacceptable stimulation to occur. When these habituated choices no longer need to be made in response to adverse conditions that no longer exist, resensitization needs to occur. The client literally relearns how to feel his or her physical body. In the Awareness phase of a session a client is constantly asked to pay attention to sensation and to consider it this body's form of speech. The therapist might ask, "Describe the tingling and where it is in your belly. Does the sensation change if you hold your breath?" Part of treatment is reacquainting the client with physical awareness and trusting that these sensations are intelligent and worthy of attention.

In the energetic body, awareness takes place through vibration. Clients pay attention to where energy flows in them and where it deadens or exaggerates. One client I worked with a few years ago was only aware of energy in her upper body. She would begin to talk about a sensitive subject and her chest, shoulders and arms would become very animated while her belly and legs would remain motionless and heavy. When she began to wake up to this discrepancy, she reported that her lower half felt asleep while her upper half felt scared and anxious. This awareness of how she was using her energetic body became the starting point for her reclamation of her sexuality and sexual identity.

Awareness in the cognitive body typically takes the form of watching when thinking occurs, and whether it seems to contribute to the client's overall movement or detract from it. It is often a very profound shift of awareness to observe the flow of thought more than the content of it, and many clients find this change of emphasis very challenging. Since thought is capable of taking a client out of direct experience and into analysis or planning, etc., the Awareness phase here is one of recognizing this avoidance mechanism when it arises. I will ask a client to notice when thoughts depress a feeling or distract him or her from a sensation. It is crucial in treatment for the client to distinguish between thoughts that support direct experience and thoughts that diminish or distort it.

In the transpersonal body, the Awareness phase works with alertness to a client's contact functions. I might ask a client to look at me and monitor how this feels, or to look at some object in the room and tell me how they are similar and dissimilar to that object, and to notice how they feel as they report this. I might ask for physical details as to how an interaction with a loved one went last week, and ask the client to notice what he/she is aware of as the story is related.

The second part of treatment is the Owning phase. This phase of labor has to do with the intensity of change, the intensifying and fully dilating contractions of delivering a transformed self. In the session, the Owning phase deals with the client finding the power and ability to move and heal herself, to find more self-regulation. There are four different mechanisms that enable the client to find this power.

Breath

The first mechanism is breath, which literally functions as fuel for movement. When the client consciously breathes more fully into an emerging body awareness, whether it be a thought, a vibration or a sensation, her breath creates a field in which the physical body can deeply feel a sensation and let it be completely "owned."

I frequently ask clients to breathe more fully into a thought, sensation or vibration that is arising. The awareness and also the process of how the awareness is habitually stopped can then become more vivid. I encourage the client to tolerate and even invite this experience to go wherever it wants to go, thus orienting the client to how the process wants to naturally occur in a complete manner, without the stoppage.

Frequently this heats things up. The client may feel frightened as feelings or movements intensify. Feelings become intense after being held back, much like water accumulated behind a dam will gush dramatically as the dam bursts. Letting the water out in waves of breath allows the energy to sequence in a friendlier manner.

Description

The second way in which the client empowers herself through the Owning phase is by describing "what is," very accurately. This requires that the client tells the complete truth about her direct experience in the moment. No withholds, no secrets, no allusions or oblique references. They will say things like "now my jaw hurts," or "I'm afraid I'm going to die," or "I hate this experience. It reminds me of my father." As they say these things they connect with their power to be completely themselves, without fear of conditional love or attention.

Quite often clients have been wounded by not being allowed to tell the truth. I have one client whose parents could not stand for him to be in pain, so they would deny he ever had any. They would say, "You are not sad, you are just tired and hungry," or "You don't need to be upset, we will take care of it." Consequently, he had a lot of difficulty in sustaining feelings that might be interpreted as negative, and would transform these feelings into confusion. The first time he was able to tell me he was angry about something he shook so violently his teeth began to clatter. I supported him to let the shaking happen, and by the end of the session he was jumping up and down yelling "Whoopee!" and grinning from ear-to-ear. He subsequently reported having more energy than he had had in years.

Feeling Feelings

Feeling feelings is the third way clients move through the Owning Phase. It is not enough to be aware of feelings, or to talk about them. If they are there, they must be felt directly in order to complete the movement that they engender. At this point, the therapist simply encourages the client to feel what they are feeling exactly the way it is, with the exact amount of intensity that it carries. This emotional accuracy is very important, as it can be harmful to arbitrarily exaggerate a feeling in order to have an intense experience. Intense experiences can often be mistaken for profound ones. Valuing intensity creates drama junkies, or people who exaggerate in order to feel or express anything.

Feeling ones' feelings has a natural complement in expression. In fact, unless the oscillatory loop of feeling and expression in the energetic body is completed, feelings remain incomplete and stored in the body until they can create another opportunity for their completion. Feelings are expressed in movement, and movement is the fourth form of fuel for empowering the Owning Phase.

Movement

Without physical movement, the other bodies do not have the support they need to sustain their own movement. When physical movement is blocked, eventually energy tends to wane. Thoughts grow sluggish, and clients are said to be depressed. Physical movement is used in the Owning Phase to keep the loop of sensation, energy and thought as a constant source of nourishment. Again, it is important to only move when there is an impulse to do so. To arbitrarily wave arms or kick a pillow does nothing to respect or contact direct experience. When clients participate with a sensation there is a natural movement that completes it. This is the movement that the client needs to find. When a feeling is felt there is a natural movement expression that accurately matches it and completes it. When an individual thinks, thoughts are given form through physical movement. Thus, movement empowers clients to act on their experience and complete it in order to make space for new energy to arise.

In a session, it is important to keep the client attentive to how their physical body wants to move with their experience and to let them make this movement. Frequently, it is the expressive movement process that is blocked in clients, and there are several different interventions that assist the client in reclaiming this ability.

INTENSIFY MOVEMENT. The first intervention is to intensify the movement. This can be used when the client is not paying enough attention to a movement, particularly an offhand gesture or postural shift. By intensifying the movement it "turns up the volume" so that they can be more awake to what the movement is trying to tell them and do for them. Intensification can also be used when a movement that looks intense is being performed in a lethargic or inadequate manner, such as shifting one's weight instead of stomping one's foot, or holding one's hand closed instead of clenching the fist. One client recently reported feeling a chronic tension in her throat that when she exaggerated it turned into choking. As she stayed with the choking she was able to move through an old near-drowning experience, and by acknowledging her fear of death and moving with it she released the tension in her throat and reported feeling less anxious in her daily life.

CONTRASTING MOVEMENT. The second intervention to promote expressive movement in the Owning Phase is contrasting. I recently asked a client who was squeezing his eyes shut to open them wide and experience what arose when he made this contrast. Contrast can give a client a direct experience of something that they are avoiding, in this case having his eyes open and available to see what was going on around him. Contrast also can bring the client in touch with an unacknowledged duality. A client may make only small movements because she has been told that large movements are ugly and brutish. By experimenting with large movement she can begin to tolerate and even enjoy the feelings that large movements create.

MOVEMENT REPETITION. Repetition is the third expressive movement intervention of the Owning phase. This is often used with clients who do not have much physical body awareness, and feel hesitant about sustaining any awareness out of fear of the unknown. Movements that appear to have some charge to them are repeated in order to allow change to be fully expressed. Repetition often transforms movements from socially acceptable gestures into meaningful communications. When a client pointed her finger at me a few years ago, I asked her to repeat the gesture until she felt finished with it. With the support of that repeated expressive gesture she was able to move through being mad at me for challenging her, to her rage at her mother who would stand very close to her and lecture her while she had to stand still and listen.

GENERALIZATION. The fourth intervention is generalization. This means that at times a movement will be confined to one small part of the physical body when it is actually being felt throughout it. By generalizing the movement to the whole body it can be accurately expressed. An example of this would be to ask a client to go from pushing one hand into the other to pushing with her whole body. This will accurately tap the energy that the client needs to experience.

SPECIFICATION. The last intervention of Owning phase movement is specification, which is the opposite of generalization. This technique is also useful with clients who are new to expressive movement, because it can help them feel safe to channel a feeling or sensation through just one particular part of their physical body. An example here would be when a client reports feeling irritable. The therapist could ask, "How would that irritable feeling come through your eyes?" (Presumably the therapist was observing some excitation or tension in the clients' eyes that would result in directing attention to that specific area).

The next phase of treatment occurs as the client sustains her direct experience. By completing processes directly the client begins to tap into the benefits of this kind of warrior-like commitment to her natural wholeness, intelligence and ability to move. This benefit takes place in the third phase—the Appreciation Phase. It corresponds to the actual delivery of the child, where it is held and welcomed and taken care of. It is the phase where the client reclaims that which was lost due to conditional attention and fragmentation—love. Love is awakened when individuals deeply witness themselves or are witnessed deeply by another and they stay in the place of contact, not abandoning themselves or another under certain conditions.

In therapy, therapists provide a basis of loving kindness throughout treatment. The client is bathed in loving attention. This does not preclude challenging them. This bathing restores the client's original birthright of unconditional care. The Appreciation Phase is the place in treatment where the client can transfer from relying on the therapist's loving kindness (like the fetus relying on the mother's body for life) to discovering their own.

Acceptance phase processes often involve the client loving himself actively. This can take the form of self-touch, self-affirmation, compassion towards difficult imprints that were taken on, and forgiveness towards people or events that forced us into those imprints. The therapist assists this by supportive touch where appropriate, active listening, and guided questions and comments that stimulate love to permeate the clients' bodies. I remember a client some time ago who allowed herself to deeply mourn the early death of her mother through all her bodies. As her sobs and movements subsided, I came close to her and when she opened her eyes I smiled and said "hi." I

took her hand and stroked it for five minutes while she rested. When she opened her eyes again, I told her how glad I was to see her, how radiant she looked, and how glad I was that she let me share her experience. She began to cry softly again, this time maintaining eye contact with me. She then stated that it felt like the first time in her life since her mother died that she did not feel alone. I encouraged her to explore the feeling of not being alone and to own it in her body. She breathed into this experience so deeply that she was able to subsequently sustain it more consistently in her daily life.

The last phase of treatment corresponds to postnatal care and the entering of the newborn into the world of gravity, air and material objects—the Action Phase. In the physical body, the transition is made by practicing moving in gravity, i.e., in the vertical, standing plane. Most of the client's daily life occurs in this plane, and any physical changes that may have happened in the session need to be experienced and integrated into the upright body. This may include walking, looking, gesturing, and breathing. The client mentioned above felt a great opening in her chest after her deep mourning. As we got back into the vertical dimension I asked her to pay attention to how she could use this expansion in her chest as she walked. She noticed that her shoulders could relax and that her arms could swing more freely, and she spent a few minutes just practicing this new walk.

In the energetic body, the Action phase transition almost always involves the client's practice of having and using more energy. The coaching of this phase involves finding new fuller breath patterns that help the energy to integrate. Patterned or locomotor movement also grounds energy, giving it a focus and a form. The Action Phase often involves moving in ways that give one's energy a satisfying place to go.

In the cognitive body, the Action Phase usually involves some talking that gets the client used to cognitively moving rather than cognitively fixating. Especially important is to practice bringing the other bodies into thinking by sensing, breathing, and moving at the same time. For instance, one can ask the client to remember what she believed about herself when she came in and while breathing and moving to sense if this still felt true. Long-held attitudes and assumptions, which are forms of fixated cognition, can be released in this manner. Clients can also spend time integrating past memories or current relationship problems that can be addressed by allowing their thoughts to have movement and dialogue with the other bodies.

In these ways, the birth of the whole client is facilitated and witnessed. The four phases of treatment most often occur in one session, but can take anywhere from a few minutes to a few years. This especially depends on the severity of the wounding in each client. Many birthings can take place over the course of treatment as the client moves through more complex issues and deeper and fuller layers of aliveness.

THE THERAPIST TRAINING CYCLE

Because I developed the Moving Cycle while steeped in an academic environment, I consistently looked for ways to coherently teach the material in an embodied form. So as the Moving Cycle developed, so did the Therapist Training Cycle, because it became obvious that learning followed the same sequence that healing did. In the Therapist Training Cycle, learning clinical skill occurs in four stages, which mirror the stages of the Moving Cycle.

Stage 1: The Witness Function–The ability to pay unconditional and varied attention to oneself and the client. Attending to the phenomenon of attention as a healing tool.

Stage 2: The Responder Function–(1) The ability to recognize when the session is in the present moment and when it is being driven by the unfinished history of the therapist and/or the client. (2) The cultivation of intuition, and being able to distinguish between intuition and projection. (3) The cultivation of therapeutic intention that honors the client, the therapist, and the community.

Stage 3: The Dialoguer Function–The ability to stay in an unconditional relationship with oneself and the client, and to use this relationship as a healing force. The cultivation of compassion.

Stage 4: The Facilitator Function–The ability to introduce technical interventions and facilitate the processes generated by these interventions in a timely, nonaggressive, and provocative manner.

Witness Function

As students enter this program, they first learn about the nature of attention through the Witness Function. For hours and hours, all we do is theoretically and experientially study forms and patterns of attention, the oscillation of attention, and the power of seeing and being seen. As described by Van Nuys (1971), students study the nature and process of their attention in order to de-automatize and rewire limited or dysfunctional attentional habits. Roberts and Vaughan Clark add: "The first step usually involves shifting the focus from external to internal awareness. As students become aware of their own inner states, they can begin to recognize important conditions which affect their learning ability" (in Hendricks & Fadiman, 1976, p. 5).

As children, part of an individual's upbringing involves being taught, both directly and indirectly, how to pay attention and what to pay attention to. Families, cultures, and religions give cues as to what is attentionally important, what is unimportant, and what is taboo. This kind of teaching can shape perceptual processes to such a degree that what is attended to becomes patterned into the nervous system, becomes automatic, and feels like reality, feels like the way the world is. Individuals will simply screen out that which perceptually disagrees with their attentional patterns. And what cannot be seen interiorly, cannot be seen in our clients.

These limitations of attention are patterns that actually form a kind of unconscious prejudice—"I'll pay attention to you if . . . , I'll withdraw my attention when you . . ."—that recapitulate the clients original wounding, in which he or she had to make deals with care-givers in order to receive adequate attention. In a healthy family system, attention to any one person is not constant, but it is uncondi-tional. Attention is for free; it comes with no strings attached that require individuals to modify who they are in order to get it. In therapy, attention can be used as a medi-cine—it can be directly applied to old wounds—which then reestablishes organis-mic wholeness through a willingness to let our focus go anywhere, everywhere it is needed.

In the program we attend to the process of attending, and we uncover any patterns of attention that limit therapeutic availability. One student realized that she began to space out every time her practice-partner got sad and began to cry. She was able to trace this pattern to her childhood, when her older brothers would persecute her if she cried. Another student found that she would get angry and judgmental when her partner exhibited joy, especially if the partner wig-gled his body with it. It took her a few weeks to realize she had male joy mixed up with sexual come-ons, arising from her happy-go-lucky father who had sexually abused her.

In these first experiences we also study the phenomenon of the oscillation of atten-tion. Attention, by its very nature, flits from one thing to another. It seems that attention needs to shift, to keep moving, to be in a state of flow in order to keep us healthy and happy (Speeth, 1982). When therapists are with a client, attention oscillates among the

client, self, and the surround. If the therapist fixates attention inward, she/he loses the client, and is of no use to him or her. If the therapist focuses solely on the client, she/he becomes immersed in the experience and loses self-awareness and the ability to con-tribute anything; becoming overly identified with the same process that is causing the clients suffering. If the therapist pays exclu-sive attention to the surround, she/he "spaces out" and again loses the ability to use attention as a medicine.

Attention naturally oscillates. Students learn to observe this flow as it goes out to the client, into themselves, and occasionally out to the environment. They learn to observe when this flow gets obstructed, for it is here that they also form patterns of limited atten-tion. Many, many students assume that they must give all their attention to the client in order to be "good therapists." It can be a shock to learn that this is actually a co-dependent state, one in which they take all their cues from the external environment. When attention oscillates, the therapist remains refreshed and centered, able to take care of him or herself. Paying exclusive attention to the client results in overwork and fatigue. Paying exclusive attention to oneself or the environment is unethical.

In the Somatic Psychology program, we train the recovery of the oscillation of atten-tion. We do this by pairing up the students, and one person becomes the mover while the other simply witnesses. The movers spend about 20 minutes moving freely and expressively in whatever way they want. This process is designed to bring up uncon-scious material; similar to the way dreams float up images, free movement accesses kinesthetic memory, physical archetypes, and suppressed feeling states. The Witness observes the mover, while also practicing oscillating attention and becoming aware of patterns of attention. Afterwards, the Witnesses report their findings to the group, and discuss what they have discovered.

The Witness function is a training tool

where students encounter any obstacles they have in seeing themselves, their partner, and the environment unconditionally. The process is related to and facilitated by meditation practice, but exists on its own as an instruction in attentional habits, their effect on perceiving others "suchness," practices that dissolve conditioned attentional patterns, and the conscious use of varied attentional states as a form of therapeutic intervention.

Responder Function

The next phase of training involves what is called the Responder Function. In this phase we use the same pairing of trainees as we did with the Witness. The seated trainee spends a few moments purely Witnessing, and then moves into nonverbally expressing whatever comes into his or her awareness. If the student gets bored, she expresses boredom, making faces and gestures that convey this; if he gets excited, he moves his excitement. The mover usually has his or her eyes closed, and does not need to be aware of what the Responder is doing. In this way, the internal responses and reactions the student has to being in a witnessing relationship are made visible and tangible and workable.

The task is to become exquisitely aware of the difference between intuition and projection. The Responder Function flushes up and deals with countertransference. The assumption inherent here is that students do not see their projections until they reveal them, and feel them through their bodies. In psychotherapies where the therapist/client relationship is valued and cultivated, this ability to identify and work with therapist projections becomes critical. In this way therapists can learn to trust their intuition. Jung (1933) defined intuition as a perception of realities that are not known to consciousness. A projection can be defined as an *assumption* of reality that arises from unfinished business stored in the unconscious. Experientially finding the distinction

between these two phenomena is crucial for any therapist.

Semantically and somatically, we work with the difference between response and reaction. We define response as the in-the-moment energies with the clients, and reaction as a state in which the student/therapist's own unconscious, incomplete issues and agendas arise and disguise themselves as feelings in the current setting. Vaughan Clark (1973) has stated that "The problem of determining when a perception is truly intuitive, in the sense that it apprehends reality, or when it is imaginary, or simply a function of personal projection, is a function of intellectual discrimination" (p. 161). This is like asking the fox to guard the chicken coop. One cannot tell by thinking whether or not thinking is accurate. The best way to begin to distinguish these two states is through the direct experience of the body. In response, the body remains open, alert, and shifting with the various energies of the interaction of therapist/client. In reaction, some part of the body (as well as thinking) goes on hold. One student found that she squeezed her eyes whenever she got reactive. Another noticed that he got a knot in his stomach. These body signals are markers that will lead us back into personal history, back to where the past upsets got withheld, and were then set up to leak out in stimulating circumstances.

Students examine in minute detail their reactive patterns, first physically, then emotionally, then cognitively. They learn under what circumstances they arise, what their nature is, how they would act out if given free rein, and what effect they have on the therapeutic relationship.

A reaction, if left unconscious, will always result in control issues. The therapist interprets the current situation reactively, she then judges it to be good/bad, acceptable/unacceptable, and lastly she tries to either control herself or the client in order to keep the goodness there or push away the badness. Therapeutic aggression is born. A student offered this example:

> I was watching the mover when I got a feeling of irritation, and a thought came into my head that he was behaving rather shallowly. I wanted to scream at him "Get on with it, will you?" There was a squeezing in my chest as I used the Responder function to shake my finger at him. As I did this, it dawned on me that that was the way my father looked when he used to rant at me. I kept at it, and a voice in my head said, "You can't yell at people," so I imagined that I would say "Perhaps you'd like to go deeper into that feeling" to my mover. But I was still shaking my finger at him. I was making that calm statement, still trying to get him to change, to do what I wanted him to do, only now it was disguised as a therapeutic suggestion.

Everyone gets reactive. It is impossible to get rid of reactions, just as it is impossible to get rid of thoughts in meditation. In the Therapist Training Cycle, we work instead on turning the garbage of reactions into the compost of curiosity, genuineness, and integrity. The Responder Function puts reactions right up in front of our, and everyone else's, faces, where they can be exposed to the light of our awareness and attention. We learn in this classroom to even welcome reactiveness, and to get curious as to its origins, its stimuli, its usefulness.

Reactiveness carries at its core an intuitive wisdom that is currently in an unusable form. Reactivity can be of tremendous use therapeutically–it is the primary fertilizer of therapeutic relationship. If I get curious as to why I tend to get mad at a client, if I take ownership of it completely, I may discover that me and my client are behaving in ways that engender this in me so that her feelings of self-disgust can be validated. I can see that I may have fallen into acting like her mother. Or I might find that I have some unfinished wounding around my own mother. I might get triggered by women with high, thin voices. Or I might be simply colluding with my client to go away attentionally at

any time things get hot between us. These realizations bring us back into the present moment, back to the nitty gritty of the current relationship. And they bring us back with more information, more ideas about how to be of assistance.

The Responder Function trains therapeutic genuineness. It transmits a value in honesty and integrity as primary ways in which lives become workable and happy. It teaches 100 percent responsibility, and disengages responsibility from the baggage of blame or burden. Responsibility as a therapist (and as a person) becomes a willingness to own and work with whatever arises, as it is. Chogyam Trungpa, Rinpoche (1983) put it wisely when he said:

> The main point is to learn to tell the truth to your patients. Then they will respond to you, because there is power in telling the truth rather than bending your logic to fit their neurosis. Truth always works. There always has to be basic honesty; that is the source of trust. When someone sees that you are telling the truth, then they will realize further that you are saying something worthwhile and trustworthy. It always works.

Dialoguer Function

The third training function is called the Dialoguer. It is here where we study and work with any grit that has been accumulated regarding relationships. For a therapeutic relationship to be powerful and safe, the therapist must maintain an unconditional presence within it. Not having conditions about one's presence is the heart of compassion. This means that the student/therapist learns to stay in the heat generated by the contact they have with their clients. They do not withdraw or withhold if they say or do something that provokes or bores us. And relationship is about sticking in there while feeling ones feelings, telling the truth, and keeping ones agreements (Hendricks & Hendricks, 1990). The Dialoguer Function trains to flush up any unconscious deals they have made to limit or place conditions on client relationships, and it assists them in learning to tolerate and welcome increased commitment and consciousness in these relationships. Through unconditional presence, they remain open and appreciative of all that arises in the client, particularly that which the client finds ugly and unacceptable about him or herself. This is the essence of compassion.

In the classroom, we maintain our pairings, but this time the Dialoguer goes out into direct contact with his or her partner. The exchange is primarily nonverbal, as this is a profound way to bring unconscious relational patterns to the light. The two simply interact spontaneously. The Dialoguers' responsibility is to stay in the heat of the interaction and physically express whatever he or she becomes aware of. It is also to study interactional patterns that arise. Common interactional patterns are codependency, withholding, deal making, and control issues. Finding the physical correlates of these patterns is of immense value. One student discovered that he tended to fold his arms across his chest and slightly lower his head whenever he got withholding with his partner. Another found that she would smile and get "touchy" when she wanted her partner to like her.

The Dialoguer, like the Responder, asks the trainee to become transparent. Whatever is made visible is made available to the light of the teachings. Even with so-called negative reactions, uncharitable moments, or critical thoughts, the function trains them to compost these into therapeutic fertilizer rather than try to get rid of them. "Whatever I try to get rid of will stick to me in the form of a disowned projection. Whatever I expose to the light can be nourished and transformed into food. Because as the trainee I am specifically told not to facilitate my partner, I am free to play in the fields of experimentation. What works and doesn't work

when I get goofy? What happened that time when I cried? What about my boredom made sense just then?" These and other questions that arise from the training functions allow the student to deeply examine his or her inner experience in the service of clinical training. When a student later begins to actually facilitate, these behavioral experimentations will fall away, yet will have performed their purpose through cleaning ones inner house, and instilling in one the experiential education values of unconditional attention, unconditional workability of arisings, and unconditional relating.

Dialoguing can be quite vivid and challenging. One student pair I observed last year made a clear discovery regarding their patterns of initiating closeness and separation. They had been sitting facing each other for about ten minutes, playing at making faces at each other, laughing and having fun. Then one got up abruptly and walked away. The other paused for a minute, and then followed her partner around the room, trying to get her to come back, to play again. As they processed this interaction, the first student realized that she had been having so much fun that a little voice came on in her head saying "You're supposed to be working now. Stop this." She had fled the interaction in a familiar way—breaking off contact abruptly as a way to manage her self-criticism. The second student also had a voice come up. When her partner left it said "You must have done something wrong to make her leave like that. Go try to make it better for her." This also exposed a familiar relational pattern—trying to make co-dependent deals with people so they wouldn't leave.

The Dialoguer helps students to expose these patterns so that they do not become unconscious therapeutic deals with clients. It also begins to teach the concepts and dynamics of couples and family therapy experientially. In addition, it transmits spontaneous strategies in play and other experiential therapies.

Facilitator Function

After much time spent in these first three functions, the trainees then take on the task of therapizing, through the Facilitator Function. It is here where the concepts and behaviors of being in service to another are studied and practiced. Experimental behaviors from the Witness, Responder, and Dialoguer are internalized, and the student focuses on allowing the spontaneous arisings in the therapeutic container to be channeled towards the healing and transformation of the client. In this light, five interventions and five intentions are introduced. The intentions offer guidelines for addressing broad therapeutic needs, and the interventions are specific cues that facilitate the filling of therapeutic needs through transpersonal values. The five intentions are:

1. **To Support**–Like an adult holding the bike seat and running alongside as a child learns to ride, supporting is an intention to provide extra energy in a client's process until they can support themselves. Example: noticing and remarking on a client's honesty until she can affirm her honest nature for herself.

2. **To Nurture**–A welcoming of the clients whole being. An affirming of their basic goodness and right to be whole. Example: "I so appreciate your willingness to keep showing up here week after week and working with your fears."

3. **To Challenge**–A refusing to collude with an addictive process, whether it be an addiction to a way of thinking, an emotional pattern, or a physical substance. Example: Calling a client on her tendency to use anger as a smoke screen for intimacy fears.

4. **To Reflect**–A mirroring of what the client is doing, a reality check. Example: "I notice that every time you talk about your father you pull on your beard."

5. **To Provide Space**–Allowing a client to discover themselves by themselves; an attentive waiting that gives the client time to explore. Example: Sitting quietly while a client's attention goes inside to feel what he or she is feeling.

Trainees learn in the Facilitator Function to notice and consciously choose intentions that are consonant with the clients' growth needs. They do this through maintaining their working pairs and practicing in mock sessions. Students also practice the interventions previously mentioned in this article–repeat, contrast, intensify, specify, and generalize.

All the above interventions are designed to liberate the energy stored in disowned parts of the client, whether that is in the body, the emotions, or the thoughts. This energy is then made available for the clients' healing and growth. The Facilitator Function also teaches that therapy is client-centered and driven, by learning to use spontaneous interactions and processes that are right there in the session. Students learn to literally facilitate on their feet, dropping agendas and working with what is uncovered when the experiential conditions of unconditional attention, unconditional honesty, and unconditional commitment are present.

CONCLUSION

The Moving Cycle continues to reveal itself and shape itself. To hold it too dear and see it as revealed truth would negate its power and our creativity. I hope and trust that my students will continue to shape it according to their witnessing experiences. In some respects, I will feel satisfied if this Cycle feels simple and obvious to the reader, taken for granted like the healing of a cut on one's finger. It should describe processes that are visible and familiar to all. It is then that therapist, student and practitioner alike can know that even though all held views are wrong, they might have relaxed enough to get this one as accurate as possible.

REFERENCES

Assagioli, R. (1973). *Meditation.* New York: Psychosynthesis Research Foundation.

Brown, S. (1994). Animals at play. *National Geographic* 186: 2–35.

Chogyam Trungpa, Rinpoche. (1983). Creating an environment of sanity. *Naropa Institute Journal of Psychology.* Boulder, CO: Nalanda Press.

Darwin, C. (1998). *The expression of emotion in man and animals.* New York: Oxford University Press.

Davis, J. & Wright, C. (1987). Content of undergraduate transpersonal psychology courses. Stanford, CA: *The Journal of Transpersonal Psychology,* vol 19, no 2.

Deikman, A. (1971). Bimodal Consciousness. *Archives of General Psychiatry,* December.

Dychtwald, K. (1977). *Bodymind.* New York: Pantheon Books.

Frager, R. (1974). A proposed model for a graduate program in transpersonal psychology. Stanford, CA: *The Journal of Transpersonal Psychology,* vol 6, no 2.

Grof, S. (1985). *Beyond the brain: Birth, death and transcendence in psychotherapy.* Albany, NY: SUNY Press.

Hanna, T. (198)7. *The Body of life.* New York: Alfred A. Knopf.

Hendricks, G. & Fadman, J. (1976). *Transpersonal education: A curriculum for feeling and being.* Englewood Cliffs, NJ: Prentice-Hall.

Hendricks, G. & Weinhold, B. (1982). *Transpersonal approaches to counseling and psychotherapy.* Denver: Love Publishing.

Hendricks, G. & Hendricks, K. (1990). *Conscious loving.* New York: Bantam.

Jordan, J., Surrey, J., Kaplan, A. (1991). *Women's growth in connection.* New York: Guilford press.

Jacobson, E. (1967). *The Biology of emotions.* Springfield, IL: Charles C Thomas.

Jung, C. (1933). *Psychological types.* New York: Harcourt.

Keleman, S. (1975). *Your body speaks its mind.* New York: Simon and Schuster.

Keleman, S. (1985). *Emotional anatomy.* Berkeley: Center Press.

Levine, S. (1987). *Healing into life and death.* Garden City, NY: Anchor Press.

Lewis, P. (1984). *Theoretical approaches to dance-movement therapy Vol. 1.* Dubuque, IA: Kendall/Hunt.

Maslow, A. (1971). *The farther reaches of human nature.* New York: Penguin Books.

May, R. (1975). *The courage to create.* New York: Bantam Books.

Murphy, M. (1992). *The Future of the body.* Los Angeles: Jeremy P. Tarcher

Perls, F. (1969). *In and out of the garbage pail.* New York: Bantam

Redmond, H. (1974). A pioneer program in transpersonal education. Stanford, CA: *The Journal of Transpersonal Psychology,* vol. 6, no. 1.

Speeth, K. (1982). On psychotherapeutic attention. Stanford, CA: *The Journal of Transpersonal Psychology,* vol 14, no 2.

Steiner, C. (1974). *Scripts people live: Transactional analysis of life scripts.* New York: Bantam.

Swimme, B. & Berry, T. (1992). *The universe story.* San Fransisco: Harper.

Van Nuys, D. (1971). A novel technique for studying attention during meditation. Stanford, CA: *The Journal of Transpersonal Psychology,* vol 3, no. 2.

Vaughan, Clark, F. (1973). Exploring intuition: Prospects and possibilities. Stanford, CA: *The Journal of Transpersonal Psychology,* vol 5, no 2.

Williamson, M. (1992). *A return to love: Reflections on the principles of a course in miracles.* New York: Harper Perennial.

Winnicot, D.W. (1965). *The maturational process and the facilitating environment.* New York: International University Press.

Wolf, E. (1988). *Treating the self.* New York: Guilford Press.

Further graduate training:

Dr. Christine Caldwell
Naropa University
Department of Somatics Psychology
2130 Arapahoe Avenue
Boulder, Colorado 80302
303-245-4845
www.naropa.edu

Chapter 17

INTEGRATIVE ENERGY MEDICINE AS A HEALING ART

ELAINE MCNULTY

GENESIS

People often ask me how I became interested in energy work. This is a question I usually avoid answering but it is relevant to this chapter in order to understand the evolution of my work. I have always been interested in a holistic approach to health and researched nutrition and natural remedies for healing in my early twenties and thirties. About 20 years ago, my husband was diagnosed with a very rare form of cancer. Very little was known about this type of cancer and the prognosis was unclear. We were devastated by the news, but rebounded with a positive and hopeful attitude. My husband was a, seemingly, healthy young man in his late thirties who exercised regularly, ate well and was a nonsmoker and nondrinker. The odds seemed to be in his favor. Over a period of time I watched this strong, robust man become physically weak and emotionally fragile from the toxic drugs used to treat the cancer. Dealing with the emotional side of the experience was especially difficult for him. All of his defenses were stripped away. He transformed from an emotionally strong person to one who became emotionally anxious just at the thought of chemotherapy. Coping with these new emotions was upset-

ting to him and destroyed his confidence and self-esteem.

I began to realize that the doctors had no other tools besides these toxic drugs. When questioned, they defended the treatments, while at the same time, admitting that they did not really know whether they could stabilize or cure his cancer. This realization, combined with lack of results, spurred me on to take charge. I bought every book I could find on cancer cures and success stories of those who had survived cancer. I took time off from work to read and do research. I began to explore alternative therapies. Visualization techniques, positive affirmations and the relaxation response methodologies, as well as concepts, such as, the mind/body connection were gaining recognition in the literature at that time. There was little or no information published on body-centered energy work. But, this was a start.

The concept of taking charge of your own healing was not in my husband's repertoire. He remained faithful to the medical model and was only minimally open to exploring alternatives. We became involved in macrobiotics and met several people who had "cured" themselves of cancer by changing their diet and life-style. These contacts led to various other people who practiced nontraditional techniques. I remember one practitioner we went to was a counselor who practiced a form of energy work called Polarity. While talking to my husband, who was in considerable pain, she positioned her hands in his energy field in such a way that deflected the pain. We both found this really amazing. She also was able to identify where all the tumors were in my husband's body. Initially, he found this very disconcerting and upsetting. How could anyone know this? We, ultimately, met up with a healer from the Philippines who had incredible healing powers. He was very intuitive and had powerful healing energy. He, also, was able to tell my husband where all the cancer was. This destabilized his prior belief system but at the same time, opened the door to spiritual and emotional healing.

This was a very arduous, stressful and painful process. When I look back I don't know how I did all that I did. My husband did not survive his cancer and died 3 years almost to the exact day that he was told the survivor statistics of his type of cancer (no one had lived more than 3 years). Although I would not wish this experience on anyone, I learned some profound truths through my own healing process.

I learned that I cannot heal anyone else. I can only support them in their own process. Healing is much more than a physical cure and can happen on many levels. Profound healing may take place on the spiritual and emotional levels but not on the physical level. Or, healing may occur on all levels even those of which we are not consciously aware. I had to accept that healing might not mean a cure or yield the exact results that I wanted, but that healing occurs nonetheless.

After my husband died, I studied with the same healer for about a year and then avidly began pursuing my curiosity about energy work and healing.

THE INTEGRATIVE PHILOSOPHIC MODEL

The foundation of my work is constructed on several beliefs. These primary beliefs evolved from my 20-year search to locate the best methods of healing. I was searching for methods that would achieve lasting results and free the individual from old patterns, physical ailments, karmic and genealogical ties, and support archetypal energies to accomplish their dreams and goals. The process of gaining greater learning and gnosis is ongoing and ever evolving.

View of the Individual

All individuals are energy beings. Individuals are energy beings as a unique microcosm and at the same time, part of a larger cosmos or universal field as a macrocosm. This energy, of which humans are comprised, is called the Life Force. This very Force keeps bodies alive. This energy is motion.

View of Health and Trauma

MOVEMENT. Motion is movement. Movement is health. Where there is no movement, there is no health. Every interaction with a person, place or thing is about an experience, an exchange of energy, either positive or negative which contributes or impacts human health in some way on a conscious and unconscious level.

TRAUMA. Second, I believe that essentially everything that people go to a healer for is about trauma and within trauma there is a message. Trauma , as defined by Webster's dictionary, is a distressful experience that results in physical and psychological shock. Peter Levine, in his book, *Waking the Tiger*, states that trauma is difficult to define accurately and therefore, difficult to recognize.

He further states that there are many experiences that would not be defined as trauma but that the body unconsciously perceives as threatening and is subsequently traumatizing (1999, p. 25).

DISTORTED AND LIMITING BELIEFS. Third, as a result of life's experience, positive or negative, the individual forms a set of beliefs about how life is. These beliefs become the filters for how the individual interacts in the world. When presented with an external event, the individual unconsciously checks out the experience or situation against these filters. These filters represent internal representation of attitudes, memories, values and beliefs, decisions, and perceptions of time and space. Based on the information in the internal representation system the individual deletes, distorts or generalizes the experience or event. The phrase or saying "What we think, we become" begins to have significance. If the distortions can be cleared in individuals' beliefs systems, and they see themselves in the world as they truly are rather than through the lens of their past histories, associations, and traumas, they can clear blocked energy that has manifested in emotional and physical distress.

Integrative Healing Work

My work integrates several therapies and creates a partnership with the client to facilitate the individual's "Remembering who they are," that is, realizing their life's purpose, and their path on this earth plane. The ultimate goal is for the Soul to find free expression through the body of the individual although this may never be explicitly stated. This is an elegant process of awakening and unfolding through which the individual rediscovers a sense of self. This process is assisted by releasing, clearing and/or healing limiting beliefs and blocked energies which have curtailed individuals from accessing their deepest wisdom, their inner resources. By connecting with who they are, remembering how to access their inner resources, living in and through the force within, and actually becoming one with that force, individuals can find harmony, balance and joy in their lives.

Clients come for all kinds of presenting issues, from managing and reducing stress to chronic issues of fatigue, illness, depression, anxiety, pain, phobias, relationship issues, physical and emotional abuse, low self-esteem, career issues, autoimmune deficiencies, overall trauma issues, feeling stuck and not knowing why, to simple maintenance of health and well-being through energy work balancing.

INTEGRATIVE APPROACHES AND TECHNIQUES

The theoretical and technical foundations of my work are based on Dr. Stone's Polarity Therapy, Guided Self Healing developed by Andy Hahn, Psy.D. and Judith Swack, Ph.D.; CranioSacral Therapy based on Franklin Sills; the Sutherland Approach and Neurolinguistic Programming (NLP). Other resources are: Reiki (3rd Degree, Master Practitioner), The Universal Calibration Lattice and Electromagnetic Field Balancing by Peggy Dubro, Certified Teacher; and ARCH, Rainbow Spirit of Transformation. My work is an integration of these modalities through which I facilitate the healing process in partnership with the client. Through these approaches we are able to access the energy field, clear and shift energy patterns which often results in profound healing.

Polarity therapy was the first formal modality that I studied and continues to be the basic foundation from which I work. Craniosacral therapy is actually embedded in Polarity Therapy and significantly changed my work. However, Guided Self-Healing added the techniques to achieve profound life changing results. It will be helpful to review the basic principles of these modalities, the concepts of how energy flows and how and why it affects our physical bodies and our well-being.

Polarity Therapy

Dr. Stone, the founder of Polarity Therapy, studied healing all over the world in search of the key to health and well-being. He knew that lasting healing was more than just a biological process but there was a missing piece. His travels eventually brought him to the Far East where he studied Chinese and Ayurvedic medicine. Here he discovered what he believed to be the missing piece. He determined that the missing link between Eastern and Western medicine was energy. His teachings and work are based on Chinese and Ayurvedic principles of energy medicine.

Dr. Stone's writings are presented in two volumes of notes that consist of many charts, diagrams, and esoteric writing about energy and health. Upon first encounter his writing was rather overwhelming and confusing. It was many years before I could actually pick up Stone's books and even read his writings and research to decipher its meaning. As I have studied various other disciplines, I keep coming back to the teachings of Stone. I now realized how far advanced he was in his thinking and appreciate the depth of his understanding of the ancient teachings.

Simply stated, Dr. Stone believed that health is the fluent and harmonious movement of energy at subtler levels. Stone said, "true health is the harmony of life within us, consisting of peace of mind, happiness and well being" (Stone, 1986, p. 20). In order to achieve this level of harmony, individuals must be aware of whom they are and make connections to this energy. Mind and body are one unit. What individuals think they become. "Mind energy creates patterns which become feeling, perception, consciousness, the root of all senses and the awareness of all sensations in and through the form of matter" (Stone, 1986, p. 19). Our life's experience, from the very moment of conception, becomes imprinted in our system.

Traditional Eastern cultures believed in treating the whole individual. They believe that there is a greater realm or larger force underlying both mental and physical planes in which there is a network of subtler relationships. To be in relationship there is an energetic interaction which is an exchange of energy between each participant. A relationship where there is movement or an active exchange is considered dynamic. One in which there is no movement is stagnant or lifeless. These relationships must be in harmony for they're to order.

The East sees the natural order, not as a mechanical process composed of multiple parts, but as a complete, whole interrelated dynamic in which man is an integral part. The wholeness is reflected in the relationships of the world and of the cosmos. The seasons, life and death; ecosystems; movement of the planets and stars, all are interrelated and interdependent aspects of it. (Sills, 1989, p. 2)

In contrast Western medicine sees things as separate. The West treats the symptoms of illness and not the cause. It breaks things into parts as separate from the whole. Generally, the West views the individual as separate from his environment, emotions and life-style.

AYURVEDA is the most ancient form of medicine in the world. It is the forerunner of all the other great systems of medicine. The guiding principles are believed to have been handed down from the Hindu gods to the great seers. The written texts of Ayurveda date back 3500 years. The concepts are incredibility complex and advanced. The concepts still form the basis of much Indian medicine today. Ayurveda is a Sanskrit word derived from two root words "Ayus" and "Vid" meaning life and knowledge respectively. Ayus and life represents a combination of the body, the sense organs, the mind, and the soul. Therefore, broadly speaking, Ayurveda means knowledge concerning the maintenance of life. Ayurveda aims to prevent illness and to balance mind, body and spirit. People are treated before illness has a chance to manifest. The Ayurvedic practitioner looks/assesses the whole person's lifestyle in order to ensure imbalances will not reoccur.

Both Chinese and Ayurvedic philosophies hold the belief that there is a greater whole or higher force of which we are a part. Dr. Stone believed that life is a reflection of that greater whole or higher power. He said that "Life is movement and movement is the manifestation of energy or that vital force" (Stone, 1986, p. 6). All manifestation depends on change. Change implies movement. For any form to come into being there must be movement. According to Chinese philosophy movement begins with a subtle pulsation from source. Stone called this movement of energy "Life Force." Others have referred to it as Chi or Prana. In order for movement to continue in motion, Stone observed that movement sets up a relationship with opposing forces or fields. This relationship is called a 'polarity.' This relationship of opposites which creates movement is called the "Polarity Principle." Polarity is a relationship that sets up movement. One pole directly opposes the other in relationship and movement is set up between them due to this opposition. This has been seen as the basic law that governs all life. Any kind of energy flow whether it is atomic, electrical energy, X-rays etc. is guided by this principle or law.

STEP-DOWN PROCESS. The Polarity Principle states that energy moves outward from the source or a source, to some completion and then must return back to the source. Dr. Stone states that the center of consciousness is the meeting place of the outgoing energy and the inflowing current of sensation (1986). This is generally referred to as the "step-down" process of spirit into form.

More specifically, the universal energy (conscious energy) emanates from a center in a "step-down" process that follows a cycle. This cycle is the golden spiral described in a subsequent paragraph. This step-down process occurs in graduated phases within a continuous process. As energy radiates outward away from source it moves towards a neutral center creating fields of force. Dr. Stone calls these fields units of *Intelligence* and *Mind.* He further states that these units of intelligence differentiate the many from the One but are still a part of the Whole or One. He equates this concept/process to bubbles in the ocean, separate but still related to the whole.

The Fibronacci progression of repeating patterns underlies the radiation of energy in nature and speaks to the organizing forces of the universe.[1] As the energy steps down into form it creates fields within fields. Each field of energy has its own resonant frequency of the step-down process of spirit into the material realm. There are fundamental resonances that are the inner vibrational basis of all phenomena (Burger, 1998).

Dr. Stone describes 5 stages of stepped-down mind energy currents. These mind energy currents build the body in embryonic life according to definitive creative patterns (Stone, 1986, p. 44). As described earlier, energy emanates from a center in an outgoing force. Burger adds that this energy follows a Golden Spiral (one of the key repeating patterns) (Burger, 1998). Franklin Sills describes the movement process as one of expansion, slowing down, exhaustion, tension and then form. This process is gradual and continuous. Stone stated in his writings back in the forties and fifties that "God Geometrizes." He was referring to these repeating patterns. Gregg Braden refers to

1. The Fibonacci progression is a mathematical sequence that is produced by starting with 1 and adding the last two numbers in progression to arrive at the next (1, 1, 2, 3, 5, 8, 13, 21, 34, 55, 89, 144, etc.) These ratios show up extensively in nature in logarithmic spirals that underlie the process of growth. Similar patterns arise in sunflowers and other plants whose leaves grow in a spiral around a central stem. Burger, *Esoteric Antaomy*, Berkeley, California, 1998, p. 144.

this in his teaching of Sacred Geometry as well as Drunvelo Melchesideck in the "Flower of Life." The same patterns are repeated throughout the universe.

HUMAN ENERGY FIELDS AND THE STEP-PING DOWN OF THOUGHTS. The first two step-downs are the causal field and the mental plane. The next five steps are elemental harmonics that underlie matter: the five elements of air, water, fire, earth, ether. The causal realm is where consciousness crystallizes as Mind. This is not a part of physical form as yet but is a layer where thoughts arise. The next step-down phase, the Astral or mental realm, is where thoughts take on feeling or the qualities of subtle emotional charge. It is here that thought and feeling step down into physical form and have a direct impact on patterns of health or disease. Many new-age texts and teachers now understand that to completely heal an issue, pattern etc. one must connect the thought and feeling to the issue or event to get to the root of the issue or trauma. The same is true for clients to manifest what they want; they must connect it with pure feeling and the intention. In other words, they must really believe in what they are asking for and clear any feelings or thoughts that are not in alignment with the intention(s). This concept of how thought steps down into the body is key to manifestation and healing.

AYURVEDIC GUNAS. Stone used the Ayurvedic model to explain the qualities of polarity relationship. The Ayurvedic system explains energy relationships as driven by three forces called Gunas. There is a neutral force which is the essence and stillness, the positive or yang force which is the driving aspect or the action and the negative force or the yin phase which has the qualities of contraction. These forces are the substructures of the Wireless Anatomy of Man as described by Stone.

As the energy pulses outward from source it goes through various step down phases, expanding outward, reaching a point of completion, and contracting, creating fields within fields until energy crystallizes into physical form. When the energy approaches physical form it moves down through the forehead or third eye forming the 6 energy centers of the chakras and the four oval fields for the elements: ether, air, fire water, earth. With each step-down, the energy becomes denser.

CHAKRAS. The chakras are the source of energy flow for the five elements (air, water, fire, earth, ether) (Sills, 1989). The chakras and the elements generate many energy patterns that support physical form. Each chakra and each element govern specific systems and physiological processes (see Figure 17-1, The three currents and Figure 17-2, The relationship of the five elements in involution and evolution in the disease process).

THE TREATMENT GOALS. The object of treatment is to remove energy blocks. Understanding the flow of energy and the step-down process, the relationship of emotions, thoughts, and feelings and the crystallization of form allows a therapist to work with an individual to facilitate healing. The wireless anatomy is the foundation of equalized current flow for health. It's unbalanced distribution causes disease—linking mental and emotional currents to physiology to bring the whole focus of man's being into therapy. Stone has said that many tools do not make a good mechanic. Skill rests in understanding the system and step-down process of energy flow.

Guided Self Healing

Guided Self Healing is a healing methodology used to work with trauma imprints and to clear/heal specific trauma structures. Guided Self Healing emanated from the innovative work of Judith Swack Ph.D. in working with phobias and her Healing from the Body Level Up technology. In her research article on trauma, Swack (1994) reports that the body does not distinguish between physical and emotional (psychological) trauma. And in fact, at the first moment

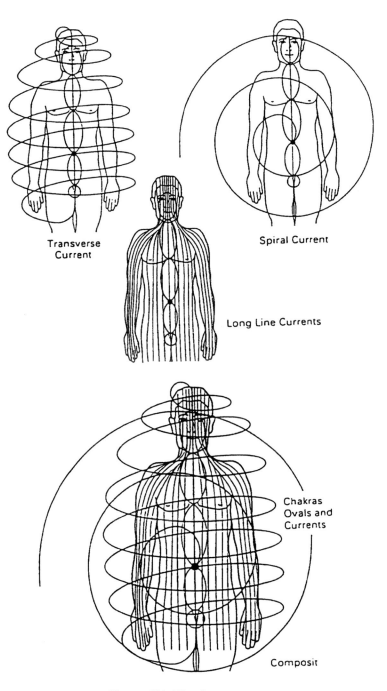

Transverse Current

Spiral Current

Long Line Currents

Chakras Ovals and Currents

Composit

Figure 17-1. The three currents.

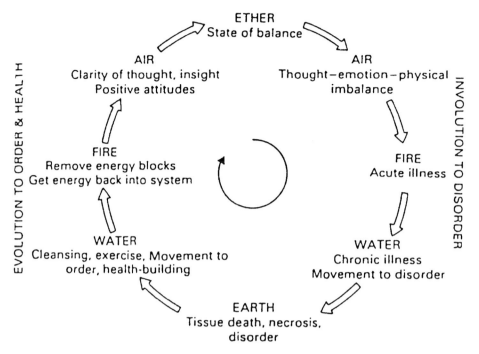

Figure 17-2. The relationship of the five elements in
involution and evolution in the disease process.

of shock, surprise, or fright, the mind and body become frozen in the experience that creates an imprint of the wound. This template formed by the imprint then becomes the basis for responding to future experiences, even after the original event is forgotten.

Andy Hahn, Psy.D. collaborated with Swack in researching various trauma patterns. Hahn expanded upon the work by mapping three centers affected by trauma: the mental, affective (emotional) and body centers. The mental center stores the beliefs that result from decisions made during the trauma. These beliefs may be about self, others, life, or God. The emotional center holds the response to the trauma and the emotions that are usually blocked. The body center holds major boundary violations which might be experienced as feeling unsafe, being rigid, shut down, or vulnerable. Each center may hold a piece of the trauma imprint. The effects of the trauma may

become splintered into what seems like separate symptoms. It is these symptoms that may be the underlying cause of illness and disease, mental disorders, autoimmune problems, addictions, compulsions, relationship problems, extreme stress, etc.

Trauma is a common fact of modern life. Many have been traumatized in their lives. Many may not even be aware of the consequences of trauma in daily life. Peter Levine's (1997) research on trauma has made a significant contribution to the understanding of how the body responds to a traumatic event. As noted above, an individual's response to a traumatic event or experience is usually associated with shock, fear and/or anxiety. The event itself is traumatizing to the nervous system. The experience creates an instinctual primitive response in the body that momentarily immobilizes the system. The individual experiences a sort of freezing effect. The longer the immobility, the greater the trauma. This freezing of the system formulates an energy pattern that remains trapped or locked in the nervous system creating a block or imprint.

The effects of tragic and violent events which the individual experiences is rather obvious, such as natural disasters, violence, serious injuries, accidents and sudden loss cause extreme stress. The effects of mild traumas are not so obvious but are still processed by the nervous system and interpreted by and stored in the unconscious. An example of mild trauma may be someone being frightened by a dog as a child, being left alone, getting lost, someone saying something unkind to us, being made fun of, not getting our way etc. All such experiences result in immobility or freezing, even if for just a moment, which creates a block in energy flow and the creation of an opinion and belief about the experience. This acts like static in the system that prevents individuals from accessing their inner wisdom.

As I mentioned previously, it is my belief that everything that people go to a healer for is about a trauma. Within each trauma there is a message. Through all of life's experiences, positive or traumatic, the individual forms a set of beliefs about how life is. These beliefs become the filters for how we interact in the world. If we can access the story behind the trauma and find the right key to unlock the immobility in the body, we can resolve the trauma, free up the energy and effect healing.

Guided self healing is a process that identifies the trauma that wounded individuals and assists them in finding the key to unlock the blocked energy and heal the wound. In the description of how energy manifests into physical form, the process of energy emanating from source or oneness stepping down into the physical form has been discussed. As this happens individuals experience what feels like a distancing or separation from this Source or from God. In other words, by entering the physical world, individuals experience God and themselves as separate in a dualistic state. This is a trauma that

imprints on the unconscious level. They may feel abandoned. They are physically and emotionally traumatized in countless ways reinforcing their sense of separateness. These represent basic core issue traumas and are extremely significant. Everyone experiences this separation as part of the stepdown process. As individuals and as a collective, humans develop many strategies to avoid any possibility of facing this separation trauma. Why is this so? Each individual has their own set of experiences as part of who they are. Embedded in these experiences are core beliefs of not feeling worthy, good enough etc. that fuel the avoidance. Individuals instinctively avoid these issues because they are afraid that what is thought might be true. For some, this might be named as the shadow side or dark side.

Guided self healing assists the individual to bring into consciousness the belief systems, the wounds, the emotional upset, and the blocked energy into the light. Individuals can now make choices that bring the deeper knowing, the wisdom, the intelligence of the system, and the part that remembers into the healing process.

Craniosacral Therapy

Craniosacral therapy is a noninvasive hands-on therapy with the primary focus of maintaining health and well-being in the human body. The health of the system is always present, never wavering, and always constant. Craniosacral therapists are trained to palpate the health of the system, assist the system in freeing up restrictions and fully access the health.

Dr. James Jealous defines the health as "the emergence of originality." "Originality expresses a complete balance of both the structure and function as intentionalized in the creation of a human being" (Jealous, 1994, p. 1).

Health or "Originality" is expressed through the body in rhythmic motions that create patterns of involuntary movement as the motion interacts with the tissues, fluids and bones of the body. There is a force within the motion that is the organizing principle. This is called the Life Force or the Breath of Life.

Franklin Sills writes:

Each person's system is a unique expression of their *history, experience and tendencies.* As we experience life, our systems will become conditioned and personalized. . . . The cells and tissues of the body will become conditioned and shaped in ways specific to a person's history. Shapes are an expression of a person's suffering and personal life journey. All of this is centered by the Breath of Life in some way and the potency is always present even within the most seemingly dense and chronic conditions. (1989, Chapter 3, Section 2, p. 1)

Craniosacral therapists palpate these shapes, identify where these pulsating rhythms are unable to express fully as health and work with the wisdom of the system in finding the health within these shapes, thus releasing the block. Craniosacral therapy deepens the practitioner's skills in listening to the very specific vibrations and rhythms of the Life Force within the body. This is possible by understanding how this Life Force flows through the body and how it impacts the tissue, fluids and bones, and feelings.

All of the methodologies described assist the client in releasing trauma from their energy fields and opening up the free flow of energy. The most powerful healing occurs when the client can connect the feelings and emotion to the original event (story) thereby healing the wounds and memories. The story does not always have to be verbal but can be expressed nonverbally through the physical body in the tissues, fluids and bones.

INTEGRATIVE ENERGY MEDICINE PROCESS

Most essential to the work is the creation of a healing space where the client can feel safe and supported. This is done by clearing the energy before each session. As practitioner it is important to stay aligned and centered. An intention is generally established for the session, based on the issues the clients practitioners bring to the session. I usually spend some time assisting them to clarify their thoughts. The intention is framed in positive terms to reflect the desired result or outcome. A brief invocation and meditation is spoken which calls on the energies, sets the intention of the clients and begins to bring the clients into their bodies and own center of balance. Then in partnership with the client, the type of work to address the intention is decided. Sometimes this is done through kinesiology (muscle testing) and sometimes this is done through discussion.

Muscle Testing

Muscle testing is a method of accessing an individual's deepest knowing to receive information not available to the conscious mind. Muscle testing is applied by asking the client to hold both arms out at a right angle to the body. The practitioner asks the client to hold their arms firm while the practitioner applies pressure to the clients' forearms. The purpose of applying pressure is to determine how the client's body responds to "yes" or "no." The practitioner asks the client's deepest knowing to show them a "yes" and a "no" response. On one of the responses the client's arms will remain firm and on the other response the client's arms will go weak and give in to the pressure. This establishes a communication system to work with the unconscious mindbody. There are specific procedures followed for holding a clear intention and ensuring truthful responses. Muscle testing has been researched as a valid technique in obtaining clear and truthful information on specific questions. David Hawkes provides extensive data and case studies on the validity of muscle testing in his book *Power vs. Force.*

In Guided Self Healing, the practitioner asks a series of questions using muscle testing to determine the specific patterns, core limiting beliefs or work which will be the focus of the session. Generally, I believe in engaging the client in their process and empowering them in their own healing. Therefore, I am partial to techniques that have the client participate more than those that would have the practitioner do the work.

CASE STUDIES

As the case studies are reviewed, keep in mind that all the work is about releasing trauma. Trauma is an energetic block often with multiple components. All the interactions and work involve energy work whether the client is on the table or not.

The following is an example of a Guided Self Healing protocol. This is the case study of a client that I work with on a regular basis with whom I usually do Polarity work. She prefers table work and tends to avoid any direct work on emotional issues. In this particular session, her intention was to establish a connection with her guidance and inner resources. She was clear about what she wanted to work on and had more energy than usual. After a brief conversation it was learned that she had a session earlier in the week and felt the work was incomplete. This was a carry-over from that session. The desire to connect with her inner guides–feel and see energy–is an ongoing concern for her. She overcompensates for her "self described" inadequacy by obsessing on tak-ing classes and learning new techniques.

When she was asked to elaborate on her intention she indicated that she has a fear of something, . . . fear of no connection (presumably with God). A secondary issue concerned her allergies. Historically, the first day of May began allergy season for her. However, she had done some significant healing around her allergies and this year did not have allergy symptoms on May 1st. She was allergy free for 15 days, but each day she was allergy free she questioned herself "Is this for real?" She expressed that she was feeling resentment towards God and felt she was being cheated out of enjoying spring. Her eyes would become watery and itchy, sinuses irritated etc. exactly on May 1st with the exception of this year. I suspected she may be experiencing some loss of this seemingly unpleasant event and pondered whether she may sabotage her healing.

Guided self-healing has a number of roles, behaviors, and patterns that can be diagnosed through muscle testing. The question is asked, "Is this being running a specific sabotage pattern?" With a confirmation of the pattern, a specific strategy can be mapped out with the client for clearing the trauma. There are a number of ways this can happen.

It was determined that she was running a sabotage pattern called a "Wounded Holy One." The pattern is from a past life in which the being was some sort of spiritual leader who broke a sacred covenant involving the evolution of the souls in their community. This is a particularly powerful pattern that many healers carry. This must be cleared at root cause (the original event). In this situation we identified where she felt the resentment in her body. This represents the blocked energy. She responded that she felt resentment in her upper body, lungs, and heart specifically. We used muscle testing or kinesiology to verify her responses by connecting with the feelings of resentment and amplifying the feelings, and the practitioner was able to guide the client to find the story.

The client was able to find the story very quickly. She envisioned a girl harvesting flowers in a large field. She was collecting herbs with the intent of helping the community. She said, "I really thought this was going to help." She was encouraged to elaborate but instead, went to a death scene where she saw a young woman swinging . . . (hanging). She said, "Oh, she's done away with." Through further questioning, she determined that this young woman was so enjoying the day and skipping through the field that she was not paying full attention to what she was picking. Someone died as a result of the wrong combination of herbs and she was held responsible. She was put to death. Part of the healing process is to gather her dying thoughts which were: a feeling of remorse and also anger with God for allowing it to happen. The being is so angry she hung on to the feelings that she carries in her energy field into this lifetime as an unresolved issue. To clear this pattern it is important for the client to recognize their mistakes and to understand how this lifetime served them. There were several interventions used to clear the remorse and anger allowing her to see she was and is always connected to God. The lessons for this being were to honor and respect the earth and to remember her connection to God.

The feelings of resentment cleared in the body and the client could make the connections from the story to the present. A person running this pattern usually has a theme in their life of being fearful of abusing power or a fear of not doing it right. It is not uncommon for healers to carry this pattern.

This case study is an example of a craniosacral and energy work. This client was approximately 50 years old and in fairly good health. She reported that she had received some bodywork a few days before which was a practice session for the practitioner. Although she felt good after the session, today she was experiencing a shooting pain in her jaw, gall bladder discomfort, and felt edgy. She had not experienced this edgi-

ness in a while. She also added that in her yoga class she felt like she could hardly breathe. She thought these symptoms might be a reaction to the session earlier in the week.

Her intention for the session was to bring her system back into balance joyfully. When I asked her "How will you know," she responded that she will feel calm and her fire will be more balanced (she was referring to the edginess she described and gall bladder discomfort).

Before beginning the session, I took a few minutes to settle into my own energetic system and center so that I could be fully present for this client. I actually do this before every session and then check in again with my system before beginning any work with a client. For this work the client is lying on a massage table on her back. The first contact I make is at the head. While honoring her system I gently make contact and cradle her head in my hands. We express the affirmation for the session and invoke this being's highest guidance and deepest wisdom to guide the session.

The next step is to develop a relationship with her bioenergy by quietly sitting with her system and listening. The practitioner listens for the health that expresses itself through the familiar rhythms in the body. The potency of her system had a gentle quality. Her system moved into inhalation and exhalation fairly quickly. This is a movement beyond the breath in which the body expresses the Life Force in a wave-like motion towards the feet and then back again towards the head. The fluids, bones and tissues move in particular recognizable patterns in relation to this movement.

As I scanned her body there was a sense of disintegration in the torso between the right and left sides around the midline. There was a faint sense of the tide, (the wave motion) in the midst of the disintegration. Still but not still. It actually felt like an airy layer beneath. Her system seemed to be organizing, moving. I was beginning to feel the fluid in the tissue in the occipital and temporal areas. As I was just listening to the system, the client suddenly expressed that she felt a pain in her temple. She suddenly felt fear. The sensation moved to her jaw, (I was not feeling any of this) and I asked her to say more about the fear. She said it was fear of pain. She was afraid that "it" (the pain) would open up. I asked her if it would be okay for her to be with that for a moment. Simultaneously she said, "Oh, the opening up is a sense of relief." When I questioned her further she indicated that she was not sure what would happen if the pain opened. She commented that she had often felt fear associated with this pain in her jaw, across her shoulders and down the center of her body. She gestured with her hands making a lateral motion across her shoulders and down the midline.

After a moment she said she felt small and was reminded of birth and prebirth. I began to feel her cranium get small in my hands. She expressed that she felt vulnerable. I invited her to remember my hands holding her head (creating a safe container for her). We talked about resources and creating a safe place. I invited her to take as much space as she needed. She was beginning to focus on what was happening. She immediately felt more relaxed as she backed off and viewed from a wider perspective. "Oh, if I give myself space I feel more relaxed." At the same time I was noticing that that there was a very slight lateral motion in the cranium in the area of the temporal bones. It is difficult to describe my impression but it seemed as if the infant just wanted to be held in this stillness. There was a sense of presence through the contact with the cranial bones but also just a sense of being. There was an organizing of the midline and a swirling motion at the base of the spine. The client stated that she was drawn to her navel. She remembers some trauma at birth around the umbilical cord. She traveled back to before she was born, experiencing the umbilical cord in its wholeness. We spent

some time here. There was a sense of calm. Nothing in particular happened, but everything was happening. I was noticing a bulging at the right temporal occipital area at the same time. The right side of the tentorium felt stretched. Then there was a lateral movement to center within the cranium. Then I had a sense of an inferior fluctuation of fluid organizing around the midline all the way down the spine. Sometime during this process the small frame shifted back to adult size. I realized that I was not sure when that happened although I felt certain that the process needed to happen.

At the right time I moved to the sacrum. After making contact her system easily moved into inhalation and exhalation. There was a strong lateral fluctuation in the pelvic region, moving into left hip, back to spine and shifting caudally expanding the energy in the sacrum. The sacrum began to feel hydrated from its center outward. As this was occurring, the client again felt pain in her jaw, and she felt a bulging on the left side of her head in the parietal area. I was wondering about the connection, trying to hold a wide perceptual field, and thinking about the embryological aspect. There was a fleeting experience of connection, but so fleeting I almost couldn't grasp it.

I held my focus at the sacrum just inviting the system to continue to find the point of balance. I made a connection to the hip with my left hand while holding the sacrum. She felt a release in her jaw. She added that her head felt funny. I continued to hold the points inviting the system to find balance. I began to feel the motion of the tides. There was a welling up at the sacrum, then a release. An inhalation, exhalation . . . with the exhalation the uncomfortable sensation in her head seemed to clear.

I ended the session with her on her side while I focused upon connecting the sacrum and frontal bone. This example is of a client releasing a birth trauma. This client may have experienced a forceps birth that would explain the shape of her experience. Given her age there may have been other interventions such as anesthesia. The body holds all of this as an experience. She cleared the fear from her jaw and could not access it at the end of the session. She felt centered, calm, the edginess disappeared and her energy shifted to a balanced state.

CONCLUSION

"The world as we experience it is a process that follows universal laws and cycles. The process of life is a flow of energy" (Sills, 1989). "The secret to learn here is for man's consciousness to remain still in the Center of Being, in its eternal Essence. Then things will right themselves" (Stone, 1986, p. 46).

REFERENCES

Braden, G. (1994). *Awakening to zero point, The collective initiative.* Ann Arbor, MI: Braun-Brumfield, Inc.

Burger, B. (1998). *Esoteric anatomy, The body as consciousness.* Berkeley: North Atlantic Books.

Hahn, A. (1999). Guided Self Healing Training Manual. A. Hahn, 115 Worcester Lane, Waltham, MA 02154.

Hawkes, D. (1998). *Power vs force.* Sedona, AZ: Veritas Publishing.

Jealous, J. (1994). *Around The Edges.* Vermont, pp.1–3.

Levine, P. (1997). *Waking the tiger, healing trauma.* Berkeley: North Atlantic Press.

Sills, F. (1989). *The Polarity Process.* Longmead: Element Books Limited

Sills, F. (1999). Seminar Three, Section 2, Point of Balanced Tension. United Kingdom: Karuna Institute, pp. 1–10.

Stone, R. (1986). *Polarity Therapy: Volume I.* Nevada: CRCS Publications.

Swack, J.A. (1994). The Basic structure of violence and loss trauma imprints. Anchor Point, March 1994. *The Magazine for Effective Neuro-Linguistic Communications.*

For further information and training in: Polarity Therapy, Guided Self-Healing, Electromagnetic Field Balancing, and Craniosacral Therapy
Contact:
Elaine McNulty MEd,RPP
emcnk@breezy.com
603-772-2453

Chapter 18

MINDBODY AND SOUL IN HEALTH, HEALING AND CREATIVE TRANSFORMATION

PENNY LEWIS

The world is only seemingly continuous, Newtonian, and material. In reality, it is discontinuous, quantum, and conscious. Such a science leads to a true reconciliation with spiritual traditions because it does not ask spirituality to be based on science, but asks science to be based on the notion of eternal spirit.
(Amit Goswami, 2001, p. 30)

GENESIS

I AM A FIRM BELIEVER that everything that individuals have experienced and been taught in their lifetime perfectly hones them for their life learning and calling. At the commencement of a nine-day professional training intensive in Transpersonal Drama Therapy, I suggested that participants group in threes with each person taking a turn, imagining themselves prior to their conception–their soul still in spirit–having a discussion with two other spirits about what womb they wanted to enter and what specific life experiences they wanted to have in order to be trained for their life calling. This spiritual reframe allows individuals to notice that even the most trying and painful of experiences, are not to be excluded from their appreciation of the wisdom and potential grace that they have accrued throughout their life.

Undergraduate courses in neuroanatomy, molecular physiology, medicine and surgery seemed useless to me at the time as I knew my interest was in the direction of the embodied arts in psychotherapy. Now as my practice, teaching, consulting, supervising and administrating has expanded and deepened into the field of integrative holistic health, I see the bigger plan and smile.

Future and current graduate students can sometimes devalue the life experiences that they have had. Raising children deserves at least a Ph.D.! Parents learn human development, individual and group approaches to communication, crisis management, psychology, and models of administration and systems theories, to name just a few as well as the engagement in a lifelong longitudinal outcome study. Others who have struggled with their own recovery understand from the inside out the difference between suffering with and without meaning. This firsthand experience can never be learned in books, academic lectures or even from listening to others.

During my early years I was taught by, apprenticed and worked along side of some of the founders of art, dance and drama therapy. At that time, there were no graduate programs in these fields. Subsequently, I founded one of the original approved graduate programs in dance-movement therapy at Antioch New England Graduate School and developed the Institute for Healing and Wellness of which one of its functions is to train alternate route students in drama therapy toward becoming Registered Drama Therapists. During this time I have always continued my learning as it is a lifelong process. The most influential training has been in Gestalt Therapy and at the C.G. Jung Institute in New York where I trained in Jungian Analysis. More recently I was asked to consult at Lesley University's Graduate Independent and Interdisciplinary Studies Department toward developing masters and graduate certificate programs in Integrative Holistic Health. These innovative programs are designed to expand and deepen holistic health practitioners skills in their practice, as consultants and administrators at a time when few programs if any exist to meet a vastly developing demand.

At a certain point in midlife, I experienced a gradual shift from the view that my ego-self was and should be the director of my life. My consciousness began to let go of outcome or at least what I thought I wanted and allowed the flow of experience to wash over me. Trusting in my calling of healing and bringing expanded consciousness to this planet, I enjoy the connection with other souls who are here for similar purpose and await what will perfectly unfold, all the while marveling at the trickster quality of the changes in what I thought was the direction my life was taking both personally and professionally.

A very wise participant in one of my workshops in Greece said to another who

needed to hold on to the specificity of an outmoded structure: "Whatever happens, that's the plan."

THEORETICAL PHILOSOPHY

View of the Individual

An individual is seen as an interconnected multidimensional mindbody-soulspirit-energetic being who is part of the totality of the Essential Eternal Source sometimes known as God or Divine Consciousness. The unique eternal essence or soul develops a personal sense of self-specific to the particular genetics, environmental and relational development of the individual. The sense of self consists of:

- Relationally cellular and limbic system-based stored history with primary caregiver(s),
- the somatic and imagistic imagining of the self or child(ren) within
- gut chemical neuropeptides which send self feelings throughout the body
- the third chakra foundationally supported by the 1st and 2nd , cared for by the 4th and expressed through the 5th
- the astral plane of the human energy field
- with the eternal Self or soul at its core.

Human growth is propelled by DNA and an inner motivating self-actualizing process that moves individuals through developmental stages throughout life span, while striving to maintain health, balance and expand Consciousness. Key interpersonal, environmental, and energetic phenomena are needed for each phase of development to reach successful culmination. Along with a sense of self that can clearly communicate what the person feels, needs and wants, and differentiate what or who is safe and approachable from what is unsafe and toxic, the individual needs to develop a conscious adult ego that can receive inner information from the self and other mindbody sources, differentiate what is inner from what is outer, and utilize adaptations and coping skills to mediate needs and function effectively in the world. This requires healthy ego, body and personal space boundaries.

As individuals evolve throughout life span, letting go of who they were in order to become who they are meant to be, a shift occurs from "my will be done" to "Thy will be done." Those self-defining aspects that have surrounded the soul diminish and the soul path brightens and becomes the conscious guiding force. Spiritual access moves the heart chakra into greater love, compassion, and intuition; and access to the transpersonal is more profoundly available though 6th and 7th chakras. Additionally, the human energy field clears of past history, balances and expands.

Health

> Health is the capacity:
> • to be fully present in the body,
> • to have cleared and balanced human energy fields,
> • to have the capacity for intimacy with oneself, others, and spiritual Grace,
> • to have functioning ego, body and personal space boundaries,
> • to have cleared the capacity for embodied spontaneous expresson.

Health is also seen as the successful integration of all previous developmental stages and the capacity to utilize all developmentally-related coping behaviors and associated roles of those stages in an adaptive manner in service to oneself, respectful interaction with others, the environment, and other co-existing realms of transpersonal reality. Successful functioning requires the ability to be fully present throughout life span life toward further evolution and growth.

Dis-ease and Trauma

Dis-ease occurs with an insufficiently developed sense of self that produces core beliefs such as:
• I am unworthy
• I am unacceptable
• I am going to be abandoned
• I am going to be smothered and lose my sense of self
• I am better than everyone and deserve special treatment
• I am shameful or guilty
• I am too much
• I am not enough
• I am a victim
• I must control everything to feel safe
• I cannot trust the world as it is unsafe and/or incapable of meeting my needs

These and other unrealistic survival-based beliefs co-exist in the astral plane of the human energy field, in the related chakras (see Figure 7-3), and produce negative self-talk, childhood survival mechanisms and addictions such as the ones listed in Chapter 5. These survival behaviors are employed instead of healthy boundaries resulting in disconnection to the self, others and the spiritual realm. Additionally, these survival self-talking complexes keep the individual from being fully present as they base their reason for being on the false assumption that the present is somehow a recreation of the past. They filter all of life through their frame, curtailing or denying any input that would discredit their version of life and the individual's relationship to it and expanding, generalizing, catastrophizing or awfulizing anything that might tangentially justify its existence. "My mother emotionally abandoned me, so I won't trust anyone in my present life." "My father always made me feel that I wasn't good enough, so I have to work harder than anyone else in order to just feel ok, but I never seem to ever feel that

I am doing enough." "As a child, whenever I asked questions or needed some attention, I always felt that I was too much, so now I make sure I'm not too much by judging everything I am about to say and do to ensure that I won't be rejected and made to feel that I am too needy for attention."

Dysfunction occurs when healthy development is arrested due to trauma within the family system or externally or the inability of the primary caregivers to create the required ontogenetic setting and associated relationship. No matter what the etiology, if the healthy integration of a particular developmental phase has not been fostered, the individual will be stuck in the stage that was not successfully completed. This "stuckness" also occurs on an energetic and cellular level and expands in complexity to repetitive behaviors and limited thinking. The role that the individual plays as well those roles transferred or projected onto others and the way in which the surrounding setting is viewed will all be based upon the core issues of the developmental phase in which they have been arrested. They repeat the theme with the associated roles over and over again unable to utilize other themes or integrate new ones (Lewis, 2000).

Thus, unresolved childhood experiences, themes and their prescribed roles interweave and repeatedly overlap recreating the past as if it were the present. The work of the mindbody, soulspirit, holistic health therapist is to not only view the client relationship as a momentary gestalt, but also to identify the repetitive phenomena and the energetic and cellular blocks. Once identified their origins can be traced back etiologically where thematic scripts along with their associated roles, childhood survival behaviors, sensations, images, assumptions and busy mind self-talk can be seen to group themselves in developmentally-based constellations. When these immature themes can be cleared from unconscious habituation, mythelogems or archetypal life themes become available to healthy children, adolescents, and adults in their unfolding personal quests and their calling on earth (Lewis, 2000). Gradually, energetic and cellular memory and blocks dissolve as the individual moves forward, step-by-step on their path.

EARLY CHILDHOOD TRAUMA. In early childhood cases where severe abandonment and/ or violation of energetic, physical or psychological boundaries have occurred, profound neurologic, somatic and human energy field trauma occurs which unconsciously can affect the rest of the individual's life. Early pre and neonatal memory is stored in the limbic system as emotional arousals without images or thoughts. Throughout life span all stimuli is first filtered through the amygdala in the limbic system of the midbrain before entering the neocortex. If any element of the stimuli is associated with prior emotionally charged memory, it will be sent to the cortex as a match. Additionally, gut feelings and other somatic emotional markers produced by liquid molecular neuropeptides in the body assign value or positive or negative reactions to stimuli effecting the individual's emotional integrity and the assessment of the safeness of others and the environment. This liquid nervous system chemically enhances or inhibits neural transmission that, in turn, modulates arousal, mood and attention.

Internally, the mindbody receives information from the unconscious housing repressed trauma, thoughts and imaginings of the individual. The mindbody, not being able to decipher the difference between real and imagined external and internal stimuli regarding safety and danger, responds similarly to both. This may include activation of the limbic system, the autonomic nervous system, the molecular and cellular emotional system, and the human energy fields.

Responses to chronic, real, or imagined danger produce the sympathetic nervous systems response of chronic stress that, in turn, reduces the functioning of the immune system. Additionally, chronic stress and imprinted trauma affect the observable quality of flow and developmentally-based rhythms of agonist and antagonist muscle systems and the shape that the body takes.

In severe trauma in which the person perceives that the external situation is a reenactment of the initial abuse, emotional hijacking occurs. The amygdala continuously refires, cutting off the capacity for cognitive reality testing in the prefrontal cortex and the capacity to learn to make adaptive decisions. Trauma is seen as being stored in the sensorimotor: ANS, Limbic, and body's peripheral nervous system both sensori and motor, as seen and held in body shape and tension areas in the body, leaving an individual vulnerable for physical trauma and illness.

Human Development

Through the theories of ego psychologists (Erikson, 1963, A. Freud, 1966) therapists have grown to understand that with each stage of life there are specific themes which manifest and dominate an individual's way of viewing and interacting in the world, requiring defined roles for that person and significant others to enact. For example, the theme of the development of trust, self-nurturing, and a sense that the environment is need satisfying (Erikson's first stage, trust vs. mistrust) is very different than the drama to be played in Erikson's second stage of autonomy where themes of power and control dominate. Dysfunction and pathology emerge when these theme-based stages have been unsuccessfully integrated due to role deviation or inappropriate setting.

Further sophistication of developmentally influenced theory emerged with the work of object relations therapists and neo-Jungians. Most therapists would agree that the origins of much of their patients' dysfunctions began the first three years of life. Ego psychologists certainly covered these years but not with the specificity of object relations' theorists such as Melanie Klein (1975), Margaret Mahler (1968), D.W. Winnicott (1971), Ronald Fairbairn (1976), et al., who held a

magnifying glass up to the intrapsychic and interpersonal threads. What they found were subtly changing empathic movement attunement and related roles within the mother-child drama which served with "good-enough mothering" to provide the child with a realistic sense of self and a constant internalized supportive and enabling object or inner mother. Somatic cellular and energetic constellations develop with each stage as well. This encoded early history occurs on a senate body level; and because of its fundamental level, is preverbal and can only be accessed somatically.

Once object constancy has been achieved, life's drama expands. Here other theoretical constructs need to be introduced, as the dramas become far more complex and diverse given the sex and dominant characterological structures of the individual. The work of Jung (1977, C.W.) and post-Jungians (Neumann, 1973, 1976, Von Franz, 1978, 1982) have taken culture's externalizations of universal life themes and characters found in myths, fairy tales, religious ritual, and stories of gods and goddesses and provided a rich view of the powerful archetypal mythelogems in the life quests and cycles of individuals. In addition, more recent investigations have further refined adult life stages (Sheehey, 1995, Moore & Gillette, 1990) expanding and enriching the understanding regarding mid-life phases.

THE THERAPEUTIC PROCESS

Awareness

Individuals' arrested developmental themes, their associated childhood survival behaviors and distorted beliefs are held like land mines in the astral plane, related chakras and soma waiting to be triggered. Additionally, they are played out in their lives through repetition compulsions, repetitive childhood patterns, and limiting distorted assumptions and beliefs originally utilized either for aborted attempts at integrating the phase or for the recreation of the trauma in order to perpetuate the familiar. These cellular body and energy blocks and thematic recreations keep them from responding adaptively to the moment. The threads of the themes and roles are gradually revealed to the patient through bioenergy-related breath, somatic awareness of sensation and body movement as well as through mind-body expressive arts techniques such as etiologically-based exploratory role-playing. These enactments may entail the interviewing of childhood survival patterns as to their origin or the elucidating of developmental themes through such venues as improvisational movement or drama, authentic sound, movement and drama, dreamwork as theater, play, and embodied sand play.

Encouragement to delve developmentally to the source of the theme and its associated role is made, through redramatization of a typical formulating occurrence. In this first state of awareness, the individual needs to get a fix on how these behaviors and interactions are internalized and projected onto their present life themes.

The Transformative Process

Mindbody-oriented dance and drama therapists have long known that it is through embodied sensory awareness and enacted experience that change can occur. Many of our patients come to us complaining that they have talked about their problems with other therapists but to no avail.

These problem patterns would be simple to change if they only existed in the empirical left hemisphere cognitive realm. In fact, much of trauma and insufficient care is stored in the soma, neurochemistry, and limbic system in bodily sensations, other sensoria and feelings.

First, individuals are encouraged to become mindful in the room—to reenter or emerge from insulation and be fully present in their bodies. Once present in their bodies, they are encouraged to notice sensation either in a solo continuum of awareness or while engaged in a rechoreography of in utero or object relations dyadic movement experience with the therapist. Additionally, we explore how they may feel safe in the room. I often will expand on the space between us and leave the room on their command to reinforce their sense of control. Attending from moment-to-moment, noticing diaphragmatic breath as they attempt to make contact with the core self, they may become aware of sensations such as numbness, nausea, excitation and notice emergent feelings such as fear, anger, sadness, and longing. During this process I monitor their level of comfort, insuring that the amygdala or the sympathetic fight, flight, freeze, faint responses have not overcharged. I do this through the somatic countertransference or what Dossey calls telesomatic connection, through high sense intuition monitoring their human energy field, and by observing their body posture, tension and shape flow, breath, and vocal tone (see Chapter 4 on the observable body).

If they are sufficiently present, not in trauma reenactment and feeling safe and in their body, I then suggest to them to allow their imagination to create images in order to personify their core gut self or inner child. The capacity to imagine taps into the realm in which healing and transformation can occur.

Creative Transformation

To understand the notion of healing and developmentally-based creative transformation in mindbody and soul therapy, the elusive phenomena of transitional space (Winnicott, 1971) in object relations theory and the imaginal realm (Schwartz-Salant, 1983-84, 1984a, Lewis 1985, 1998b, 1993, 2000, Turner, 1969) in Jungian theory need to be explored.

Winnicott's transitional space and the imaginal realm described by Jung in the

Mysterium Conunctionis (Vol. XIV) have a common experiential link. In both cases the individual is experiencing the moment in a realm that lies between reality and the unconscious. It is akin to the world of "pretend" play in childhood. This is the realm where the internalized origin of the threads of repetitive dramas lie. Thus, in order to transform them, the patient and/or group and therapist must all enter into the bipersonal field of the imaginal realm in a fully embodied, enacted manner.

The Bipersonal Energetic Field Between Client and Therapist

Individual depth work allows for the mindbody subtle nuances associated with early object related trauma to be monitored from moment-to-moment by the therapist and responded to through her subtle body and vocal responses, co-creating within the bipersonal energetic field, a transitional space of healing. The role of the therapist is paramount in healing early stages of development; for just as no infant could evolve a sense of self without the attentive ministerings of the attuned mother, no adult can do so either. Additionally, just as children know if their parents truly love and know them deeply, clients, as well, are not fooled by therapists "going though the motions" of acting like they care. Thus the role of the therapist is that of genuine care and concern seeking connection (relational model), contact (Gestalt model), and genuine intimacy.

This means that the therapy room can become a nursery for old pathological scenes to be reexperienced. Here, classic psychodrama techniques and structures are exceedingly helpful, particularly in the recreation of history, confrontation and antagonist transformation (Lewis, 2000). Then redramatization of healthy development is possible between the patient and myself or within a group.

Individuals' further development is, of course, also curtailed when early phases have been disrupted. In these situations, it is not so much the "re" enacting but providing the needed developmentally-based setting for the patient to integrate higher levels. Again, this is not so much empirically provided as it is liminally and creatively provided. Once childhood development is integrated, jungles are created for a hero to confront and individuate his or her inner instinctual beast. From a Jungian archetypal perspective, this means that numinous energy can enter the room through the embodied personification of a goddess or spontaneous enactment of a ritual dance or rite of passage. The therapist's repertoire of roles extends to all possible enabling and destructive characters in human development as described by the individual in their personal history or by individuals through culture's history in myths, fairy tales, literature, religious liturgy and other manifestations.

Being cognizant of adult stages of development allows the therapist to encourage and give meaning to archetypal life themes that emerge from the imaginal realm. For example, understanding the death, dismembering and putrefying alchemical cycle of the heroic quest can provide the needed support and encouragement for the patient to undergo this sometimes frightening but necessary mid-life rite of passage (see Chapter 8: Sacred Alchemy).

Being in the Moment with the Creative Void

The third stage in the therapeutic process unfolds naturally. Clients observe, sometimes in retrospect, how their behavior has changed. They have choice as to whether or not they want to repeat an archaic dramatic theme or be possessed by a distorted belief from a busy mind, and they no longer are fixed in an unconscious replay of a childhood role. They live in the moment with mindful presence, cleared human energy fields and spontaneously respond to the many realms of existence. They experience subtle but profound change in their life and the manner in which it is lived.

MINDBODY AND SOUL TECHNIQUES IN THE INTEGRATIVE MODEL

The Internal Drama

Reclaiming preverbal memories that lie in the body and bodily sensations allow both the client and therapist the ability to reconstruct early prelanguage experiences. Winnicott has stated that many memories are "preverbal, nonverbal and unverbalizable" (1971, p. 130). Since many memories of trauma and misattunement occur prior to language, they are often held in unconscious somatic schemata and the primitive limbic system that can only be recalled by slowly increasing awareness of acceptable levels of sensations, feelings and imaginal embodied reconstruction. Asking clients to imagine journeying inside their body and personifying sensations, feelings, viscera and other body parts begins to create a dramatic communicational bridge from the clients' early history to the present.

Core to the formation of a sense of self is the suggestion for clients to journey to their solar plexus to find the core of who they are or the child within. Relating to the imagined child allows for the clearing of abusive history and the beginning of healthy reparenting or co- parenting with my entering into the bipersonal imaginal realm.

The Use of the Somatic Counter-transference or Telesomatic Connection

Another aspect of the internal drama is the technique of the somatic countertransference. Based upon phenomenological research (Lewis, 1981), I began to conceptualize this bipersonal dialogue between therapist and client. I was further encouraged when I began my analytic training in 1984 at

the C.G. Jung Institute of New York. Jung (CW vol. XVI) in his "Psychology of the Transference" discussed an unconscious to unconscious connection between the patient and therapist. Jung suggested that not only are patient and therapist communicating on a conscious to a conscious level or, as in psychoanalytic work, from the patient's unconscious to the analyst's conscious level; but that there is also a direct unconscious to unconscious communication going on all the time. The therapist thus receives from the unconscious of the patient into her body unconscious and can send back to the patient's unconscious as well either through the conscious ego or the unconscious. In this realm, attending to the somatic countertransference it is possible, for example, to imaginally create dramas which heal inner child(ren) and transferred negative objects (Grotstein, 1981; Jung, 1977; Lewis, 1988a, 1988b, 1992, 1993, 2000; Racker,1982, Schwartz-Salant, 1983-1984; Stein, 1984). The therapist may receive the patient's abusive childhood survival mechanisms such as the inner critic, false mother addiction or nonattuned parent from the patient's somatic unconscious and, may imaginally utilize themes from fairy tales or myths to heal and transform these feeling-charged personifications while still in the therapist's body vessel.

With others, their infant self may be imaginatively received for love and healthy gestation to be retransferred when the patient is ready. This form of projective identification has proven highly successful. Again, just as clients do not benefit from having a new role superimposed on them, it doesn't work for the therapist to conjure up what she/he *thinks* the character should act like. Nor am I suggesting something akin to Stanislovsky "method acting." I imagine I am playing the role of my patient's symbiotic good mother and; based upon what the inner child needs that I receive from the client's unconscious, I imagine a corrective drama. Because this unconscious to unconscious connection travels both ways, this imagining can be received by the patient's unconscious. This imagined enacted dialogue has a powerful effect and is always received by the patient. I have had many confirmations of this through patients' dreams, poetry, drawings or statements, such as, "I know you've been holding me all along" or "my inner child feels your constant encouragement of her assertion" (Lewis, 1984, 1993, 1994).

Rechoreography and Redramatization of Object Relations

Healthy infant and toddler care is conducted on a relational sensorimotor level. Mahler (1968); Kestenberg (1965); Stern (1985); Winnicott (1971) et al., discuss concepts such as attunement, rhythmic synchrony, holding and handling by the mother as conveying to the infant relatedness, appropriate boundaries and a sense of trust, safety, identity and internalized other. All of these are crucial in the foundation for healthy development. They are learned *in vivo* through the actual enacted experience and cannot be conveyed by the "talking about them." Therefore, the thematically-based developmental redramatization of the mother/child embodied relationship by the patient and therapist is often a *sine qua non* of transformation.

Here, the empathetic mindbody movement therapist can attune her posture and movement to the changing ontogenetic nuances of movement she has visually or tactilely received from the client:

- the in utero movement,
- the early symbiotic rhythmic sucking,
- the differentiating patting or massaging biting and chewing rhythm,
- the ambivalent twisting rhythm and playful distancing of the practicing phase, or
- the vis a vis vertical external boundaried assertions of the rapprochement phase (see Chapter 4: Tension Flow Rhythms).

These bipersonal dyadic dance-movement therapy experiences can tap into molecular-cellular memory opening the client to foundational developmentally impaired relationally based sensations, movements and feelings. These, in turn, can be slowly transformed as the client embodies their fetal, infant, or toddler self with the therapist as the developmentally sensitive and loving healing parent. Here the therapist's body position, movement and tone of voice is crucial, and needs to be developmentally attuned to the phase the individual is embodying (Lewis, 1987a, b & c, 1990, 1993, 1999, 2000).

The Embodied Psyche Technique

As in Chapter 5, the embodied psyche technique engages the client in an externalized personified role-play of the different voices they hear inside their head. In one-to-one work, I personify a variety of intrapsyche complexes that the person needs distance from. If they are part of a group, various group members take on the different roles and may be arranged in an initial sculpture. Each personified complex is given a signature statement and gesture. The client can observe and is then asked, "Is this the way you want your psyche to be?" If the answer is no, then the drama therapy process continues with the person role-playing parts of their psyche with whom they want more connection: the ego, child self, healthy boundaries, soul, animus/a or shadow aspect with others or myself playing those complexes that need to be externalized and depotentiated: survival mechanisms, addictions, and toxic introjects. Role reversal by the protagonist is encouraged with complexes to be empowered and drawn into closer relationship to the ego.

For example, the embodied psyche technique was utilized in an ongoing drama therapy group at a men's long-term residential treatment center for addictions. Men were paroled to the sight due to battering and drug-related crimes. Each group would commence with the premise and goal: "Recovery is the capacity to connect to oneself, others and the Higher Power. Addictions and out-dated survival behaviors attack this connection. They need to be replaced with healthy boundaries." Making a case for drama therapy I add, "We believe that it is often more helpful to see what's happening and to experience change rather than just talk about it."

In the second group of a series of eight, 18 men were asked to each connect to their core self/ inner child and see what feelings, needs and wants emerge. Matt, three months into the program, responded, "I want to be respected, to be loved, to be seen and missed." He then reported feeling confused. His inner confusor complex clearly didn't want him to connect to himself. If that occurred, the "confusor" survival behavior would be out of a job. Matt picked one of the men who was particularly connected to himself to be his inner child; another man who knew his own inner confusor volunteered to portray Matt's complex. Another older man volunteered to be his addiction: the pill pusher. Interviewing Matt, I came across another inner voice: his internalized father complex who would repeatedly trash him and tell him that he was worthless. In short order, after interviewing Matt as his dad, another resident heard the familiar senario and volunteered. Finally another resident was selected to be his ego/inner adult. Matt then told them what to say and with some more directing on his part, he sat back to watch.

His father began, "You're no good. You'll never be any good. You're a f...-up." Then his addiction began, "Who needs him. Who needs anybody. Let's take some of these pills and feel good." His inner child responded, "No please see me. I don't want those pills." His inner confusor, blocking access and interrupting his inner child and aligning himself with his addiction, said, "Your confused. It's just all too confusing. Don't feel anything; the feelings are way too confusing. Just take the pills."

"That's it!" he exclaimed with some amazement, "That's just what it sounds like in my head." "Is that how you would like your head to sound?" I asked. "No" was his emphatic response.

He was then instructed to take his ego's place and his complexes began their litany. Doubling his addiction, I exposed what I call the belly-side of this complex. "What do you mean you don't want me anymore? I have to have your attention. I live off you. I'll lose my power over you if you pay attention to your core self. You'll get stronger and I'll get weaker. I don't like that." "Tough!" was his response. Doubling his inner confusor, I say, "We'll go now, but we'll be back when you forget to connect to yourself or when things get tough." "Yeah," pipes up his addiction, "You can't get rid of us." With very little repetition he was able to shut his father, addiction, and survival behavior up. He then joined his child, and they gave each other an enthusiastic special handshake.

Other groups at this residential center had residents representing themselves encouraging the protagonist to come out from under his tough guy needless and wantless survival behavior to relate and feel their support. On occasion, an emissary from the Higher Power has been enacted (typically by one of my interns as being in control is a larger-than-life issue for these men and generally not encouraged).

In individual work, the mindbody creative arts therapist role-plays the survival mechanisms, negative introjects and any addictions. The languaging is always the same. First the therapist attempts to sway the ego of the client into believing that it is a caring mother surrogate, then the devouring self-gratifying power hungry side is revealed.

One woman, having struggled with anorexia, began work with me. She reported that her throat felt blocked. I wasn't sure whether her throat was keeping others from entering or herself from expressing. Interviewing the block it appeared that it was both. It was neither safe to express herself nor had it been healthy to let in others. Since it is vital for a client to feel safe in the therapy container, I began shifting my distance from her in the room. She needed to feel her boundary and my respect of it. What became clear, however, was that there was present in her astral human energy field imprints of individuals who had violated her space. These energetic trauma memories of emotional and physical violators would contaminate anyone who came within two feet of her body. I asked permission to enact these holographic energy forms which barred the possibility of interpersonal intimacy. "I still have you trapped. You are mine. No one else can be with you. I will contaminate them if they come near you, and cast a spell over you, so you cannot tell that they are safe. Don't trust Penny. Don't trust anyone."

I then de-roled and placed a large pillow between us infusing it with the contaminated energy of the pervasive abusive objects. From this point we worked gradually, with her always in control, to clear the toxicity and create a safe bipersonal field between us (Lewis, 1987, 1993).

With couples, the projections and particularly the parental transferences are role-played by the drama therapist. In one instance, a man's dark internalized mother complex was transferred on to his partner. He saw her as controlling and withheld from her. She, in turn, transferred on to him her unavailable internalized father whom she felt never really saw her. Role-playing both transferences while placing my body between them allowed them to begin to see the other. In a witch-like tone I said to the man, "All women are controlling. They want to take you over and feed from your accomplishments. Stay away from her, you're mine. I will blind you to her gentleness and love for you." To the woman I say, "All men are cold, unavailable and care only about themselves. No man will ever want to see you and love who you are. Besides, this one is imprisoned in a witch's spell." Playfully they dip and sway to get to each other, finally shoving me out of the way.

Hence, drama focusing on enacted personifications of the inner child self, intrapsychic survival mechanisms, addictions, and other split off aspects of the psyche as well as the internalized parents can be embodied by both client and therapist; and, if in group therapy, by group members in service to healing. This technique allows for externalized viewing by the client and the therapist as well as for the needed transformation of the psyche. Through dramatic process needed shifts in psychic energy distribution and placement of the complexes can occur in relation to the ego.

Dreamwork as Theater

Dreamwork as theater, embodied art and sand play work are creative transformational techniques based upon the premise that the purpose of dreams and other art expressions are not only to inform but also transform the dreamer/artist (Lewis, 1993a, 1993b, 2000). For this reason, dream and art interpretation is found to curtail the full value of this unconscious expression. If a dream is interpreted, it serves to separate the dreamer from the dream. It has the same effect as interpreting a work of art would. In both cases the observer looks at and intellectually assesses the work rather than experiencing it.

With dreams that are symbolic in nature and emerge from the personal unconscious, the technique of dreamwork as theater can be used. This technique keeps the dream and the dreamer in the imaginal realm. The dreamer can then understand the dream though the experience of it and can frequently use dreams as vehicles of transformation.

Dreams are one of the avenues into the unconscious that can be of invaluable help to someone engaged in recovery or individuation. Dreams can symbolically identify parts of the self that have remained unavailable to the ego. They can be "red flags" brought forth to tell the individual that they are in a toxic situation or relationship or generally going in the wrong direction in their sacred path. When an individual is in therapy or analysis, the unconscious often presents the dreamer with symbolic information pertinent to their process. Typically, these dreams come from the personal unconscious. But occasionally they emerge from the transpersonal archetypal unconscious. These are what Jungians call "big dreams." Their purpose is to expedite the therapy process by providing profoundly compelling experiences often of a deeply spiritual nature.

In addition to symbolic dreams, individuals can also have flashbacks during the dream cycle. These are typically not symbolic but the reexperiencing of actual prior traumatic events. There are occasions when the individual will have nightmares that are partially symbolic and partially from a real recollection. The specific symbolism utilized is typically created at the time that the abuse was suppressed, and can be of archetypal proportions.

Individuals may also have visions, visitations, or psychically-related events. Because there are very different types of phenomena that can occur during dream cycles, it is very important to be able to distinguish among them. For example, many women upon first encountering their inner masculine, may dream that some strange man is chasing them. In the dream they fear for their life or that they might be raped. Interviewing the pursuer it is discovered that this inner male is angry with the dreamer for not paying any attention to him, so he decided to make his presence known. Communicating with this aspect in the imaginal realm results in his softening and becoming more compellingly attractive to the dreamer. A union frequently ensues that is filled with all the romance and loving pleasure that could be hoped for. Flashbacks, even if couched in a layer of symbolism, have a very different feel to them. Attending to the somatic countertransference, the therapist may pick up fear or have a dark foreboding sensation. Noticing any primitive survival mechanisms such as

deanimation or dissociative responses exhibited by the client indicates the possibility that this may be a flashback contra-indicating the technique of dreamwork as theater.

In the dreamwork technique, the individual is asked to become different characters, inanimate objects, or atmosphere in the dream. I then interview the dreamer as the personification. At times dialogues ensue between two characters or aspects of the dream. If the dream is too scary, I further separate the dreamer from the dream by having them pretend that the dream is a movie in the process of being filmed. I suggest that the actors and crew just took a break and that I am an entertainment newsperson interviewing the dreamer who is cast in the role of the dream/movie character or scriptwriter.

At times the dream appears to have a beginning and middle but no ending. After interviewing the characters I suggest that the client imagine an ending. Since the responses and story endings emerge from the imagination, there are no "wrong" responses as the dream has come from the same source (Lewis, 1993a, 1993c). Dreams invariably reflect history that needs to be revealed or new life themes and the associated shadow and animus/a aspects that seek recognition and integration. Dreams can be altered through the imaginal realm to give the dreamer an experience of greater individuation. After interviewing the characters I suggest for the dreamer to imagine the dream in a way that supports the awareness that has occurred in the dramatization.

The role of the therapist is to assist in the enacted recreation of the dream. Upon entering the dream, characters can be interviewed, understood, claimed, transformed, and integrated in service to recovery and individuation. Themes and plots can unfold a map of a person's entire therapy process, and the archetypal can profoundly reconnect an individual to the many layers of Spiritual Consciousness.

One person, in the dark night journey of

the soul, had a series of archetypal alchemical dreams. She fought not to let go of what she had known in the past. But in the end, as Jung said, the decision was made over her head and despite her ego. She let go of her life as she knew it and moved into the liminal realm. She dreamt that a bomb had exploded outside her home. When she went out, everything was in devastation. She knew she would be dead soon from radiation poisoning. In the next dream a male (not anyone she knew, but clearly her animus) had been shrunk and lay in a small casket. She wanted to reanimate him but to no avail. Utilizing dreamwork as theater, she gestured as if she were disrobing, and climbed into the coffin. Lying down on the floor, she reported feeling at peace for this first time. The next week she dreamt she was in a church that had the reputation of being filled with the grace of God. She reported that the church was packed but that she was able to lie down on the pew. Before she closed her eyes with the rest of the attendants, she saw a large black man enter the church carrying an automatic weapon. She feared for her life and the lives of others. She stayed frozen, afraid to attract attention to herself. With her eyes closed she heard him walking up the aisle and stop in front of her. The next thing she felt was his kissing her heart. She awoke with a start. She lay down in the therapy space and asked him, "Why did you do that?" "You are doing the right thing," he commented in a wise voice, "but if you leave, I will have to shoot you." She commented, "God's grace comes in unexpected ways. I know I must stay in this gestating death. I do not know who I will become when I arise, but I know I am on my spiritual path."

Sand Play

Sand play sometimes called "the world technique" is a Jungian technique in which an individual moves or shapes sand in a box or arranges small symbolic figures in the sand. Usually individuals allow their imagination to select from figures that range from animals (magical, domesticated or wild), human figures (all ages and character types), environmental objects (trees, containers, walls, stones, shells, etc), dollhouse furniture, vehicles, sacred icons, and other small objects of symbolic significance. Often the result is a symbolic representation of their psyche or a map of their developmental, psychological and spiritual journey. These figures are then given imaginal life and the small sand space is treated as a world in and of itself. The figures are interviewed and converse among themselves with the sand play arrangers playing all the parts. Because the sand play arrangers stay within the imaginal realm, they can experience the transformative power fostering healthy growth as they come to understand the symbolic meaning through the experience of living in it (Lewis, 1993a).

The role of the drama therapist is to assist in the recreation of the dream or sand play world. On occasion I too enter into the dream, art or sand play world to further reveal the meaning and foster development. The experience of being in the bipersonal field can be expanded to include others in a group and can serve to continue to extend the drama of the developmental themes or related characters (Lewis, 1989, 1992, 1993a&b).

In doing so, characters can transform for the purpose of integration or union. Developmental themes can unfold a map of a person's entire life journey or therapy process, and the archetypal life themes can propel the individual through adult life stage process.

Art, Poetry, and Journaling

Other forms of creative arts therapies such as art, poetry and journaling are employed when externalizing the inner process is beneficial. Here individuals can allow their imagination to express what their consciousness may be less aware. Distancing themselves in this way allows for the possibility to become mindfully nonattached but compassionately curious at the same time. In these venues they may be able to be introduced to a feeling or part of themselves in a way that allows them to heal and reintegrate what is truly a part of their being. Interpretation is inappropriate here, as it is a left brain activity. Staying in the imaginal realm with the client, dialoguing and, in some instances, embodying part of the art or written material allows individuals digestible portions of the arts expression for integration.

Authentic Sound, Movement and Drama

Authentic Sound, Movement, and Drama is a technique of active imagination that was first identified by Mary Whitehouse (Lewis 1982, 1986, 1996). It is an experience of "being moved" by the imaginal metaphoric realm of the unconscious. The technique of authentic sound, movement and drama began its infancy in 1966 and reached full form in 1971. About this time I heard of Mary's technique of authentic movement and so decided to employ the name she had created. But the technique is slightly different than Whitehouse's classical approach as those who trained with her teach it. In the Whitehouse approach, participants engage in the technique with the therapist acting as stationary observer. The therapist is identified as a "witness" who is not encouraged to interact on a movement level with the mover(s). Additionally, classical authentic movement is based upon a somewhat parallel process group style. Although interaction among the participants is not taboo, it is also not considered an integral part of the work. Authentic sound, movement and drama however encourages the interaction between therapist and individual mover when it supports relationally-oriented healing and developmentally based growth. Additionally, it advocates group interaction in which individuals can co-participate in each other's

imaginal realm. Group members are encouraged to spontaneously transfer or project any role onto any member. Thus, one member may transfer his engulfing space-invading parent onto another member and explore separating and maintaining healthy boundaries by finding and embodying the part of him that, although still in instinctual animal-like state, can growl and snarl. While the other person may project her distancing biting, snapping childhood survival pattern on to the man who is transferring on to her.

In her case, she may attempt to soothe him, telling him there is no reason to be so snappy and angry. While, he in turn, viewing her as attempting to cajole him back into enmeshed complacency, continues to growl. Thus, each are reinforced positively: he in claiming his differentiating instinctual self, she in claiming her core self and desire for externalizing and attempting to transform her off putting survival mechanism.

Authentic sound, movement, and drama is employed with individuals and with groups. Some movers prefer silence; others prefer white noise such as ocean or wind recordings, while others prefer the many New Age tapes available. With those individuals who are unfamiliar with authentic movement, I will offer an initial guided imagery to assist them into a deeper imaginal state.

Some individuals feel various sensations and are moved in response to them. Most, however, create imagistic environments and move and sound within them. These can be recreations of the past that emerge from the unconscious realm to be consciously known or reclaimed by the enactor, or they may be new experiences that are unfolding for the individual to embody and integrate into their personality.

Authentic sound, movement and drama is a meditational practice and has been considered as a contemplative discipline for decades. Being fully present in the body allowing sensation, feeling and image to move the individual while the ego observes allows for the individual to honor what their being needs to experience to achieve clearing and balance. People often feel refreshed even though they may have begun the process in an exhausted state. Although no EEG's have been hooked up to an authentic mover for documentation, the induction into an altered state is documented through numerous qualitative studies.

Access to the numinous and Grace is also a common experience. As participants surrender to the movement, images and transpersonal human energy field connection, a profound healing is provided through the presence of the divine. At these times individuals may be lying still in a deep trance or engaged in a repetitive archetypal movement or spontaneous soul song. When this occurs, all in the room including myself are healed and blessed as well. It feels as if every molecule of my being is being bathed in Light and love–truly an indescribable bliss.

Theme-Based Improvisational Sound, Movement and Drama

Theme-based improvisational movement, sound or drama is similar to the above technique. The only difference is that a suggestion is made by the therapist that is then taken by the patient into the imaginal realm.

For example, I have frequently offered the suggestion to explore a developmentally based thematic process that has emerged in a dream or in their life to increase the individual's experience toward adaptive integration.

Ritual Dance and Drama

Ritual dance and drama taps into the archetypal universal pool of transformational theater. The creation of sacred dance and dramatic rites of passage, typically carried out in communities, help honor and support the transition from one developmental stage to another. Additionally, ritual has been employed throughout the ages as a means to connect to the sacred, to feel a part of all nature and the eternal. Ecstatic dance moves the participant into community with others transforming them all into one mind, one body, one human energy field with Divine Consciousness.

Recovery of the Inner Child(ren)

With severe physical abuse the core self can become lost and fragmented into many inner children. This occurs when the abuse is so horrifying that the experience is thrown into the unconscious, typically with the child self still surrounded by the abuse and the perpetrators. The individual survives by casting the event(s) into the unconscious, but often at the expense of maintaining a connection to the child(ren) within. The split-off part of the self then remains in a freeze frame of the abuse until the individual reclaims the memory and separates the part of the self from the abusive event. Additionally, memories are lodged in the human energy fields and the sensorium of the body.

RESCUING THE INNER CHILD(REN) FROM ABUSE. The parts of the self that have been abused must be located and subsequently rescued by the adult ego in order for the person to feel safe enough to begin to talk about the event along with the many associated feelings. If the person does not first rescue the child, adolescent, or adult self who suffered the abuse, they will retraumatize themselves when they delve into the perpetration. If an individual was repeatedly abused throughout childhood, the inner children may be of different ages.

Often the key to unraveling the mystery lies in the bodily sensations, but eventually these cues will lead to the imaginal realm. When it does the rescue may be enacted in a group or imagined in an inner drama. The individual is asked to imagine the traumatic event just prior to the event happening (retraumatization through the reexperiencing of the event is unnecessary and abusive).

Then the individual is asked as an adult to enter into the scene and take the child out to a safe place such as their heart or a previously created sanctuary. This technique, first made popular by Bradshaw, allows the person to retrieve his or herself from each abusive event. In one group drama, the protagonist had one group member literally take the member who was playing her child-self out of the drama therapy space into my garden while she confronted the abuser.

Where the abuse is severe, resulting in dissociative responses, embodiment through drama may be initially too powerful. Arts media, such as art, sand play, story writing, and journaling which externalize trauma-based phenomena can provide the needed distancing. These external symbols may be personified and interviewed by the therapist. With the needed healing and transformation carried out externally first, primitive survival behaviors and flashbacks are less apt to be triggered. The client can then internalize the drama therapy process when it is safe to do so.

PLACING THE CHILD(REN) IN A SAFE PLACE. Thus a safe, place may be a picture or a physical representation of the child in a serene or loving setting. Externalized for a period of time, they can then be reinternalized after sufficient healing. Many clients have given me figures of mothers and children to be left in special "safe places" in my office while the transference heals their mother through my nurturing and supporting of their truth and healing. These figures are then reclaimed by the client when the healing of the inner mother, now capable of protecting them, is complete.

RESCUING THE CHILD(REN) FROM SURVIVAL BEHAVIORS. Primitive survival behaviors such as dissociation (when the soul leaves the body), deanimation (when the child is placed in suspended animation), and multiple personality dissociative states (when the ego complex is cast out of consciousness while inner children of different ages and personalities take over), are often present with severe repeated physical abuse. In these instances, the inner children must feel safe enough to be fully present in an embodied manner along with the attention of the inner adult ego. With multiple personality disorder, the therapist must be the appropriate parent to each alter and help to develop interrelationships among the inner children and the inner adult ego.

Everything stops when a person leaves his/her body. This typically only occurs when the individual is having a flashback early on in the recovery work. Often this disabling process is what brings them into treatment. Speaking and moving minimally, the therapist asks concrete safe questions. I once spent much of an hour supporting the individual being aware of her body noticing reality based nontriggering stimuli from moment-to-moment; while, through the somatic countertransference, intuiting an imaginal drama that would coax the frightened self back into my client's body.

Deanimation may be enacted as a survival behavior. "I will keep your inner child frozen in numbness for eternity. Aren't I a caring protector? You do not ever have to pay attention to your core self. No need to ponder what you truly feel. I will make sure you sense that you feel or want or need nothing." Often the inner child(ren) feel a false sense of safety within this survival mechanism, but with unconditional love and care, they can be retrieved.

HEALING AND REINTEGRATION OF THE CHILD(REN). Through embodiment or giving voice to a picture, photo, dream, sand play figure or other external representation, the child(ren) begin to be healed. One woman dreamt that a child had been found wounded and starving in a comatose state with maggots crawling on her. I encouraged her to reenter the dream and pick her up. She wouldn't do it. She felt disgusted by the condition of the child. Asking permission to enter her dream, I moved over and cradled the dream image. The woman began to cry. I picked the maggots off her and began imaginally to give her liquid. Then I bathed her in healing waters. By this time the woman had moved closer. I said to her, "Look she is beautiful. She has your eyes." The woman was then able to receive her into her arms and heart.

Archetypal Enactment

At the center of each complex within the psyche is an archetypal core. Often the recovery and individuation process clears personal history allowing the archetypal energy to be accessible to the individual. The experience of the archetypal is a sacred event. All present are healed when the numinous enters the holistic therapy space. Through art, sand play, dreams, authentic and improvisational drama, individuals can access and experience its power to shake loose any disconnection to the archetypal's transpersonal power to heal and bring consciousness.

The process of individuation fosters various inner masculine and inner feminine aspects previously waiting in the wings of a person's psyche to enter and be claimed. Often the negative qualities manifest if an individual keeps their personal relationship to the archetypal out of the civilizing influence of consciousness (see Figures 5-4 and 5-5 in Chapter 5).

An example of the integration of these techniques can be seen in a workshop that brought individuals to an island in Greece for a spiritual journey of self-exploration employing daily embodied sand play, dreamwork as theater, and archetypal enactment. Daily female archetypes were invoked through Greek goddesses for theme-based dramatic experiences.

One evening Persephone, the daughter of the Earth Mother Goddess, Demeter was invoked. An innocent girl (Kore), she was abducted by the god of the underworld and eventually transformed from being a victim to becoming the queen of the underworld. Through this process she moved from

unconsciousness into being one who had psychic abilities and became a charismatic guide for those who journey into death.

Many women and men's *animae* have suffered victimization in their lives through their experience of being abused either by their family, perpetrators, and/or the culture. The capacity to let go of this view of being a victim and to claim the power of womanhood with all its wisdom and capacity to venture into the cyclic realms of death and rebirth is key for some. In the sound, movement drama experience, men and women let go of who they were in service of claiming greater wholeness. A tenor, who had come from generations of African American Baptist ministers, began leading the group in a wail. All members joined in until the group became the wail, speaking-moaning of their suffering and loss as they dropped to the floor, surrendering to the pull of symbolic death. I shrouded each one as they ritually experienced their life force leave their bodies. They then floated into a gestating pregnant timelessness. After a period of time, they experienced reanimation and gradually arose renewed with a greater access to divine wisdom.

A man said of this experience, "I thought that Persephone was a goddess only for women; I realize I am a Persephone. My innocence was ravaged, I was forced to leave a deep connection to the safety of my mother, but I see now what I have received in the hellish place of my despair. I have my own power in my recovery." A single, middle-aged woman said, "I have not wanted to let go of my innocent Kore (Persephone before she claimed her queenship). I felt that I would be thrown into the disposal heap of 'older women' when it comes to men. They do not want powerful women. But I finally see that unless I claim my wisdom and intuitive abilities; I might as well stay in suspended animation under this shroud you put on me. If a man only wants a Kore, I wouldn't want him!"

A couple came to me. The wife complained of volatile abusive outbursts from her husband. Working first with solution-focused role-play, the behaviors were arrested. He then began individual recovery work with me in which he found his core inner child frightened and rageful at not being seen. Healing the relationship between his adult self and child also bought about a clearing of his mother complex. Through my involvement in co-parenting, his mother was transferred into me for healing. At one point I needed to switch his hours twice in a week. He responded to this break in the consistency of the holding environment by missing his next two appointments. When he finally came in, he experienced permission to be appropriately angry. I not only received his anger but also reflected how this inconsistency affected him at a deep level. In the next hour, he came in and stretched out in an open posture. He reported feeling safe. He noticed two trees outside my window. I respond by saying, "Once upon a time, there were two trees. . . ." He continued this derivative story about relationship. At the end, he expressed love for me. I responded, "You have given a part of yourself to me. She is your inner feminine. I will hold her, but she is yours and belongs with you." I began feeling his anima. She was genteel, wise, loving and compassionate–goddess-like. I suggested he dialogue with her, which he did and left with her in his heart. The following week, he reported experiences of being at one, fully present with those around him, with nature and his involvement with it. He had been offered promotions that would bring him power and status. He declined as he served a different God. He called his inner feminine Grace.

Distance Intention and Energy Healing

Holding clients' highest intention is part of my practice as a transformational creative therapist. Sending health and healing is a discipline of mine whenever a client comes to mind and heart. Trained as a Reiki Master I

also send energy; and at times, when my clients distress is producing physical symptoms, I will, with permission, focus my hands on their chakras and human energy field.

Mindfulness Meditation

Before and during every session I center and place myself in a mindful meditative wakeful consciousness. I also meditate with many of my clients. With some, it is a weekly initial practice to help bring them into themselves, the room and present awareness. If someone is focused on the past or future, no transformation can take place. With others, who because of ADHD or defensive flight have lost the moment, I may interrupt their imbalance and suggest they bring themselves into the moment and follow their diaphragmatic breath noticing without judgement or editing what sensations, feelings, and thoughts come up. In other instances, I may encourage mindful meditation, then after a few minutes ask them what they truly need and want right now. With some, the meditation itself becomes the transformational process. This is carried out either through classic sitting meditation, moving meditation, sustained eye-to-eye contacted presence with me, or noticing from moment-to-moment their inner sensations and feelings or the subtle changing nuances of the river and tree-lined field in front of their view in a Gestalt continuum of awareness. Often these moments have produced profound grace and pivotally changed individuals lives.

THE ROLE OF THE MINDBODY SOULSPIRIT THERAPIST

It is the role of the therapist to create and hold the temenos or sacred container of the holistic health setting. The mindbody and soulspirit of the client need to be cared for in their interrelated totality. It order to do so, holistic health practitioner/therapists must be connected to their own mindbody and spirituality. Any personal recovery work needs to have been delved into in depth. This is due to the fact that unresolved history and associated assumptions and survival behaviors are carried on an energetic, unconscious as well as psychological level telesomatically affecting the bipersonal energetic field between the client and practitioner/therapist.

Practitioner/therapists must be on their own spiritual path. Their work in relation to the client is carried out with a sacred mindful relationally oriented compassionate presence. Attending from moment to moment, as there is so much to be aware of:

• The human energy fields
• The body posture and movement behavior
• The tone of voice
• Explicit verbal content including underlying assumptions, beliefs, and survival behaviors
• Symbolic or metaphoric content
• Sensations, feelings and images received telesomatically into the therapist through the somatic countertransference
• Nonverbal communication: clothing and grooming are indirect statements about self-image
• Their level of presence in their body
• Their response to you verbally and nonverbally including developmentally associated transferences and projections
• Information intuitively received or channeled on behalf of the individual
• Moment-to-moment information from the client regarding internal somatic sensations, feelings and images

With so much to influence and draw upon, the therapist/practitioner cannot afford to lose attention! This requires the therapist not to be attached to outcome. If there are agendas floating around in the therapist's mind, they will most certainly affect the level of intimacy that can be attained. Having a meditational discipline is key here. Each session with a client is to be considered a meditation. Clients frequently say that they feel such peace in my presence. Years of meditation and the discipline of mindfulness-based wakefulness allow me to be both nonattached and nonjudgmental as well as loving and deeply caring.

Some professionals have licensure, others do not. Regardless, becoming aware of standards of ethical practice in existing holistic health fields such as counseling can help inform a practitioner regarding issues of confidentiality, boundaries of competence, informed consent, dual relationship and mandated reporting. No matter where we are we represent our profession and the field of holistic health. Thus mindfulness must extend beyond the meditation cushion and the consulting room.

Who's the facilitator? As part of my training in Jungian Analysis, I was taught that it was the patient's unconscious and not the analyst who was the authority. Thus, it is the unconscious with its access to the trauma held in the personal unconscious and the spiritual connection through the archetypal unconscious which provides the subject matter and the direction. My role is that of midwifing consciousness. I encourage the process but also make sure that the birth is not traumatic or too swift. I frequently use the metaphor of "having an appropriate amount on your plate." Too much material from the unconscious and the person can become overwhelmed with recycling from the amygdala producing emotional hijacking. On the opposite pole, overworked survival mechanisms can keep a person from having any access to the unconscious and result in the person living in a psychic desert without any ability to find the well spring of potential awaiting them. With too little on their plate, they go through life starved for a connection to themselves and depth of meaning. Thus, the therapist/practitioner must also be facile at moving in and out of the imaginal transitional space allowing the power of the imagination to heal. The therapist must be able to move through developmentally-based roles. They, even with the same client, may become for example, a mother to an infant, toddler, child or adolescent; a playmate, beloved projected contrasexual animus/a, despised projected shadow aspect, or a wise man, woman or shaman (see Chapter 5 and Lewis, 1993, 2000).

APPROPRIATE POPULATIONS FOR THE MINDBODY AND SOUL CREATIVE TRANSFORMATIONAL APPROACH

Because the approach is by definition developmental, all ages from infancy to aging and dying are appropriate. Those with most all forms of emotional disorders as well as stress-related distress and chronic and life-threatening diseases have experienced transformation and healing. Additionally, those in spiritual crisis and life stage transition have benefited as well. This approach has been used with individuals, couples, mothers and children and groups of all ages in private practice, clinical and organizational systems settings.

MINDBODY SOULSPIRIT TRANSFORMATIONAL CASE EXAMPLES

Healing From and Through Breast Cancer with Dreamwork as Theater

Kate was a highly respected professional woman in her job when she was hit with the diagnosis of breast cancer. The tissue was found in her axilary lymph nodes as well. By the time she had come to see me, her oncologist had put her on a chemotherapy regime. The chemo was to be followed by radiation, followed by surgery, followed by another round as needed. This allopathic treatment plan was to span a year of her life.

Kate, now in her forties, had excelled in whatever she did much to the surprise of her mother who gave her such self-affirming beliefs as: "You've done nothing in your life but go to school; what do you know. You should never get married or have children, you would be horrible at it." All these damaging statements were projections of her mother's own inability, and produced core beliefs in Kate that she wasn't good enough and that there was something fundamentally wrong with her. Her father was an exciting, dashing manic-depressive who committed suicide in her early twenties. Her assigned role in the family was to feel everyone's unspoken feelings and to speak out as best she could for the underdog. This family script evolved into her calling in life working for the underprivileged and disenfranchised.

In an initial dream, she asks her mother to see her beautiful flower garden she has created. Her mother responds with disinterest. She then goes to an airport to see me. She wants a bag at a store there but is unable to purchase one for herself. She finds me and we go to some bleachers, and she watches me with two clients. The first is mourning the death of her husband and the second, although pretending that everything is fine in her life, is being held by me while I am chanting Om. Using dreamwork as theater, I go with her to buy the bag, symbolic of the inner feminine, that she wanted. We mourn the death of her inner masculine from the abuse of her mother and the betrayal of males in her childhood. Her unconscious had plotted the course of the healing: Support to find and value her inner feminine self, the resurrection and reclaiming of the inner masculine and the experience of the archetypal healing mother.

The next week she brings in a recurring dream: "I am in my childhood home, there is an angry male mob outside, I am afraid and I can't wake my husband up." Her inner masculine in multiple form was struggling to be let into her life. I encouraged her to dialogue with the leader of the mob. She and I role-play the dialogue. I reverse roles with her when it is relevant for her to come to understand the meaning of the dream through the experience of the character. I begin as her, "you're frightening me what do you want?" Kate as the mob leader, "We want to be let in, you have shut us out long enough." I respond, "Well look at you, you're loud, angry and unruly–of course I would shut you out. You would make a mess out of my life and me if I let you in." Kate as the mob leader, "You don't look like your life is in too great shape." I respond, "Well you certainly can't help me." "How do you know that, you've shut me out for so long."

This dialogue begins the possibility of reclaiming a relationship to her inner masculine. Research has shown that the "fighters" have a statistically greater chance of cancer survival. I sent her home with homework to continue to dialogue with this inner masculine figure toward the goal of his becoming a protector or lover.

In the third session after I suggested she might consider the breast cancer support group that was offered at her hospital, we began to look at all the "great ideas" people have for her. I immediately apologized and commended her on her ability to speak out about what she needs. This moved her to tears, but then her guilt at speaking up for herself began to attack her. Personifying her guilt, I then spoke directly to it, "Oh guilt, who invited you? Or did you just think you could come in here and rob Kate of her capacity to honor and care for herself. Why don't you go and try to convince that angry mob (referring to last weeks dream) that you're here in Kate's best interest."

Kate and I then experience several moments of real intimacy. She shared that she had difficulty trusting people. I respond that that would be a normal response given her childhood.

We then shift our focus to the beautiful trees and river view out the picture window in front of her as the presence of the moment filled us with grace.

The session opened from here. Meditation and presence fills the room. She remarks that her holistic health program looks unlike anyone else's. "I just sit in reverie and do nothing; just be." Yoga initially felt too uncomfortable for her as her image of instructors was what I call "the pretzel people"–nothing she felt she could identify with. Instead, she began with a stretch class. I, in turn, deeply affirm her clear boundaries about knowing just what she needs.

Just a month later, her life-long reoccurring dream changes. She dreams she is in a house, but she is not afraid of the darkened rooms and the adolescent male driving by. She reports that life has slowly turned around for her. "Things that would have bothered me before are not bothering me." She now wants to ask an older sibling to help her remember her childhood. She speaks about the possibility of creating a new family of friends and colleagues. A week later she has ventured into the yoga class that I had spoken about with a loving–"nonpretzel"– Kripalu teacher. She said she had experienced such bliss in this class and remarked how accepting the teacher was. I had known of Barbara's heart and goodness as she was part of my referral collective, but one of the most important aspects of Kate's healing was attuning and valuing her needs and timing. No existing holistic health breast cancer program would have been more helpful than Kate's sense of listening to her own needs and personality in service to creating her own program. She reports in the third month that her heart felt more open.

In the next session she comes in with a beret covering her "chemo hairdo." Bringing in humor we laugh at the thought of her being confused as member of a gang which uses berets as their identification. She dreams she is in a huge courthouse. Men were running around strangling women. One man comes to strangle her, but two women come from the shadows and step on him. He then changes his mind and invites her to New York City.

New York, she associates was where she was heading in her young adulthood, but got rerouted instead. As the male she says, "I was just doing what the other men were doing." Knives, swords, guns and penetrating weapons are usually associated with male energy. Poisoning, strangling and smothering are more associated with female energy. The patriarchy and her mother's inner masculine had kept her from being spirited, speaking and following her dreams.

She reports that she was offered a job. In the past she would have taken it, but now she was aware of the level of stress it produced in her body. So she was able to honor herself. Speaking out she declined the position, as she knew she was heading in a different direction.

Now her reoccurring home dream continues to transform. In the next week she dreams she is in a house with her mother. Kate is telling her how to shut the doors (put up good boundaries) in order to protect them. Then there appears a beautiful blue and gods and goddesses appear. She feels transformed in their presence. She reports that she continues to feel deep calm and peace at the end of her yoga classes.

Her breast and lymph node surgery was emerging on the horizon. She expressed fear at being under the knife. She states that she is relieved that I don't try to reassure her but let her have her real sense of being violated. She reports the following dream: "I am flying and then I crash into the water. I walk into a forest and meet a hermit with a daughter. The hermit says, 'You can stay here with me for a while. Then you will find your way.' She then finds herself in a jungle in a community of people who believe that nature heals. They say, 'We exist together and come and go without pressure. We are like one web. The lush green is sacred, spiritual.'"

After reporting the dream, I encourage her to image these places before, during and after the surgery.

Her energy healer had suggested to her to give individuals in her life a chakra color to send to her while she was in surgery. She asked me to send red the root chakra color. At the time of her surgery, I was teaching a dance-movement therapy class at Antioch University. I asked all my students to imagine being red and then to send it into the circle allowing it to combine; we then sent it to her. When she returned from the surgery, she reported feeling incredible peace. Although the nurses said that most would feel nauseous post-op, she had no such symptoms and could eat solid food. Additionally, she said that her highly intuitive husband had seen red and green (the color her energy healer had chosen) very clearly and powerfully.

The surgeons felt that the margins were clear. She said to me, "I remember some time ago in this room when I felt the cancer left me . . . right down my arm and we both knew I was cancer free." We talked frequently being moved to tears about how her spiritual faith had expanded from the inside out, and about how she waited for the crystallization of her path and how she will serve. She thanked me for knowing that what she needed was not to jump into the classical holistic health breast cancer program, but to encourage and acknowledge her own path–to be still and mindfully present.

During termination our discussions ventured into the bigger picture. She says, "I used to be personally fearful. This work has changed all that. Now I am concerned for the world." I liken her process to a monastic retreat. Leaving who she was, experiencing the loss of roles and personas, going into a liminal meditative realm like suspended animation, now she is slowing emerging like the rebirth cycle of spring. Before ending her unconscious wanted her to heal and reclaim aspects of her core self.

In the one month follow up she brings in the following dream: "My husband drops me off and tells me to go through a tunnel. I proceed and these children start climbing over the walls and pulling at my suitcase. I wake up screaming" I suggest that I role-play her and she the children. As the children they report that they want the fuzzy and warm things in her suitcase. I respond as her but with an added aspect of healing as I felt in the dream she had treated these inner child selves as her mother had treated her. Thus, I respond with love and care, "Oh little ones, I'd love to share what I have with you come with me and you can have whatever you like. I am glad you have climbed over the walls because now I have these warm fuzzy things to take care of you with." Now tears come to her eyes as she begins to experience the healing. Her unconscious knew that she was ready to nurture her inner child selves. She just needed a little help.

In the last session of the process she says, "I've had an epiphany. If I am going to die, I don't want people to say 'she struggled with cancer for years.' I want to get on with my life."

I respond, "We are all going to die. What is important is to be fully present in life."

Healing Cancer from a Shamanic Frame

A man returned to therapy with me after a diagnosis of cancer was made with a removal of a metastasized tumor. With chemotherapy about to begin and the possibility of his own mortality facing him, he wanted to understand more deeply what his path was. Having been raised Protestant he reported having had very little interest in anything religious or spiritual.

For the several sessions synchronistic phenomena would occur during his therapy hour in the form of animal appearances never before seen out my office window. In his second session two seals appeared at river's edge in front of us. Within a shamanic frame, the unusual appearance of animals may suggest that the individual may need to receive information from those creatures who are in a deeper connection with the nature of things on how to unfold one's own nature. With this perspective in mind, I suggested he enter into the imaginal realm with

the seals and dialogue with them. "Be harmonious with nature, and joy and pleasure will be yours," was their response.

In the next hour, he looked up to find a magnificent 8 point stag in the meadow out front who appeared and stayed for his hour only. I knew from my research that the stag is one of the major power animal of shamans and is a symbol of Christ (Lewis, 1993). Through dramatic dialogue with the buck he received, "Get rid of fear. This is filling your mind with useless thoughts. Get off your butt. Don't waste time looking for outside guidance through books. Be open now."

In the following hour, he reported a dream, "I am in a medieval inner courtyard–like a circular paddock. The stag goes through a big dark wooden door. I feel I'm supposed to follow, but I don't want to. Then I'm aware there is a huge male figure dressed in white robes. He is laughing." He role-played the white figure who is clearly a trickster psychopomp. He told him he must go through the door. If he didn't, all his suffering from the chemo will have no meaning.

He returns a month later racked with pain and nausea from the chemo. Placing my hand over his third chakra, I cleared his nausea from his energy field utilizing Reiki. He reported seeing two hawks facing in opposite directions on the same branch in the front of my office. He lay down and I suggested he connect with the hawks. During this time I saw soul energy moving from his body. He later reported that the hawks helped him leave his body. "Now I know I have a body; I am not a body." "Yes," I responded, "It is easier for people to be willing to have out of body experiences if they are in physical pain."

Three weeks later he returned with the following dream: He is in monk's habit leading a group in the wilderness. He comes upon a rock impasse. Before him appeared 5 angels. Each sent him their names: Love, Compassion, Truth, Understanding, and Humility. He extends his hands and radiant beams of light emanate. He then told me he is not religious and feels unworthy. I instructed him to ask the angels. He stretched out his arms and then began to laugh. "They say that is beside the point." he reported. I then instruct him to reenact his dream. During this drama he began to cry. "This may sound corny," he reported later, "but to touch people . . . we're all suffering . . . to touch with kindness. . . ."

After a hiatus in which he was recovering from the chemo, he returned. I suggested he imagine and reconnect with the animals that had appeared to him. Moving about the room he reported, "The hawk is circling above and the stag is entering a forest." "Follow him" I responded with a sense of knowing which comes from opening myself to divine guidance on behalf of my clients. He came to a circular clearing with a 20-ft. stone circle and a fire in the middle. He saw many faces in the fire. "Step into the fire" I heard myself say with assurance. He stepped in and reported, "I'm looking out. Everything is dark. I sense there is something beyond, something green, but I'm afraid of the dark." My insistence was to no avail. At this point all the electricity in my office went off and stayed off until he left. By this time, an appreciation of the nonrational, nonempirical was clearly present, for his response was to laugh knowingly; and to apologize.

In the next session, I returned him to his incomplete journey. He stepped in the flame and reported a dark hole in the middle not dissimilar to the earth entry descent points in shamanic journeying. Reminding him to let go off his fear, he was able to descend down. The hole got smaller and still embodying the visualization, he crawled until he reported seeing large teeth in front of him that kept him from proceeding. He said finally, "You know this is funny but if I were a snake I could slither right through." "Be a snake" I responded. He proceeded and learned he could shape shift.

In his last session he reported that the president of his company wanted to place him in a managerial position, one in which he would be speaking nationally. But he told me he was afraid of what he would say. "They might ask questions that I don't know the answers to." I responded, "Ask the angels." The angels say, "It's not what you say. It's your being, your compassion and your love which is the message." He then said to me, "All my life I've always judged myself as being a 'jack of all trades master of none'. I've never reached the pinnacle of accomplishment in any field. Now I realize this is not the direction at all. It is not what you do; it is who you are." "Yes," I responded, "Manifesting your soul is truly the most important accomplishment."

Expanding Beliefs from a Christian Fundamentalist Frame

Another man began work with me with a highly defined religious faith. He was concerned about engaging in psychotherapy with someone who was not of his church and proceeded to ask me several questions about my beliefs. Attuning to his religious faith I employed a Christian frame. I responded that we would work within his beliefs. He then asked me if I believed in the existence of evil. "Absolutely," I responded. He then reported going to a well-known spiritual healer of his faith. Kneeling in front of her he prayed for generational healing. Through the somatic countertransference (Lewis, 1993, 1996), I began feeling deep sadness and pain. He continued saying that he was prayed over and that the spiritual healer saw a chalice in his throat. At that moment my throat went into spasm; breathing and speaking become difficult. "The same thing happened to the healer he said, I feel terrible; what should we do." "Pray." I responded. I then looked heavenward. Tears—neither his nor mine—flooded my eyes. Through his prayer, this sensation released. He then added that the cup had claw-like feet and shared family history that gave meaning to the image. From this experience a trust in our relationship developed, and he deceased in asking any further questions regarding my beliefs.

The therapy focused upon healing from a shame-based childhood with a controlling unattuned mother and extended into the reenactment of his childhood relationship with his mother in his present life. In one session I drew his attention from his head-based intellectualization into his body and there, he described a bottomless pit in which he felt like he was falling forever. I responded that there was no one that held his core self as a child, and that he needed to catch the child within. He catches the child but, with only his parents as role models, he became irritated at his child self and did not want to continue holding him. I then asked, "Could Jesus hold you holding your child?" He responded. "I didn't think I needed him." I responded within his religious frame, "What hubris!" i.e., to assume that he didn't need Jesus.

He then realized that his view of God was contaminated by his experience with his parents and a highly judgmental minister. I suggested he use baptismal water to clean his personal associations so that God's love could emerge. He reported that this was difficult. I responded. "Open your heart to God. Let God's love fill you and connect you." He then rose, expanded his chest and extended his arms, an expression of bliss emanated from his countenance as he walked around the office-studio. In the next session he reported he had gotten a book entitled "Your God is too small."

Healing from Trauma through a Spiritualist Frame

The last example required a greater willingness to expand and join with another's religious/spiritual view than any other client that I have had. For three years I had to push and expand my beliefs and face my fears regarding what was for me highly unusual

circumstances. I had heard of my client prior to her beginning recovery work with me. She was a well-known highly respected healer and psychic. I pondered what it would be like working with someone who channeled spirits; what information would she receive; how would this affect the therapeutic frame? Carl Jung had felt that unless both the analysand and analyst are healed no healing occurs. I believe that unless both the client and therapist learn and grow from the therapeutic relationship, no growth occurs for the person seeking help. I knew without a doubt that I was going to grow from this relationship and that my consciousness–particularly spiritually–would have to expand.

The embodied arts of drama and dance-movement are often the most powerful as the person is experiencing the healing process as it is happening. But with this client, childhood physical and sexual abuse had repeatedly violated her body boundaries, and in her case as with others, embodiment was too powerful as it can literally send the individual out of her body triggering the childhood survival pattern of dissociation. Thus, arts media that externalize trauma-based complexes was far more appropriate. Through art, poetry, story writing, and journaling, my client could distance herself from the events; then personifying different aspects, she could interview them and begin to put the pieces together in a way that didn't tear her apart in the process.

DISSOCIATION AND SPIRITUAL CONNECTION. Where abuse is physical either through torture in war-torn countries, from a traumatic accident, from a progressive debilitating disease, or from beatings or sexual assault, some individuals elect to leave their bodies through dissociation in order to survive. Some stay fairly close to their bodies often floating above and viewing the events cut off from their feelings. Others elect to leave the proximity of their bodies and access a different realm–a realm where everyone is in spirit. When these individuals return many of them maintain a spiritual connection and are identified as psychics, mediums, and channels. In the past these individuals were burned as witches; later they were told they were insane; today they are accepted and respected by many.

With individuals who have suffered severe repeated physical abuse it is often an all or nothing. Either their survival mechanisms have clamped their childhood shut and the person can't remember anything, or the flood gates are open with flashbacks of the traumatic events invading their dreams at night and their waking life as well. When the latter happens the triggers for this flooding can be what someone says, the tone of voice, the surroundings, a smell, a portion of their body which experienced the trauma being stimulated in some way or just the overwhelming readiness of the unconscious to pour forth. At these times I attempt to ground adult ego consciousness to help it from drowning. Thus, instead of encouraging access to the unconscious, I focus on the nonimaginal. Slowing separating sensation, from feeling, from thoughts can reduce the impact and cultivate a mindful observing ego that understands that they have thoughts and feelings, but are not the thoughts, feelings and sensations. Additionally, concrete practical reality-based left brain discussion along with interpretation ensues with the goal of compartmentalizing some of the flooding and holding it in abeyance until their "plate" is less full.

Since the abuse occurred over many years her core child self was fragmented into many children of different ages. All of these inner children needed to be rescued from the trauma within which they were frozen in her now emerging memories. This took several weeks. My client consulted with her guides and reported that they helped in the rescue and subsequent creation of a safe holding environment.

Sometime later she brought in a dream about a child that had no skin. The experience of being skinless is a frequent metaphor of individuals who have had their body boundaries violated. My client wrote in her journal:

> I had a dream about a child with no skin. She was raw. Penny asked me to try to relate to the child. I took away the covers and surrounded the child with Light. I could not have a conversation with this child; I could only heal her. Penny asked me to be this child. The child was frozen with stark terror: stuck; iced up. I did not like doing this. I felt numb and then I felt the mothering part of me emerging wanting to help this baby. Drawing the healing process brought forth an angel holding the child.

Once her inner children were freed from the abuse memories, they needed further releasing from her childhood survival patterns that attempted to protect her. Individually each child self emerged from an imagistic wall and frozen numbness of her past. Each child told her story and was loved and received by my client and myself. I would often put the drawing of the child on my lap as if I were holding the actual child; and with my client speaking for her, she would tell us what she wanted us to know.

Once her present lifetime cleared sufficiently, very different but very specific visual images began to appear in her flashbacks. Only these images were not of this lifetime. They were of a child in a Nazi prison camp who's job it was to shove hacked up bodies into the ovens. She put herself in front of a bullet when she realized she would have to shove her own sister into the flames.

Reincarnation was a concept that I had accepted as a distinct possibility, but actually engaging in past life therapy. . . . I had willingly left this form of therapy to those "new agey" therapists lest I might be labeled as a quack. Now I had to look at my own prejudice against acknowledging this spiritual truth of this woman and continue to assist her in her own recovery process. I had to have the courage to step out of the traditional world view of acceptable Judeo Christian beliefs and join with this woman. I felt I went through a process described in the quote from Jung earlier in this book: "The ego never lacks moral and rational counter arguments which one cannot and should not set aside so long as it is possible to hold on to them. For you only feel yourself on the right road when the conflicts of duty seemed to have resolved themselves, and you have become the victim of a decision made over your head in defiance of the heart."

Thus, honoring and respecting her process, we began to help heal this beleaguered child. She began drawing her. The writing on the picture read, "Blood ran between the bricks–like earth worms running from the fires of hell."

Parallel to the emergence of this child came another hidden in a cave-like surround who later came to be know as "The Butterfly Soul Child."

An excerpt from one of her many poems speaks to the powerful spiritual belief that began to grow in her.

My adult self responds:

but ME-THE ADULT SOUL has feet
which, bare and complete,
penetrate into rich soil
to stand firm against
ridiculous invasion
and hold up high
rescued bodies and souls of US
from that rotten
cement floor
to GOD
and, tell all the pained ones
about the POWER OF GOD
that I am finding in ME.

I give the children a mirror
to show them their own Light.
Don't be afraid, little ones.
You are in "the remembering."

The Angels and all gentle spirits
guide us, help us, and
some people of the earth
love us and heal us too.

Come away from the fires of pain
to my garden where
my feet are whole
and planted among the flowers.

I AM THE ADULT SOUL AND I HAVE
    THE POWER
OF GOD IN ME
I AM THE BUTTERFLY CHILD SOUL
There is fresh air-sunshine-loving transformation here.
Come little ones,
My arms are long and wide enough to hold
    you.

One of her last drawings was of the soul now emerged from the cave bringing her child self of the past life into the light. She looks down at her feet now healed from the torture. There remain other souls from those who died in the holocaust still in the cave not yet ready to emerge. It was after this drawing that synchronistically individuals began calling my client for readings. Many of them said that they knew they had died in the prison camps in their immediate past life, and needed to heal and connect more deeply with what they are meant to do.

Throughout her work with me she channeled drawings and messages into her journal from her spiritual guides. Toward the end of the work one guide sent her the following message:

Breathe with conviction, yes. Breathing with compassion is better. Just breathing in this moment is best. Compassion is the salve you seek to relieve your pain. It is also the rock that you search for to hold you securely above the floods of time. Sometimes the winds may temporarily cool the surface and cause you to wonder where you are but it is your understanding of the fire within and trust in its eternal light that will keep you on your path, your rock of truth. Compassion is the heat of the soul. Let it be your breath and the foundation of your life for every moment and every second of your existence.

Compassion is a very powerful soul voice that automatically seals boundaries and allows the soul voice to be heard. It is powerful medicine for accumulated pain and does not allow anger and fear to dwell for very long in anyone's life. Anger and hatred are the defense mechanisms of the ego. Compassion is the way of the soul and the only way to spiritually respond to life. You have learned about anger and hatred from many lifetimes, especially during the life in the German camp. You have carried that deep bitterness into this life for healing. Do you wish to continue carrying its heaviness further? Life is not as complicated as it seems.

If you dwell on sickness you will become it. This is the lesson that you have to learn, that beyond all of the physical and mental violence there is still the soul, and the soul cannot express itself if it is surrounded by hate and fear. The real work is the clearing the energy that surrounds your center of love. If your energy field is filled with your soul's compassion and the gentleness and strength of its love, you will have what you need to feel safe in your life. As I said before, this is not a weakness, it is the power of God becoming your presence (Lewis, 2000).

In summary, when my client left her body, as many do during physical abuse, she reaffirmed a connection with souls that are in spirit. That connection maintained through her life has for some time evolved into her life's vocation. What was a means of escape in childhood has become the foundation of her livelihood and the means through which she serves Divine Consciousness and her fellow humans.

The arts, drawing, story writing, journaling, poetry, and dramatic embodiment were crucial to the healing process. They provided the vehicle with which to enter into the unconscious both personal and universal-archetypal; they provided the vessel within which to rescue, heal, and transform; and they provided the means by which the spiritual could enter matter and be known.

CONCLUSION

From my training as a dance-movement, drama therapist, and gestalt therapist, I have come to respect what emerges on a somatic level. From my training in Jungian Analysis I have come to absolutely trust what emerges from an individual's unconscious. As I venture into the imaginal somatic realm with my clients it has continued to be affirmed that the symbolic and metaphoric have their own reality which must be respected as that which emerges holds the key to healing. There is no question that my work with clients has forced me to expand my existing belief system. For what has emerged from their experience of the truth also demanded of me and particularly of my rational analytical empirical left brain to extend my view of reality. My work with these individuals required me to not just nod at some beliefs but be able to work within them and through them.

There is no question that spiritual beliefs through institutionalized religions and commercial packaging of neo-transpersonal systems were scooped up, projected and transferred into, ripped apart, devoured and regurgitated. Integrative holistic health and healing has begun to establish a body of knowledge about the union of the healing process and spiritual/religious beliefs. These transpersonal phenomena may resonate with the individual's stated beliefs or may emerge from the symbols, themes, movements, and sounds of the archetypal expressive arts process. It is therefore vital that the holistic health practitioner and therapist have an ecumenical transpersonal world view.

Further in the beginning of civilization the doctors of healing were also the priests and priestesses of their community. It is thus vital for the therapist to not only expand tolerance and acceptance of various cultures spiritual traditions, but also be able to be a vessel for and manifest the transpersonal in service to the patient's own connection to the transformational power of spiritual consciousness.

SUMMARY

In summary, this mindbody and soul creative transformational model focuses upon recovery from the past toward being fully present in the moment able to be intimate with themselves, others, and the sacred. When individuals are mindfully present, they become stress hardy capable of rebounding through life's ups and downs. Presence supports clear human energy fields. Additionally, spiritually-based dance and drama therapy supports individuals as they continue throughout their life undergoing adult life stages, deepening their understanding of the meaning of life and their role in it, and expanding their spiritual Consciousness.

REFERENCES

Arts in Psychotherapy Journal. (1992). Vol. 15, No. 4.

Barber, T. (1976). *Advances in altered states of consciousness & human potential.* New York: Psychological Dimensions, Inc.

Boorstein, S. (1991). *Transpersonal psychotherapy.* Stanford, CA: JTP Books.

Carter-Haar, B. (1975). What is psychosynthesis? *Synthesis,* Vol. 1, No, 2, pp. 115–118.

Edinger, E. (1982). *Ego and archetype.* New York: Penguin Books.

Goswami, A. (2001). Quantum Yoga. In *IONS Noetic Science Review,* June-August, no. 56.

Harner, M. (1982). *The way of the shaman.* New York: Bantam Books.

Jung, C.G. (1969). *The archetypes and the collective unconscious.* CW, Vol. 9 part 1. Princeton, NJ.: Princeton University Press.

Jung, C.G. (1963). *Mysterium coniunctionis.* CW. 14. Princeton, NJ: Princeton University Press.

Jung, C.G. (1969). *Symbols of transformation.* CW Vol. 5. Princeton, NJ: Princeton University

Press.

Lewis, P. & Johnson, D. (2000). *Current approaches in drama therapy.* Springfield: Charles C Thomas.

Lewis, P. (1993). *Creative transformation: The healing power of the arts.* Willmette, IL: Chiron Publishing.

Lewis, P. (1996). Depth psychotherapy in dance/movement therapy. *American Journal of Dance Therapy,* Vol. 18, 95–114.

Lewis, P. (1986). *Theoretical approaches in dance-movement therapy,* Vol. II. Dubuque, IA: Kendall/Hunt.

Lewis, P. (1988). The transformative process in the imaginal realm. *Arts in Psychotherapy,* Vol. 15, pp. 309–316.

Lewis, P. (1992). The transference and countertransference in arts psychotherapy. *Arts in Psychotherapy Journal,* 15.

Smart, N. & Hecht, R. (1982). *Sacred texts of the world: A universal anthology.* New York: Crossroad Publishing Company.

Walsh, R. & Vaughan, F. (1993). *Paths beyond ego the transpersonal vision.* Los Angeles: Jeremy PTarcher/Perigee Books.

Bibliography

Books

Lewis-Bernstein, P. (1975). Editor. *Therapeutic process movement as integration.* Columbia: ADTA.

Lewis-Bernstein, P. & Singer, D. (Eds.). (1982). *The choreography of object relations.* Keene: Antioch University.

Lewis, P. (1986). *Theoretical approaches in dance-movement therapy,* Vol. I. Dubuque: W.C. Brown-Kendall/Hunt.

Lewis, P. (1987a). *Theoretical approaches in dance-movement therapy,* Vol. II. Dubuque: W.C. Brown-Kendall/Hunt.

Lewis, P. and S. Loman, Eds. (1990). *The Kestenberg Movement Profile: Its past, present and future applications.* Keene: Antioch University.

Lewis, P. (1993). *Creative transformation: The healing power of the expressive arts.* Willmette: Chiron Publishing.

Lewis, P. (1994). *The clinical interpretation of the Kestenberg Movement Profile.* Keene: Antioch New England Provost Fund.

Lewis, P. (1999). *Schopfennshe Prozesse. Kunst in*

Der Therapeutis Chen Praxis. Zurich/ Dusseldorf: Verlag Pub.

Amaghi, J., Loman, S., Lewis, P., & Sossin, M., Eds. (1999). *The meaning of movement: Developmental and clinical perspectives in the Kestenberg Movement Profile.* Newark, NJ: Gordon & Breach.

Lewis, P. & Johnson, D. (2000) *Current approaches in drama therapy.* Springfield, IL: Charles C Thomas.

Articles and Chapters

Lewis Bernstein, P. & Cafarelli, E. (1972). An electromyographical validation of the effort system of notation. *Writings on body movement and communication,* Vol. II. Columbia: ADTA.

Lewis Bernstein, P. (1972). Range of response as seen through a developmental progression. *What is dance therapy really?* Barbara Govine (Ed.). Columbia: ADTA.

Lewis Bernstein, P. & Bernstein, L. (1973-4). A conceptualization of group dance-movement therapy as a ritual process. *Writings on body movement and communication,* Vol. III. Columbia: ADTA.

Lewis Bernstein, P. & Garson, B. (1975). Pilot atudy in the use of tension flow system of movement notation in an ongoing study of infants at risk for schizophrenic disorders. *Dance Therapy–Depth and Dimension.* Delores Plunk (Ed.). Columbia: ADTA.

Lewis Bernstein, P. (1975). Tension flow rhythms: As a developmental diagnostic tool within the theory of the recapitulation of ontogeny. *Dance Therapy–Depth and Dimension.* Columbia: ADTA.

Lewis Bernstein, P., Rubin, J. & Irwin, E. (1975). Play, parenting, and the arts. *Therapeutic process movement as integration.* Penny Lewis Bernstein (Ed.). Columbia: ADTA.

Lewis Bernstein, P. (1980). Dance-movement therapy. *Psychotherapy Handbook.* Richard Herink (Ed.). New York: The New American Library Press.

Lewis Bernstein, P. (1980). A mythic quest: Jungian movement therapy with the psychosomatic client. *American Journal of Dance Therapy,* Spring, Vol. 3, No. 2, pp. 44–55.

Lewis Bernstein, P. (1980). The union of the Gestalt concept of experiment and Jungian active imagination within a woman's mythic quest. *The Gestalt Journal,* Fall, Vol. 3, No. 2, pp. 36–46.

Lewis Bernstein, P. (1981). Moon goddess, medium, and earth mother: A phenomenological study of the guiding archetypes of the dance movement therapist. *Research as Creative Process.* Columbia: ADTA.

Lewis Bernstein, P. (1982). Authentic movement as active imagination. *The Compendium of Psychotherapeutic Techniques.* Jusuf Hariman (Ed.). New York: Charles C Thomas.

Lewis Bernstein, P. (1986). Embodied transformational images in dance-movement therapy. *Journal of Mental Imagery,* Vol. 9, No. 4, pp. 1–9.

Lewis, P. (1987b). The expressive therapies in the choreography of object relations. *The Arts in Psychotherapy Journal,* Vol. 14, No. 4, pp. 321–332.

Lewis, P. (1987c). The unconscious as choreographer: The use of tension flow rhythms in the transference relationship. *A.D.T.A. Conference Monograph.* Columbia: ADTA.

Lewis, P. (1988). The transformative process within the imaginal realm. *The Arts in Psychotherapy Journal,* Vol. 15, No. 3, Fall, pp. 309–316.

Lewis, P. (1988). The dance between the conscious and unconscious: Transformation in the embodied imaginal realm. *The Moving Dialogue.* Columbia: ADTA.

Lewis, P. (1988). The marriage of our art with science: The Kestenberg Profile and the choreography of object relations. *Monograph 5.* Columbia: ADTA.

Lewis, P. (1990a). The Kestenberg Movement Profile in the psychotherapeutic process with borderline disorder. *The KMP: Its past, present application and future directions.* Lewis & Loman (Eds.). Keene: Antioch University Publishing.

Lewis, P. & Brownell, A. (1990b). The Kestenberg Movement Profile in assessment of vocalization. *The KMP: Its past, present application and future directions.* Lewis & Loman (Eds.). Keene: Antioch University Publishing.

Lewis, P. (1991). Creative transformation: The alchemy of healing, individuation and spiritual consciousness. *Shadow and light: Moving toward wholeness.* Columbia: ADTA.

Lewis, P. (1993). The use of reflection, reciprocity, rhythmic body action, and the imaginal in the depth dance therapy process of recovery, healing and spiritual consciousness. *Marian Chace, Her Papers, 2nd Edition.* Sandel, S. Chaiklin, S. & Lohn, A. (Eds.). Columbia: ADTA.

Lewis, P. (1993). Michael Jackson, Analysiert Mit Hilfe Des. Kestenberg-Bewegungsprofils in Tanztherapie. Hormann, K. (Ed.). *The application of the Kestenberg Movement Profile and its concepts.* Zurich: Beitrage zur Augewandten Hogrefe.

Lewis, P. (1992). The creative arts in transference-countertransference relationships. *Arts in Psychotherapy Journal,* Vol. 19, No. 5, pp. 317–324.

Lewis, P. (1993). Kestenberg Movement Profile interpretation: Clinical, cultural and organizational application. In *American Dance Therapy Association Proceedings.* Columbia: ADTA.

Lewis, P. (1993). Following our dreams: Dance therapy as transformation. In *American Dance Association Proceedings.* Columbia: ADTA.

Lewis, P. (1994). Die Tiefenpsychologisch Orientierte Tanztherapie. In *Sprache der Bewegung.* Berlin: Nervenklinik Spandau Publication.

Lewis, P. (1996). Depth psychotherapy and dance-movement therapy. In *American Journal of Dance Therapy,* Vol. 18, No. 2.

Lewis, P. (1996). Authentic sound movement and drama: An interview with Penny Lewis. Annie Geissinger, Interviewer. In *A Moving Journal.* Providence: Vol. 3 No. 1.

Lewis, P. (1996). The Gestalt movement therapy approach. In Tsung-Chin, Lee (Ed.) *Dance Therapy.* Taipei, Taiwan: Publisher identified in Chinese Characters. In Chinese

Lewis, P. (1996) Authentic sound, movement, and drama: An interactional approach. In Robbins, M. (Ed.) *Body Oriented Psychotherapy,* Vol. I. Somerville, MA: Inter-Scientific Community for Psycho-Corporal Therapies.

Lewis, P. (1996). The Kestenberg Movement Profile." In Robbins, M. (Ed.) *Body Oriented Psychotherapy,* Vol. I. Somerville, MA: Inter-Scientific Community for Psycho-Corporal Therapies.

Lewis, P. (1997). Multiculturalism and global-ism in the arts in psychotherapy. In *The Arts in Psychotherapy Journal,* Vol. 24, No. 2, pp. 123–128.

Lewis, P. (1997). Appreciating diversity, commonality, and the transcendent. In *Arts in Psychotherapy Journal,* Vol. 24, No. 3.

Lewis, P. (1997). Transpersonal arts psychotherapy: Toward an ecumenical worldview. In *Arts in Psychotherapy Journal,* Vol. 24, No. 3.

Lewis, P. (In process). An embodied relational model: The use of the somatic countertransference and intersubjectivity within the affective-imaginal realm. In Robbins, M. *Body Oriented Psychotherapy,* Vol II. Somerville: Inter-Scientific Community for Psycho-Corporal Therapies.

Lewis, P. (1999a). Healing early child abuse: The application of the Kestenberg Movement Profile. In Amaghi, J., Loman, S., Lewis, P., et al. *The meaning of movement: Developmental and clinical perspectives of the Kestenberg Movement Profile.* Newark: Gordon & Breach.

Lewis, P. (1999b). The embodied feminine: Dance and drama therapy in women's holistic health. In Olshansky, E. (Ed.) *Woman's holistic health care.* Gaithersburg, MD: Aspen Publishers, Inc.

Further training:
Integrative Holistic Health Studies MA and Certificate Programs
Lesley University
Department of Independent and Interdisciplinary Studies
Dr. Penny Lewis
29 Everett Street
Cambridge, MA 02138
617-868-9600

Alternate Route Graduate Certificate Program in Transpersonal Drama Therapy:
Co-Directors: Penny Lewis Ph.D., ADTR, RDT-BCT and Saphira Linden MA, RDT-BCT Jointly located at the Institute for Healing and Wellness, Inc. in Amesbury and Omega Theater, Inc. in Jamaica Plains near Boston. The program has relationships with Antioch-New England Graduate School and Lesley University. Contact:

Dr. Penny Lewis
27 Merrill Street
Amesbury, MA 01913
Telephone: 978-388-3035
Fax: 978-388-5757
Email: *drplewis@seacoast.com*
www.dramatherapy.com

**Masters in Dance Movement Therapy
with a Counseling Minor**
Antioch-New England Graduate School
Masters in Dance Movement Therapy
Program
40 Avon Street
Keene, NH 03431
603-357-3122

Chapter 19

EPILOGUE

It is hoped that you, the reader, have been stimulated to affirm and expand the ways of knowing that have shaped your beliefs in integrative holistic health. I encourage you to speak out regarding your own philosophy that informs your work and the practice of those to whom you would refer.

Whatever your role or vision of a role in alternative and complementary medicine, be it practitioner, consultant, referral source, supervisor, teacher or administrator, *you* are creating and defining the field of integrative holistic health. Bring consciousness to the biggest picture of health, healing and transformation that you can envision for your clients, staff, students and most importantly, for yourself. For we have only just begun to comprehend the possibilities.

INDEX

Dharma, 105

Dhyana, 105

Diabetes, 35, 96

Dialoguer function, 291–292

Diarrhea, 15

Diet, 13, 15, 65, 79, 112, 140, 145, 150, 155, 164, 165–167, 190, 218–219; conscious eating, 218–219; diet direction, 83, 145; building diet, 83, 145–164; balancing diet, 83–84, 145, 164; cleansing diet, 84, 145, 164

Differentiation phase, 36, 40–41, 51

Displacement, 46

Dissociation, 62

Distant intention and distant healing, 7–8, 128–130, 156, 159, 166–167, 326

Dopamine, 18, 19, 31

Dossey, L., 6, 122

Drama therapy, 61, 68–70, 73, 215–216, 314–336

Drawing, 60 (see Art therapy)

Dreams, 60, 153; dreamwork technique, 67, 73, 114, 319–321, 328–332

E

Eastern spiritual traditions, 101–106

Eating meditation, 190

Edwards, H., 125,127

Ego, 37, 46, 68; ego boundaries, 39–41, 46, 142, 144, 164; ego mediation, 44; ego psychology, 57; ego-self axis, 107, 143

Einsteinian medicine, 6, 140–161, 207 (see Energy medicine)

Electrostatically shielded room, 7, 88

Embodiment as a technique, 59

Embodied psyche technique, 68–72, 317–319

Emotion, molecular, 17–18, 25, 28, 163–164

Emotional hijacking, 26, 27, 64, 139, 149, 315

Emotions, 28, 139

Empathy, 29, 39

Endocrine system, 18, 25, 28

Endorphins, 18, 20, 28, 35

Energy, 50; energy healing, 295–301, 326; energy medicine, 6, 7, 18, 22, 58, 86–102, 120, 155, 161, 163–167, 206, 220, 295, 319; energy diagnosis, 120–124, 150, 157; human energy field, 50, 140, 141, 145, 311; universal energy field, 132

Enlightenment, 105, 111, 117, 129, 146, 156

Era I medicine, 6–7, 12; era II medicine, 6, 7, 9–23, 24–34, 35–56, 58, 112, 138–161, 163–167; era III medicine, 6–7, 29, 103–118, 120–134, 141–162, 163–167

Erikson, E., 200, 313

Eros, 57, 111, 114

Ethical standards, 182, 183–184, 326–327

Evaluation of practitioners, 181–185

Exercise, 35, 166, 191, 212, 218–219, 220, 231–235

F

Faith, 21, 60, 98, 104, 146–147

Family systems, 200–201

Fasting, 219

Fatigue, 82, 150, 230, 297

Fear, 96, 148, 149, 231, 233, 297

Feldenkrais method, 260–262

Fever, 113

Fight/flight/fear/faint responses, 10, 14, 17, 33, 48, 92

Finances of wellness centers, 267–268

Fixation, 36, 37–38, 39, 41, 42, 43, 54

Flashbacks, 49, 320, 333–334

Flow, 37–56; free flow, 46; bound flow, 47; even flow, 47; flow adjustment, 47; high intensity, 48; low intensity, 48; abruptness, 48–49; graduality, 49; shape flow, 49–56

Forgiveness, 144, 147, 156, 166, 213

Freud, A., 57

Freud, S., 18, 27, 57

G

Gender stereotyping, 43, 44

Gerber, R., 6, 86–102

Gershon, M., 27–28

God, 106, 110, 116, 117, 121, 127, 146, 150–151, 165

Grace, 64, 103, 118, 332

Green, E., and A., 205

Groff, S., 108, 202–204, 281

Grounding, 96, 101

Guided self healing 297, 300, 302–303, 305–306

Guides, 106, 167, 210 (see Spirit guides)

Gut feelings, 18, 27, 39, 47, 92; enteroceptive sense of self, 39

H

Hands-on-healing 128

Hanh, Thich Nhat, 280

Hannaford, C., 31

Harvard University Medical school, 6

Headaches, 14, 15

Charles C Thomas
PUBLISHER • LTD.

P.O. Box 19265
Springfield, IL 62794-9265

- Bellini, James L. & Phillip D. Rumrill, Jr.—**RESEARCH IN REHABILITA-TION COUNSELING: A Guide to Design, Methodology, and Utilization. (2nd Ed.)** '09, 318 pp. (7 x 10) 3 il., 5 tables.

- Brooke, Stephanie L.—**THE USE OF THE CREATIVE THERAPIES WITH CHEMICAL DEPENDECY ISSUES.** '09, 300 pp. (7 x 10), 33 il., 3 tables.

- Johnson, David Read & Renee Emunah—**CURRENT APPROACH-ES IN DRAMA THERAPY. (2nd Ed.)** '09, (7 x 10) 11 il.

- Luginbuehl-Oelhafen, Ruth R.—**ART THERAPY WITH CHRONIC PHYS-ICALLY ILL ADOLESCENTS: Ex-ploring the Effectiveness of Medical Art Therapy as a Complementary Treatment.** '09, 220 pp. (7 x 10), 67 il., (12 in color), $37.95, paper.

- McNiff, Shaun—**INTEGRATING THE ARTS IN THERAPY: History, Theory, and Practice.** '09, 272 pp. (7 x 10), 60 il.

- Wilkes, Jane K.—**THE ROLE OF COMPANION ANIMALS IN COUN-SELING AND PSYCHOTHERAPY: Discovering Their Use in the Ther-apeutic Process.** '09,172 pp. (7 x 10), 2 tables, paper.

- Correia, Kevin M.— **A HANDBOOK FOR CORRECTIONAL PSYCHOLOGISTS: Guidance for the Prison Practitioner. (2nd Ed.)** '09, 202 pp. (7 x 10), 3 tables, $54.95, hard, $34.95, paper.

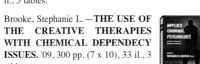

- Horovitz, Ellen G. & Sarah L. Eksten—**THE ART THERAPISTS' PRIMER: A Clinical Guide to Writing As-sessments, Diagnosis, & Treatment.** '09, 332 pp. (7 x 10), 106 il., 2 tables, $85.95, hard, $55.95, paper.

- Kocsis, Richard N.— **APPLIED CRIMINAL PSYCHOLOGY: A Guide to Forensic Behavioral Sciences.** '09, 306 pp. (7 x 10), 4 il., 2 tables, $65.95, hard, $45.95, paper.

- Moon, Bruce L.—**EXIS-TENTIAL ART THER-APY: The Canvas Mir-ror. (3rd Ed.)** '09, 284 pp. (7 x 10), 51 il., $64.95, hard, $44.95, paper.

- Richard, Michael A., William G. Emener, & William S. Hutchison, Jr.— **EMPLOYEE ASSIS-TANCE PROGRAMS: Wellness/Enhancement Programming. (4th Ed.)** '09, 428 pp. (8 x 10), 8 il., 1 table, $79.95, hard, $57.95, paper.

- Brooke, Stephanie L.—**THE CREATIVE THERA-PIES AND EATING DISORDERS.** '08, 304 pp. (7 x 10), 20 il., 2 tables, $64.95, hard, $44.95, paper.

- Geldard, Kathryn & David Geldard—**PER-SONAL COUNSEL-ING SKILLS: An Inte-grative Approach.** '08, 316 pp. (7 x 10), 20 il., 3 tables, $49.95, paper.

- Junge, Maxine Borowsky— **MOURNING, MEMO-RY AND LIFE ITSELF: Essays by an Art Thera-pist.** '08, 292 pp. (7 x 10), 38 il, $61.95, hard, $41.95, paper.

- Kendler, Howard H.— **AMORAL THOUGHTS ABOUT MORALITY: The Intersection of Sci-ence, Psychology, and Ethics. (2nd Ed.)** '08, 270 pp. (7 x 10), $59.95, hard, $39.95, paper.

- Wiseman, Dennis G.— **THE AMERICAN FAM-ILY: Understanding its Changing Dynamics and Place in Society.** '08, 172 pp. (7 x 10), 4 tables, $31.95, paper.

- Arrington, Doris Banowsky— **ART, ANGST, AND TRAUMA: Right Brain Interventions with Devel-opmental Issues.** '07, 278 pp. (7 x 10), 123 il., (10 in color, paper edition only), $63.95, hard, $48.95, paper.

- Daniels, Thomas & Allen Ivey—**MICROCOUN-SELING: Making Skills Training Work In a Multicultural World.** '07, 296 pp. (7 x 10), 12 il., 3 tables, $65.95, hard, $45.95, paper.

- Olson, R. Paul—**MENTAL HEALTH SYSTEMS COMPARED: Great Bri-tain, Norway, Canada, and the United States.** '06, 398 pp. (8 1/2 x 11), 10 il., 65 tables, $89.95, hard, $64.95, paper.

5 easy ways to order!

PHONE: 1-800-258-8980 or (217) 789-8980

FAX: (217) 789-9130

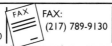
@ EMAIL: books@ccthomas.com
Web: www.ccthomas.com

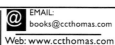

MAIL: Charles C Thomas • Publisher, Ltd. P.O. Box 19265 Springfield, IL 62794-9265

Complete catalog available at ccthomas.com • books@ccthomas.com

Books sent on approval • Shipping charges: $7.75 min. U.S. / Outside U.S., actual shipping fees will be charged • Prices subject to change without notice